The Gravest Show on Earth

BOOKS BY ELINOR BURKETT

A Gospel of Shame:
Children, Sexual Abuse, and
the Catholic Church
(with Frank Bruni)

The Gravest Show on Earth:
America in the Age of AIDS

THE
GRAVEST
SHOW ON
EARTH

America in the Age of AIDS

ELINOR BURKETT

HOUGHTON MIFFLIN COMPANY

BOSTON · NEW YORK · 1995

For information about permission to reproduce selections from
this book, write to Permissions, Houghton Mifflin Company,
215 Park Avenue South, New York, New York 10003.

For information about this and other Houghton Mifflin
trade and reference books and multimedia products, visit
The Bookstore at Houghton Mifflin on the World Wide Web
at http://www.hmco.com/trade/.

Library of Congress Cataloging-in-Publication Data
  Burkett, Elinor.
  The gravest show on earth : America in the age
  of AIDS / Elinor Burkett.
      p. cm.
  Includes index.
  ISBN 0-395-74537-3
    1. AIDS (Disease) — Social aspects — United States. I. Title.
  RA644.A25B868 1995
  362.'969792'00973 — dc20   95-9021
                                    CIP

Printed in the United States of America

MP 10 9 8 7 6 5 4 3 2 1

Book design by Melodie Wertelet

CONTENTS

Acknowledgments   vii

INTRODUCTION   Mad Dogs and Medicine Men   1

ONE   Pomp Without Circumstance   19

TWO   Evidence to the Contrary   53

THREE   Magic Bullets and Bottom Lines   77

FOUR   Riding the AIDS Gravy Train   109

FIVE   AIDS Inc.   141

SIX   Color Bind   169

SEVEN   Vaginal Politics   191

EIGHT   The Immaculate Transmission   215

NINE   Lights, Camera . . . Death   242

TEN   Pill Pushers and Policy Makers   255

ELEVEN   The Enemies of the People   286

TWELVE   Strike a Pose   315

Sources   353

Notes   357

Index   377

ACKNOWLEDGMENTS

No individual ever authors a book alone. Books, like the ideas in them, reflect a complex series of interactions, observations, relationships and experiences that form a unique consciousness.

Three of the individuals whose influence is stamped most heavily on this work are dead. Enrique Bertheau, Juan Faedo and Miguel Chinchilla shared their deaths with me. In so doing, they offered me the profound gift of a series of lessons in fear, pain and morality, as well as the courage and grace about which so much is written. Mostly they taught me about honesty — for when your life is narrowing to fewer and fewer weeks, and to increasingly confined spaces, truth emerges from the ruins of banality with extraordinary clarity. If I no longer mince words, nor tolerate those who process truth in their Vego-Matics, it is because I have learned, in the most profound way, that there simply isn't any time.

Members of the Miami AIDS community created a home for me during my four years in that muggy city, supporting me both professionally and personally. What peace I maintained in the tempest of death and dying I found at Body Positive Resource Center, which became my family. My deepest gratitude goes to Doris Feinberg, my sister in grief, who created that refuge for so many of us struggling to survive the epidemic. My thanks to John O'Hara, the former director of Body Positive, who brought us all the grace of his special brand of Christian love and to Ernie Lopez, Body Positive's current director who was always ready with a kind word, a cup of coffee, a perfectly timed party. His is a talent and grace every city needs. To the late Jim Pruitt, who stayed alive despite the odds so he could make the world a kinder and more just place for the men and women suffering from AIDS, I give my thanks and my greatest admiration.

I am also grateful to four physicians who have earned a special place in my life. Drs. Ross Abrams and Sam Denmeade of Johns Hopkins University kept me alive, and sane enough to tell this story. Saying thank you seems an insufficient offering in return for what they have given me. Dr. Judith Ratzan of Mount Sinai Hospital on Miami Beach and Dr. Nancy Klimas of the Veterans Administration Medical Center shared both life and death with me and showed me the art of medicine as well as the science.

Six friends and colleagues eased my way into writing about AIDS at a time when journalism declared it an irrelevant pursuit. It has become rare indeed to find editors who support writing about what is important in an age when writing about what is not has been defined as the appropriate strategy for marketing the nation's newspapers. My thanks, then, to Lois Uttley, who saw me in a newsroom long before I'd ever seen one; to John Doussard, who allowed himself to see a compelling story; to Susan Olds, who fought to get it into the paper; to the nation's finest executive editor, the late Janet Chusmir, of the *Miami Herald*; and to Lisa Bankoff, my agent, who vowed to peddle this book on Fifty-seventh Street if necessary; and to Dawn Seferian, my editor at Houghton Mifflin, who made that unnecessary.

In the act of writing a book, the author spends years hounding people for interviews, documents, reactions, memories and every other sort of help. The list of those who generously shared their time and insights with me appears in the notes. I would, however, like to acknowledge the extraordinary assistance of Shepherd Smith, the nation's least likely AIDS activist. A Republican and a Christian, Shepherd is the type of man liberal reporters fail to contact unless they are seeking a hostile quote; they do him, and themselves, a disservice. Mark Harrington always has been willing to answer a question or offer an insight. I would like to express both my thanks and my respect, which he has earned through his endless willingness to think.

And then there are my friends, my family, who put up with me through pedophile priests, marriage, lymphoma and AIDS. Few people have been as blessed as I with friends of patience, humor, insight, stubbornness and love. Thanks to Joel Rapoport, friend, maid of honor and researcher extraordinaire, with whom I have shared so much happiness and so much grief; to Frank Bruni, my favorite coauthor, now my favorite editor and a gifted friend; to Robin Haueter, for endless phone numbers and an inexhaustible willingness to keep pushing me; to Joe DeCola, whose wisdom has graced my life and kept it on an even keel; to Robert Jones, whose impatience with my long complaints was the origin of this book; to Jim Fouratt, with whom I have shared so much history; and to Ivan Bernstein, who grows and grows even while retaining his wonder, and in the process helps me stay in touch with the wonderment of life.

Finally, I would thank my husband, who married into a world filled with frail bodies and memorial services, campy drag and demented humor. It has been a long journey, Dennis, from death to hope and a mountaintop.

The Gravest Show on Earth

INTRODUCTION

Mad Dogs and Medicine Men

I started living with AIDS in 1988, when I moved from New York to Miami's South Beach, a neighborhood teetering on the brink of trendiness. Once elegant Art Deco hotels that had become seedy rent-by-the-weeks for elderly Jews and impoverished Hispanics were being claimed by developers intent on returning them to their former glory. Madonna and Versace had yet to establish beachheads, but South Beach was on the verge of becoming America's own Riviera.

It was also becoming a cemetery, but that was a trend of which the local news media — which I had just joined — seemed oblivious. The gay Cuban men who served drinks and food in the bars and restaurants catering to the first wave of artists, models and club kids were missing work, hospitalized with strange pneumonias that no one discussed. Sunday afternoon tea dances offered by gay bars were peppered with comments about why Enrique didn't go out anymore or about the dark spots on Juan's face.

Nobody talked about AIDS, but that was hardly surprising. By the late 1980s, America seemed intent on ignoring dozens of problems, from crumbling highways to the burgeoning number of homeless. The truth of poverty, racism and corporate greed was disguised in euphemism. The reality of a plague was a mere whisper.

But the silence shrouding AIDS was more deafening in Miami than in other epicenters of infection. Miami wasn't squalid enough to provide a convincing backdrop for a plague. Trim young bodies in skimpy bikinis and sundresses paraded along Ocean Drive. Even the senior citizens sported tans as they carried tennis rackets to the courts.

By the time the first young victims of a new virus were being buried,

Miami had also become the Cuban miracle, a sleepy backwater converted into the capital of Latin America by the drive of almost a million immigrants intent on proving Fidel Castro wrong. Ultramodern skyscrapers had begun to shade a downtown that just a decade earlier looked like a provincial city in the Dominican Republic. The port of Miami was packed with cruise ships competing for docking space with cargo ships signaling the city's arrival as the import-export center of Latin America.

No one was eager to acknowledge the misery beneath the makeup: that the young men driving Jaguar convertibles around town were paying their cellular phone bills with drug money; that the black community had missed out on the 1960s and still languished in virtual segregation; that the lack of a state income tax had left education, medical care and a wide range of social services on the level of that of rural Mississippi.

Miami, of all American cities, excelled at illusion.

The epidemic leached into a city of taboos, the most important of which forbade unpleasant truths. Miami was certainly not unique in its aversion to reality, but it enforced compliance to fantasy with singular viciousness. Those who didn't understand the city's first commandment — Thou shalt not speak the truth about certain issues — needed only to hear about the Miami radio announcer who had dared to praise some of Castro's reforms and was blown up, and left paralyzed, in response.

AIDS touched all of the city's rawest nerves. It first hit Little Haiti, a community still scarred by the terrors that had been Haiti's national history. It then grabbed hold of gay men whose nascent attempts to organize themselves had careened from a stunning victory in 1977, when Dade County commissioners passed one of the nation's first anti-discrimination laws, to a demoralizing defeat in the face of the anti-gay hysteria whipped up by Anita Bryant. AIDS began to claim African American men, who pretended to be heroin addicts rather than admit to homosexuality.

The virus spread through a city with no meaningful history of free speech; denial reached fever pitch. What Hispanic and Haitian tradition did not quiet, a brand of Catholicism still untouched by the liberalizing precepts of Vatican II did. So when the first young Cuban men succumbed to the new disease, their mothers maintained their decorum and insisted that their sons had been devastated by cancer. When the first young Cuban women developed the odd pneumonias, no one dared talk about how common bisexuality was among Hispanic men.

On the surface, the city responded brilliantly. Largely because of the efforts of a young physician, Dr. Margaret Fischl, Miami's only public hospital developed a research program that quickly became one of the nation's principal AIDS research sites, well funded by the federal government and pharmaceutical companies. Across the street, the Veterans Administration Medical Center reached out to its infected constituency — mostly the homeless and the drug addicted — with a treatment program so sophisticated that the well-insured fought for access to its services. A group of lesbian and gay physicians responded to their community's need almost instantly, setting up specialized AIDS practices and keeping abreast of even the most experimental treatments.

Two brothers, both infected with HIV, talked their parents into converting their popular sports bar into Body Positive, an AIDS resource center where gay men could go for seminars on new treatments, advice on everything from housing to Social Security, or a cup of coffee and an hour of comfort. A young Puerto Rican graduate of an overseas medical school opened a center to promote AIDS awareness in the Hispanic community. And the city's Haitian population formed its own AIDS coalition to mobilize Haitian physicians against the epidemic and to fight the branding of Haitians as "high risks" for AIDS.

But as with so much else in AIDS, these were little more than illusions.

Fischl's research did not live up to its well-publicized promise. Repeated studies showed that AZT, the drug whose merits she had allegedly proven, was toxic and arguably ineffective. Haitians, targeted early as a "risk group," refused to heed that early warning. All the attention given to their beleaguered community was simple racism, their leaders argued, and they turned their energies to saving their ethnic reputation rather than their lives.

Sonia Singleton, a black debutante from Palm Beach who had recently been released from a drug rehabilitation program, joined the Body Positive team intent on breaking the silence about the swath AIDS was cutting through the city's black neighborhoods. She was cheered at nurses' conventions and on World AIDS Day, but she was not welcome on the pulpits of Miami's African American churches.

Body Positive was racked by three years of the same kind of infighting that divided AIDS service organizations all across America; it didn't succumb, but it barely survived. And the Hispanic AIDS center became a constant source of suspicion when it moved out of a poor minority neighborhood into an affluent Anglo suburb. When the local chapter of the AIDS activist group ACT UP received $25,000 from a national fundraising campaign, it held no demonstrations. It bought no newspaper ads, printed no eye-catching fliers, forced no change in the city's policy of ignoring AIDS. ACT UP used the money to buy certificates of deposit. The People with AIDS Coalition kicked one long-time member off its board after he missed the group's annual retreat. The fact that he had been caring for his best friend, who was dying of AIDS, was not deemed a valid excuse. Refugees terrified that immigration officials would discover that they were HIV positive and deport them refused to seek medical assistance. Quacks peddling everything from lemons to electric therapy treatments preyed on the vulnerable, untouched by state health enforcement officials.

And the party continued on Miami Beach, where Gay America went to take a vacation from safe sex.

During my first year or two in the city, I thought the problems were unique to Miami — and vowed to shake things up. I naively thought that if I told the truth the problems would disappear. I was seriously deluded. The problems weren't so much indifference to the plight of the sick as a dozen competing agendas — political, economic, scientific and social — that had nothing to do with the growing number of obituaries of thirty-five-year-olds. But that truth, about AIDS and America, unfolded slowly in story after story.

Reporting on AIDS is not a plum assignment. Newspaper editors and publishers are indifferent, if not hostile, to the beat. Most readers don't want to hear about what they are sure is somebody else's plague.

Like most major American dailies, my paper, the *Miami Herald*, had followed AIDS from the mystery and fear of the first cases to the discovery of HIV. Following the pack, the daily paper had run a series of stories after Rock Hudson returned from Paris, gaunt and dying. It treated readers to the predictable round of "Is a heterosexual breakout imminent?" analyses, then pretty much dropped AIDS as an ongoing issue unless Sophia Loren hosted a glitzy social event or some government agency sent out a press release that demanded translation into plain English.

"All the good AIDS stories have been written," the *Herald*'s city editor, John Brecher, told editors and reporters anxious to increase coverage of AIDS. No one was willing to buck him in order to prove him wrong.

Despite the widespread assumption that homophobia was the driving force behind the media's seeming indifference to AIDS, Brecher was not some screeching bigot reveling in the demise of gay men. Nowhere in the nation did news executives huddle in their offices rubbing their hands in delight at how their refusal to cover AIDS might increase the death toll. No doubt most editors and reporters weren't comfortable talking about, not to mention writing about, homosexuality. But they weren't much more comfortable with other forms of sexuality either. Sex, after all, had yet to go prime time. America is the land of doublespeak, and these were straight white men who couldn't even talk about menstruation.

Like editors and television producers all over the country, Brecher exercised his news judgment, which was inevitably colored by his personal experiences. AIDS was not part of the daily landscape of white, middle-class America; it wasn't the central topic of conversation at the cocktail parties where news executives gathered. Ergo, it couldn't be very important.

Other major dailies — *Newsday* and the *New York Times,* the *Washington Post,* the *San Francisco Chronicle,* the *Los Angeles Times,* even the *Wall Street Journal* — had AIDS reporters. But not by editorial fiat. Unlike most beats in American journalism, the AIDS beat was created from the bottom up, or the outside in. The government had not declared AIDS a national emergency worthy of coverage, so it fell to reporters convinced that something awesome was happening — a plague that promised to reshape American society — to badger management into submission. Or it fell to gay men with clout to guilt-trip liberal editors into attending to their concerns.

Miami had neither.

There were numerous gay men in the *Herald*'s cavernous newsroom, but none was sick, and none talked openly about sick friends, lovers or relatives. Some might have had more than a passing interest in the disease that was felling their friends and being discussed obsessively in their community, but AIDS was never mentioned when writers gathered in the paper's cafeteria at lunchtime or for late-night drinks after work. Young men on their way up knew better than to push too hard to write about AIDS; Brecher could be a mighty foe.

And the local gay community didn't complain. Instead of demanding more coverage, they carped about what little coverage there was.

That was the national norm. Reporters who chose to cover AIDS were subjected to incessant complaint, even harassment, by an increasingly shrill activist community.

From Miami, I watched the attacks on Randy Shilts, the first mainstream journalist to make the epidemic a hard-hitting beat. Shilts should have been a hero: an openly gay man writing about his community for a San Francisco newspaper. But he cared too much about the truth, and certain truths were off limits in AIDS reporting — most important, any careful examination of the sexual practices of gay men. Shilts refused to sugarcoat reality to make it more palatable to straight society. Gay strangers actually spit at him when he walked through the Castro. In bars and stores he was accosted and branded as an Uncle Tom and a traitor. Even when he was close to death in 1993, Shilts remained bitter at the reaction. "I was telling the truth and they didn't want to hear it. They tried to shoot the messenger."

My colleagues in the gay press weren't spared the wrath of the AIDS thought police. In July 1990 the *Washington Blade,* that city's gay weekly, was stormed by nine activists from ACT UP who were irate that the paper had not lent its editorial support to their national boycott of Miller Brewing Company. Miller's crime was contributing to the war chest of a mortal enemy, Jesse Helms. *Blade* staffers might have supported the boycott, but the paper had a policy of running no editorials. That fact was ignored.

It was impossible not to feel the pressure to follow the activist agenda. The expectations were explicit; they arrived in the mail or by fax, in a long list of "Buzz Words" that reporters were told to avoid. The term "general population" was verboten because it "implies that some groups of people (in particular, gay men, lesbians, people of color and intravenous drug users) are less valid members of our society than others," one handout explained. "Every person with AIDS is part of the 'general population.'" Calling people with AIDS "victims" was declared the ultimate breach of political correctness: "It robs them of their dignity as individuals and belittles their struggle to survive and lead full lives." The fact that the preferred term, people with AIDS, or PWAs, was long and awkward was deemed irrelevant, as was the fact that people with cancer or muscular dystrophy have never been referred to as PWC or PWMD.

Most of the activist rules were unwritten. I discovered that you were never supposed to ask an AIDS patient how he got infected only when I posed that question and was promptly upbraided for my offense. I sought counsel from my friend Frank Bruni, a gay reporter at the *Detroit Free Press,* who related the safe rule he'd learned. "It is considered unseemly to ask people what their risk behaviors were or how many partners they had," he told me. "If you do, you'll be accused of playing the blame game."

Even if I'd been more inclined to subservience, I would have run into trouble anyway, because the rules were constantly changing. For months after I began writing about AIDS in Gay Miami, I heard complaints that I was treating AIDS as an exclusively homosexual epidemic. So I wrote about the mother of two hemophiliac sons who had died of AIDS and about a New York teenager infected with HIV during a one-night stand with a bisexual bartender.

"How dare you focus on aberrations," I was chastised.

"You quickly came to understand that you could never please AIDS activists," says Bruni, who is now his paper's movie critic. "No matter which tack you took, it was the wrong one. I've never met a population of activists more intent on feeling aggrieved."

The pressure I felt was nothing compared to the stress put on gay male reporters on the beat. They were members of a community with a clear political line on AIDS. They crossed the line at peril to their social standing; they toed the line at peril to their professionalism. "For a gay male reporter, there was an incredible pull to this beat, and an extra danger," says Bruni. "You wanted to cover AIDS because it was a tangible way to help your community, but there was also a constant nervousness. You worried that you were treading on ground where you could easily lose your professional credibility. You always worried that by arguing for the urgency of this disease, you'd be given a little less credibility in the newsroom because you were part of the group that naysayers believed was suffering alone.

"At the same time, there were stories you were hesitant to do. I remember a few years back being at a newsroom seminar and the topic of AIDS and gay issues came up. The paper had been extraordinarily supportive of AIDS coverage, and I mentioned that the best undone story was on the resurgence of unsafe sex. I talked about the new sex clubs and the sexual practices of the younger generation that hadn't seen their peers die.

"My editor's face lit up with a wow. I knew at that moment that I could have gotten the time and travel money to do the story, but I never pursued it. I was hesitant to do a story that would give comfort to our enemies, that would immediately be hated by my friends, that would be questioned every time I went to a gay social event. On balance, I made the wrong decision. I chose to protect the community from critics rather than holding gay men's feet to the fire."

Many gay male reporters went even further, involving themselves so closely with the AIDS activists whose antics they covered that their professional detachment was open to serious question. During the Sixth International Conference on AIDS in San Francisco, Frank Browning of National Public Radio wound up in bed in a threesome with two leaders of ACT UP Los Angeles. The *Los Angeles Times*'s Victor Zonana, now the spokesman for Health and Human Services Secretary Donna Shalala, left the conference with a new boyfriend: a heavyweight in ACT UP New York.

Another land mine on the AIDS beat was the Christian right, which didn't want Gay America to be written about as anything but a sin-ridden freak show. Some readers were offended by explicit discussions of sex or intravenous drug use. When I wrote a long magazine piece about the plight of the gay Cubans who'd escaped Castro's oppression in 1980 only to be decimated by AIDS, one Cuban radio station in Miami branded me a racist. "This American woman, a supposed expert in Latin American affairs, insists that thirty thousand faggots came on the Mariel boatlift," one commentator declared. "There have never been thirty thousand homosexuals on the entire island of Cuba."

Over the years, my copy was subjected to microscopic examination, but that scrutiny was mild compared with the hypersensitivity that greeted every word written or spoken by reporters in San Francisco and New York. No one took a worse beating than Gina Kolata, a science and medical reporter for the *New York Times*. Kolata never covered AIDS full time, but when she arrived at the *Times* in 1987, she began writing about the disease and quickly became the darling of New York's AIDS activists. Every word Kolata wrote was applauded. "I was inundated with phone calls telling me how wonderful I was, how fabulous," says Kolata. "It was really strange. Nobody calls reporters to tell them they are terrific, so I assumed it was just a way of buttering me up."

In fact, Kolata didn't run into trouble early on because her first AIDS stories meshed with the activist agenda: reports on new drugs in development, on how women were being ignored in drug trials and on the importance of broadening the definition of AIDS. "Those stories fit with their idea of political correctness," she says. "I didn't write anything advocates wouldn't have liked."

Then Kolata fell off her pedestal when she wrote about the deaths of patients in an underground study of a Chinese cucumber root called Compound Q, said to have almost magical powers against AIDS. The head of the study, Martin Delaney of San Francisco, declared war, insisting in a letter to the *Times* that Kolata had misrepresented the study and that Compound Q had had nothing to do with the deaths.

Two months later AIDS researchers complained to Kolata that activists' demands that patients be allowed to take drugs still undergoing testing would destroy their studies — and with them any chance to discover how effective those drugs might actually be. Kolata believed in the tried-and-true approach to drug testing. She ran with a front-page story, "Innovative Drug Plan May Be Undermining Testing."

All hell broke loose. Kolata was vilified by ACT UP New York, whose members feared that her story would make the FDA more timid in opening up access to experimental drugs. Young men would die, they claimed, and it would be Gina Kolata's fault. Suddenly senior officials at the National Institutes of Health joined activists in berating Kolata. One of her primary sources, Dr. Douglas Richman of the University of California at San Diego, complained that he had been misquoted. "I was shocked," Kolata says. "I knew I was right, that the story was accurate. But Richman didn't want to make enemies among gay men, so he backed away from what he'd said. None of them want to make enemies among gay men. I don't care if I make enemies. I only care about the truth."

When Kolata continued to call the shots as she saw them, activists declared war on her. She was targeted as "the worst AIDS reporter in America" on stickers plastered on *Times* news boxes around the city. The *Village Voice* picked up on the dispute when Robert Massa, an HIV-positive gay reporter there, wrote a story about Kolata called "Unfit to Print."

Most sane reporters would have forgotten about AIDS. Kolata didn't need it; she had plenty of other things to cover at the *Times,* from cancer to mathematics. And her editors gave her their full support. "If I only wrote about AIDS, maybe they would have questioned me," she says. "But I write dozens of articles in other areas and no one ever complains. So they had to ask, How come when it comes to AIDS I'm suddenly so terrible?"

Kolata admits that she was tempted to give up. "I did feel like saying, Who cares about this subject, forget it, I'm not doing any more AIDS stories. But I wasn't willing to give activists that power. I didn't want them to think that their being vicious would change the way we report. I wasn't willing to give them the satisfaction of thinking they could intimidate me."

They tried to intimidate me, too. One day in 1990, I received a phone call from a gay attorney begging me to write about a gay bathhouse in Miami. I was shocked. In cities like New York and San Francisco, gay bathhouses — which are about sex, not cleanliness — had been closed down or regulated to death in the mid-1980s. I had never heard of a bathhouse in Miami and had assumed such local institutions had disappeared as they had elsewhere. Intrigued, I began to ask around about a place called the Club Body Center and was drowned out almost before I could articulate a question. "Leave the baths alone, they are none of your business," said Roland Funk, president of the People with AIDS Coalition of Dade County. (Funk died of AIDS three years later.) "Writing about the bathhouse will only make straight people hate us more. Do you want to promote gay bashing?"

One evening, a young man with AIDS cornered me after a weekly AIDS information exchange, where patients received updates on the latest treatments. His face contorted and turned purple as he spat out, "You homophobic bitch. Leave us alone. You just don't want gay men to have sex. You have no respect for our civil rights. Why don't you pick on straight sex clubs — or do you think they're just fine."

A male colleague from the *Herald* and I forged ahead nonetheless, and on February 12, 1991, told readers about a festive Saturday night at Club Body Center. My colleague had witnessed orgies disguised as "safe-sex workshops," daisy chains of unprotected anal and oral intercourse. Just as alarming was what he didn't see: condoms, sex information or warning posters.

It was a tough story to print in a family newspaper. When we were finishing the final edit, I spent an entire evening in the office of the managing editor, surrounded by other editors and lawyers — all straight — discussing anal intercourse, the risks of swallowing sperm and the relative advantages of different brands of lubricants. Could we print the phrase "daisy chains of anal and oral intercourse" at the top of a story on the front page? Should we simply tell readers that a local "safe-sex instructor," who regularly invited his students to perform oral sex on him, had Kaposi's sarcoma on his genitals, or should we say straight out that he had cancerous lesions on his penis?

No wonder newspapers don't want to print stories on AIDS, I thought as I left the session.

The day after the story appeared, a group of activists demanded a meeting with the publisher and harangued him about the safety of oral sex without a condom. "I've sucked more than a thousand cocks and I'm not infected," one activist shouted. Gay college professors pronounced in high-minded language on the importance of the bathhouse for "courtship and socialization." Letters to the editor accused us of bigotry. The national gay press picked up the story after the owner of Club Body Center complained to national lesbian and gay organizations that the *Miami Herald* had launched an attack on the gay men. I was "outed" as a "bitchy dyke from New York." My assailants got it half right: I can be a real bitch.

The experience reminded me how expendable the truth is when a wider agenda is being pursued. After all, Gay America was simply emulating Senator Jesse Helms, who attacked AIDS prevention programs for his own bigoted ends, and Ronald Reagan, whose exegeses on the State of the Union managed to omit anything embarrassing.

But the upshot of the *Herald* piece caught me totally off guard. Humiliated by their own inaction, the Dade County commissioners passed an ordinance prohibiting unsafe sex in public facilities like bathhouses. Under intense pressure from gay leaders, the county agreed to allow places like Club Body Center to remain open, but required owners to enforce safe-sex measures. Failure to do so meant closure and jail. In Miami, that owner was John "Jack" Campbell, a powerhouse in the Florida Democratic party. I suspected that his connections had offered him protection. I naively assumed that the ordinance would change that.

Eighteen months after the ordinance was passed, two gay activists decided to see how life had changed at Club Body Center. They found business as usual: rooms with mattresses and beds where men had sex, no condoms, no safe-sex information, no monitors patrolling the halls to enforce county regulations. When the activists complained to the county, a health department attorney filed suit to close the place down. He even got state's attorney Janet Reno, now the U.S. attorney general, to sign on to the suit. But the day before their scheduled court appearance, the activists received a call informing them that Reno's office had made a deal. The club would install windows on the cubicle doors and improve the lighting. It would also remain open.

Strangely, Reno seemed proud of the deal and used the records of the case in congressional hearings on her confirmation as attorney general. The incident supposedly demonstrated her tough stance on pornography.

Only once did the criticism of me become personal. In the summer of 1990, after watching activists stage a mock trial of Dr. Margaret Fischl at the Sixth International Conference on AIDS, I wrote a story for the *Herald*'s Sunday magazine about why the young Miami physician had become the target of so much contempt. Shortly after it ran, the publisher received an eight-page diatribe from Martin Delaney, the San Francisco AIDS activist who had attacked Gina Kolata and others in the press. Unable to point out any errors of fact in the piece, he argued that I had exposed Fischl because my sibling had died of AIDS while under her care. As it happens, I have only one sibling, an HIV-negative sister in upstate New York. The truth, however, didn't seem relevant. Nor was it relevant to Fischl's employer: the University of Miami repeated the same charge in a letter to the *Herald*'s attorney.

Working the AIDS beat taught me how easily truth becomes a casualty of competing interests, commercial and political — inside and outside newsrooms. Tales of corruption and opportunism were ignored because editors didn't want to upset local universities. The politics driving public health and research was never exposed because so many of the nation's medical reporters were closely linked to the medical profession and were so dependent on official sources for continuing information that they didn't approach their beat with the hard, skeptical edge applied to industry or politics — or they were so enmeshed with the activists that they lost all distance.

Sensationalism sells more TV commercials and ad space than dry medical reports, so research results were often blown out of proportion, to the detriment of public understanding. At the International Conference on AIDS in Florence, Italy, in 1991, for example, Dr. William Haseltine, a top AIDS researcher at Boston's Dana-Farber Cancer Institute, presented data showing that cells lining mucous membranes — in the vagina, the anus, or the mouth — can be infected with HIV and can then transfer the virus to the bloodstream and the lymph nodes.

During a press conference after his session, reporters ignored all the serious implications of Haseltine's work and grilled him instead about the dangers of kissing. "Deep kissing," with an exchange of saliva, could be a risk, Haseltine admitted, adding that the risk was extremely low. There was, in fact, no evidence that anyone had ever been infected by a kiss, shallow or deep. But television news created a media circus around the theoretical possibility, broadcasting the alarmist message: "New evidence presented revealing that HIV can be transmitted in a passionate kiss."

Dozens of stories didn't make it into newspapers or onto the air because they might have offended the sensibilities of the PC police. Gay America's romance with illicit drugs and the resistance to safe sex among young gay men who saw AIDS as a way to avoid "becoming old trolls" have never been fully explored. No mainstream newspaper has yet delved into the homophobia of Black America or the devastating effect of AIDS on the already beleaguered black family. Too controversial. Too accusatory. Too negative.

No one has written about the number of gay priests dying of AIDS or the number of Catholic hospitals that refuse to give out information on condoms. Should these hospitals continue to receive public funds if they are unwilling to follow such an accepted standard of care? The issue is never raised.

Society reporters cover the endless round of parties, auctions, horse shows and performances billed as AIDS fundraisers. In June 1993 they followed Elizabeth Taylor and her monied friends across the Atlantic to Venice for the Art Against AIDS Gala, at the sixteenth-century Palazzo Volpi on the Grand Canal. They wrote breathlessly about Robert Rauschenberg's turquoise suit and shirt, complete with the tie pin in the shape of a moth which he had cast in silver over the creature's dead body. They never mentioned how much of the money raised at these events wound up paying caterers rather than helping people with AIDS.

Reporters have turned a blind eye to stories with real significance because they don't know what to make of them or how to handle their implications. A compelling example is the accuracy of the two tests used to screen for HIV infection. These tests — called the ELISA, which is used for preliminary screening, and the Western Blot, which is used to confirm positive ELISAS — have consistently been reported to be highly sensitive to the virus. Such sensitivity is essential with a disease in which the stakes are so high that individuals testing positive have been known to commit suicide upon receiving the dire news. Yet over the past two years, teams of researchers in the United States and Australia have demonstrated that both tests tend to produce positive HIV results with troubling frequency when those being tested do not have HIV, but have tuberculosis, leprosy, malaria, even certain types of influenza.

Neither test isolates HIV itself. They both react to the presence of antibodies, the immune system's foot soldiers that attack invading pathogens. Recent research suggests that the tests confuse HIV antibodies with antibodies produced to fight other viruses or even bacteria.

The implications are revolutionary — and throw innumerable elements of AIDS research and accepted wisdom into doubt. No journalist has confronted this.

By the time I left the *Herald* in 1992, I had come to understand that politics, greed and utter stupidity were making a mockery of the war against the epidemic. AIDS never got a chance to be simply a disease. It was too busy masquerading as a scourge from God, a comment on the nation's sexual practices, an opportunity for homophobes and heterophobes, even a shot at a Nobel Prize.

It was a multi-billion-dollar growth industry and an epistemological battle between its victims and the press over whether silence really equaled death. It was cure-mongers hawking $50,000 miracles in the slums of Haiti, suburban Jewish mothers turned drug smugglers by the wasting away of their sons and dying young men transforming fear of mortality into anger. It was corruption in the nation's research laboratories, sloganeering disguised as public health policy and vanity run riot. It was a classic case of blaming the victim — along with his physician, scientists, promiscuity, government indifference, bureaucratic incompetence, self-indulgence, homophobia, racism, permissiveness, the homosexual lobby and God — for the havoc of a minuscule virus.

As I took note of all this, I began to see both the epidemic and the nation through a different lens. AIDS had become a plague without end because of what could not be said in America.

The war against AIDS was a mess from the start because the virus crept into the nation along with Ronald Reagan and the feel-good eighties. It was "morning in America" — who wanted to gasp at this nightfall? American optimism could not be questioned, and American invincibility could not be tarnished. The unsightly was banished or simply ignored.

The epidemic's first victims were members of a community reveling in its own feel-good moment. Gay America, at least the urban, clone culture where AIDS first hit with deadly accuracy, had been feeling great, and ignoring the consequences, since gay liberation declared its independence from guilt and its right to the pursuit of unlimited pleasure. The loss of that right to a deadly virus seemed impossible. Gay men suffered the pain of fag jokes, bashing and harassment, holding on to unbridled sexual pleasure as the one silver lining. The clouds were growing more ominous; the silver lining was looking like a noose. It must be someone's fault: scientists in a biological-warfare laboratory, a government conspiring to murder homosexuals, public health officials skewing the message to impose prudery and heterosexuality.

I began to see AIDS as a lens through which the flaws of the nation were magnified. It revealed America's need to blame someone rather than to accept tragedy and cope with the truth of our relative powerlessness against nature. It shone a light on Americans' need to define themselves by membership in victim groups, competing for most-victimized status and the financial and psychic benefits that carried. AIDS provided a glimpse of a society more comfortable with fairy-tale villains — human or viral — than the reality of sluggish scientific progress and the complex interaction between behavior and infectious agents.

Who wanted to deal with the complexities of needle exchange when the easy answer was that drugs are bad, junkies weak and saying no, along with jail enlargement, can solve the problem? How could a nation still clinging to the myth of the missionary position cope with a crisis demanding front-page discussion of anal intercourse and classes for adolescents in the techniques of safe-sex negotiation?

AIDS was a challenge America proved inept in confronting.

Early in the epidemic, I joined the liberal crowd in blaming the Reagan-Helms crowd for that reality, as well as a wide range of other AIDS-related evils. The president never spoke about AIDS; research wasn't funded adequately; the nation remained indifferent to the crisis. Helms whipped up the Christian right, so AIDS became more an opportunity for moralizing than for safe-sex education. Ordinary people — the mythic mainstream Americans — didn't care about AIDS because they weren't falling sick and because they couldn't care less if gays and addicts were wiped off the face of the earth.

In that lexicon of blame, there was never enough money, interest or goodwill.

But by 1994 Reagan and Bush were out of office and Bill Clinton had met virtually all the activists' demands, from a souped-up Office of AIDS Research at the National Institutes of Health to regular consultation with the gay community on all AIDS-related matters, from an enormous increase in federal AIDS spending to the airing of public service announcements that encouraged condom use. A task force of scientists, activists, pharmaceutical company representatives and government officials had been appointed to critique the nation's search for drugs to help the dying. An AIDS czar had been appointed. Discrimination against the infected had been outlawed at the federal level. And the president was talking about AIDS candidly, regularly and with palpable compassion.

Yet activists continued to screech — at the drug companies, at the president, even at each other. They had somehow operated on faith that if Clinton were elected, their friends would live. When their friends continued dying, leaders nitpicked Clinton's every move, although their real complaint was that he had not pulled a cure out of his hat. They pointed their fingers elsewhere, too: at scientists who were the pawns of greedy pharmaceutical companies, at government agencies rife with egotists and incompetents, at directors of movies about AIDS that weren't explicit enough.

Much of that gospel of blame was based on cold, concrete fact. Much of it was true. But all of it ignored an even larger, more difficult truth. This is what they couldn't face: AIDS is not caused by avarice, indifference, opportunism, careerism or homophobia. As best we know, it is caused by a virus (from the Latin for "poison"), an exquisitely primitive form of life that does not care about politics, money or the Nobel Prize. A virus is programmed to care about only one thing: survival.

And survival is no easy feat for a microorganism that has no reproductive system. Instead, viruses need to infiltrate the cells of humans or other animals, take over their basic structures and turn them into reproductive factories. The irony is that viruses also tend to make humans and animals sick. And if the beings they infect die, the viruses within cannot survive.

Viruses have evolved hundreds of different strategies to get around the perils to their survival. Some, like the viruses that cause measles and influenza, are so infectious that they can spread across entire cities within weeks. Others, like HIV, use stealth and persistence, remaining hidden inside their hosts — and transmissible — for decades. Those strategies have defeated centuries of human medicine. No existing antibiotic can annihilate the smallpox or chickenpox virus. No scientist has figured out how to kill a virus without killing every cell it has infected. The only defense humans have against viral diseases is their own immune system.

That reality is almost impossible for most people with AIDS — indeed, most Americans — to face. After years of struggle against the scourges of malaria, smallpox, tuberculosis and polio, we have become comfortable in the assumption that science can defeat anything nature throws at us. Before AIDS humbled us, we had blithely assumed that epidemics were historical footnotes or Third World nightmares, not something that could happen in postmodern America.

But nature is not benign, medicine is not invincible and acts of political will are irrelevant to that equation. "You can't shout a cure out of a test tube," one AIDS activist, Mark Harrington, said recently in a confession few of his colleagues admire. Nor can you coax it out with dollars. Cures most often come from scientific serendipity, from leaps of imagination by scattered researchers, by accidents or chance. Until or unless some new Einstein has a flash of insight, scientists can do little more than plod along with their research, splicing genes, measuring viral burden, dissecting lymph nodes and placing drops of drugs in petri dishes of HIV-infected tissue.

It is the harshest of all truths, but the only force left to blame for the continuing roster of deaths and infections is a virus — a virus that continues to defeat the most massive research effort ever mounted against a single disease.

And who wants to yell at a virus?

I slouched toward this position with trepidation, for it runs smack up against AIDSthink, a constellation of fears and assumptions that may or may not have been warranted in the first years of the epidemic but that have defined it for more than a decade. These assumptions have remained relatively unchallenged — even unexamined — because one of the clearest and strongest tenets of AIDSthink is that anyone who does not hold these truths to be self-evident is an enemy of the suffering masses.

But a plague demands casting aside, at least temporarily, pettiness, politics and ignorance, or what a friend of mine with AIDS calls "over-inflated egos, preening peacocks and the hope of a Nobel Prize."

What follows, then, is no heart-rending account of the shrunken faces of the dying. Those stories have been told. They have promoted education and stirred compassion, but they have done nothing to force Americans to look into the mirror and see the nation on the brink of a new millennium. The reflections aren't pretty. They suggest that we have become a country of small-minded, self-interested issue surfers who hide from passion in rhetoric and wall ourselves off from our neighbors by taking refuge in the lowest common denominator. Our failure to treat AIDS as a disease, pure and simple, is one of the dozens of deadly mistakes that we've made for more than a decade.

This book is the account of that debacle. It is a story of science run amok, of backroom deals between activists and government bureaucrats, of biotechnology companies manipulating stock prices by manipulating research results. It is a tragedy of bungled research, scientific and activist vanity, the dangers of political correctness and, finally, the price more than a million Americans are paying for a nation's folly.

ONE

Pomp Without Circumstance

June 20, 1990. More than twelve thousand activists, scientists, politicians and social workers from across the globe were streaming into San Francisco for the Sixth International Conference on AIDS.

But the big news was who wasn't coming.

Robert Gallo, the nation's leading AIDS scientist, had been scheduled to deliver a major address, to roam the halls with an entourage hanging on his every word, as he had done at every other international AIDS conference. But seven months before the event, the officially designated codiscoverer of HIV had been accused of scientific fraud in a sixteen-page *Chicago Tribune* article that alleged that deception, backstabbing, media manipulation, forgery and political intrigue had earned him that title. He wound up as the target of an investigation on charges that he and his colleagues at the National Cancer Institute had wasted years on a self-serving and misguided crusade to prove that an earlier Gallo discovery, a human leukemia virus, was also the cause of AIDS. When they had failed, and realized that French scientists were on the verge of solving the most important medical mystery of the era, they had allegedly appropriated the French discovery for themselves. Gallo's detractors, and they were legion, delighted in the humiliation of a scientist with the debating style of a construction worker and an ego that made even empty lecture halls feel crowded.

On the eve of the conference, Gallo sent a terse telegram to the organizers of the San Francisco meeting. Detained in Moscow, he informed them. Regrets.

Larry Kramer didn't bother with such formalities. He was too busy pouting. The grand old man of AIDS activism had recently declared that America had lost the war on AIDS, and he called on gay Americans to shed blood — preferably heterosexuals' — in the streets of San Francisco. The city's police force panicked; local AIDS officials pleaded. "For God's sake, Larry, accept the responsibility of your position as the most famous AIDS activist in America and retract your call for violence around AIDS," wrote the executive director of San Francisco's Mobilization Against AIDS. "You are putting our community in an even more dangerous position than it is already."

ACT UP's media moguls fretted over their organization's image and opted for a tactful deification of their creator, asserting, "Larry Kramer is a hero of this movement." But not a single one of them volunteered to follow him onto the battlefield.

If the AIDS wars could be reduced to just two individuals — to two figures who have both dominated and symbolized the vanity fair that is AIDS in America — they would be Robert Gallo and Larry Kramer. The world's most infamous AIDS researcher and the world's most infamous AIDS activist, alter egos of almost mythic proportions who have trained all their own neuroses onto the epidemic and defined it as a frenzied dance of ego.

Gallo, who has been running for a Nobel Prize since leaving medical school, is the quintessential scientist on the make. For two decades he's reached for the pinnacle, and fallen short. He's pushed the field of retrovirology forward in laboratory techniques and concepts, but the one great discovery that would mark his place in the annals of human science has escaped him, despite his constant claims to the contrary. He has won the Albert Lasker Prize, America's most prestigious biomedical award, but the Nobel gold has always gone to somebody else.

Gallo is an often vitriolic man with the scruples of a street fighter. But when he is accused of making premature announcements or fudging data, his face softens, his voice actually quivers, his shoulders curl in. "Why me? Why do they persecute me?" he asks plaintively.

Larry Kramer is a second-rank author whose primary accomplishments prior to AIDS were his novel, *Faggots,* and his screenplay for *Women in Love.* Kramer has never gotten over the fact that his father mocked him as a sissy, that his mother was overprotective and that his beloved brother Arthur wanted to cure him of homosexuality. Still caught up in adolescent neediness, he turned to the gay community and Hollywood for love and acceptance. Gay America dismissed him as an embittered troll. Hollywood held out the carrot, even nominating him for an Oscar, but both adulation and the Oscar eluded him.

AIDS has given Kramer a new forum. He attacks the plague, and all those he deems responsible for it, with prose as subtle as a brickbat. Anyone who dares disagree with his insistence that AIDS is a holocaust — the intentional murder of gay Americans — is written off as a modern Adolf Eichmann. In quieter moments, Kramer becomes less shrill. Why me? he asks. Why don't they listen to me?

For Robert Gallo, AIDS is a battle to save a sagging reputation; for Larry Kramer, it is a battle to earn the moniker of the man who saved Gay America. For more than a decade, they've slashed and burned their way through the byways of the epidemic. Neither Gallo's nor Kramer's reputation has been enhanced by their efforts.

Larry Kramer's first public foray into AIDS was a quiet and modest appeal for money. He wasn't angry, he was afraid. It was the summer of 1981, and gay men were dying of an odd cancer and an even odder pneumonia. No one was quite sure what was happening. "It's easy to become frightened that one of the many things we've done or taken over the past years may be all that it takes for a cancer to grow from a tiny something-or-other that got in there who knows when from doing who knows what," he wrote in the *New York Native.*

It was the wrong way to appeal to his community's conscience. Gay Americans were having a party and didn't need Larry Kramer to suggest that the morning-after consequences might be lethal. To many, the plea sounded like Kramer's whining yet again about the wages of gay sin. In his 1978 novel, *Faggots,* he'd aimed his caustic wit at gay men who'd come out of the closet only to escape to self-imposed ghettos where sex overwhelmed love. Being right about the perils of one-a-night stands, two-a-night stands, five-a-night stands didn't make him popular with the gay A-list. But the not so old curmudgeon wouldn't have been comfortable with popularity. It simply wasn't his shtick.

Faggots sold extremely well, forty thousand copies in hardback. But gay reviewers asked readers to boycott the book. The Oscar Wilde Memorial Bookshop, in New York City, refused to carry it. Kramer became persona non grata on Fire Island, Gay America's favorite playground. "Self-hating homophobe" was the kindest criticism leveled at him.

He charged ahead anyway. On Labor Day weekend, 1981, Kramer and a small band of gay men canvassed Fire Island to raise money for research into the new gay cancer. Brochures were dropped on the front steps of every house in the Pines and the Grove. Tables were set up in the harbors of both communities, with banners reading, "Give to Gay Cancer." On Saturday night, from midnight to 8 A.M., the men stood in front of the Ice Palace, a popular gay disco, asking for help. They collected $126. The weekend total was $769.55.

Kramer began using his telephone, his favorite weapon. I'm Larry Kramer, he said, "the Yale University grad who had been the assistant to the presidents of Columbia and United Artist Pictures, who'd won an Academy Award nomination, who lives on Washington Square Park and had a lot of money in the bank." No one returned his phone calls — not Hollywood's most infamous queers, not New York Mayor Ed Koch, not even Koch's lowliest assistant.

No one appreciated him. They would all be sorry.

Robert Gallo was too busy basking in scientific "I told you so" to notice the first stirrings of the new epidemic.

Gallo had been on the staff of the National Cancer Institute since 1965, when he took a job as a clinical associate right after finishing his residency at the University of Chicago. Although he'd studied medicine at Thomas Jefferson University School of Medicine in Philadelphia, Gallo wasn't headed for a career caring for the ailing. "I don't have the benevolence of some who are made to be with patients," he says. "I don't like something I can't control, and you can't control the fact that many of these people are dying. There are too many failures."

Instead of patients, Gallo was working with strange organisms called retroviruses, which seemed to be genetic mirror images of their cousins the viruses. In 1910 an American pathologist named Francis Peyton Rous had proven that retroviruses could cause cancer in hens. Other scientists showed they could be equally lethal to other animals. Gallo was convinced they were the cause of disease in humans as well.

For years no one could find retroviruses in human beings. After 1971, when Richard Nixon declared war on cancer, everyone was looking for them. The allure was enormous: isolate a cancer-causing virus, develop a vaccine, and you'd become the most celebrated scientist of the century for consigning malignancies to the dustbin of medical mysteries solved by the genius of science.

In 1970, two scientists in different parts of the country had stumbled on the elusive key to the retroviral puzzle. Howard Temin of the University of Wisconsin and David Baltimore of the Massachusetts

Institute of Technology discovered an enzyme they called reverse transcriptase, which allowed retroviruses to seize control of the genetic machinery of the cells they infected and turn them into reproduction factories.

When Temin and Baltimore made the obligatory presentation of their discovery at the National Institutes of Health, Gallo sat in the audience, riveted. Temin and Baltimore had found reverse transcriptase in mice and chickens; Gallo vowed to find it in human beings. Temin and Baltimore won the Nobel Prize for identifying an enzyme; Gallo would win it for discovering a way to cure cancer.

Within months, Gallo announced that he had found reverse transcriptase in human leukemia cells. The discovery was not widely hailed; no one seemed able to reproduce his results. But Gallo was the National Cancer Institute's leading researcher on viral causes of cancer. He was charming, well connected and rose quickly to the directorship of the largest laboratory at the National Cancer Institute in Bethesda, Maryland.

Throughout the early seventies, Gallo kept refining his test for locating reverse transcriptase. With each publication, the snickering grew louder. "If there's all that reverse transcriptase out there, where are the human retroviruses?" his skeptical colleagues asked.

Gallo was not easily dissuaded.

Then, on a Saturday in January 1975, Gallo convened the big guns at the National Cancer Institute to announce that he had done it. He and his colleague, Robert Gallagher, had isolated a human retrovirus that he was calling HL-23 from the blood of a leukemia patient from Texas. The discovery of what was believed to be the first human cancer virus was, as Gallo is fond of saying, one of those "Eureka" moments. He was intent on playing it to the hilt. The discovery was plastered across American newspapers, without any independent scientific confirmation. Gallo's Nobel seemed at hand.

His moment of glory lasted less than a year. Scientists across the globe rushed to verify his finding and came up with . . . monkey viruses. Cells from baboons, gibbons and woolly monkeys. His colleagues gleefully lectured Gallo on the dangers of contamination, as if he were a graduate student. He refused to concede. Maybe the patient was also infected with a baboon virus, he suggested. When no one bought this odd explanation, he began spreading rumors about sabotage in his lab.

Eventually Gallo, who can't stand to lose even a friendly game of softball or tennis, retreated to his lab in defeat. HL-23 was widely renamed "the human rumor virus." Researchers began looking for defective genes rather than retroviruses as the cause of cancer.

Robert Gallo clung to them as to the Holy Grail.

Finally, at the end of 1978, while examining a lymph node from an Alabama patient with an unusual T-cell cancer, researchers in Gallo's lab found reverse transcriptase. Calm down, they told themselves, remembering the ignominy of Gallo's earlier announcement. For almost two years they grew huge quantities of what seemed to be a retrovirus. They checked and rechecked to make sure there was no contamination. They looked for the retrovirus in other cancer patients and found it in two of them.

Robert Gallo's vindication was at hand. In December 1980 he published the first in a series of papers in the *Proceedings of the National Academy of Sciences* to announce the discovery of the first human retrovirus associated with cancer. It was Gallo's most unsullied moment of glory, one that sealed his reputation as the father of human retrovirology. The only sticky matter was what disease his new pathogen, called HTLV, human T-cell lymphoma virus, actually caused.

While Gallo was looking for a disease to marry to his new virus, the Japanese were looking for a virus to wed to a new disease. In the fall of 1977, physicians in Japan had identified a new type of cancer, an adult T-cell leukemia unlike anything they had ever seen. They also thought they'd found a retrovirus in a tissue sample from fishermen dying of the new cancer. They were calling it ATLV, adult T-cell leukemia virus. When Gallo made his announcement, the Japanese researchers sent blood samples to Bethesda to see if their ATLV might be HTLV.

In March 1981, just as Larry Kramer was beginning to feel the chilly premonition of disaster in New York, Robert Gallo boarded a plane for Kyoto, where he announced that he had found a disease to match his virus: HTLV was the cause of the Japanese fishermen's cancer. The Japanese were not surprised. When genetic sequencing was done to compare ATLV and HTLV, they turned out to be identical.

The Alabama man had not died from that T-cell lymphoma after all. HTLV kept its initials, but was quietly changed to human T-cell leukemia virus. The Japanese were given barely a mention in Gallo's publications on the discovery.

Nobody wanted Larry Kramer to be president. He was too confrontational. He was an outsider among the Important Homosexuals needed to raise money and recruit volunteers for their new group. The small band that had canvassed Fire Island the previous Labor Day had been meeting for months in Kramer's living room, and in January 1982 they formed the Gay Men's Health Crisis to mobilize New York City's gay community around the terrifying new disease. Kramer didn't mind not being the president. The man chosen was in the closet, so Kramer knew that he himself would wind up being the group's public face.

But from the first there was dissension. Kramer is better at founding organizations than at working within them. No one has ever accused him of possessing tact or a talent for compromise. He began by alienating everyone with his insistence on preaching safe sex. "I am sick of guys who moan that giving up careless sex until this blows over is worse than death," he wrote. "How can they value life so little and cocks and asses so much? . . . I am sick of guys who think that all being gay means is sex in the first place. I am sick of guys who can only think with their cocks."

Stop moralizing, the other GMHC board members cautioned. What if there isn't an infectious agent? You can't tell gay men to turn their backs on hard-won sexual freedom. Every man must make his own decision. Just give out information, don't preach.

They were essentially asking him not to be Larry Kramer, a postmodern version of an Old Testament prophet who had warned of pestilence and plague even before they had struck. He certainly wasn't about to stop now that gay men were dying. Soon he was roaming New York, posting AIDS warnings on the doors of gay bathhouses and shrieking from every available soapbox, "All it seems to take is the one wrong fuck."

Next Kramer began the delicious business of identifying enemies and denigrating them. He wasn't discriminating. The mayor wouldn't meet with him? The mayor was a pig. The *New York Times* wasn't covering AIDS as he thought proper? The *Times* was homophobic. Ronald Reagan, the National Institutes of Health, the straight media, the Centers for Disease Control, the *New England Journal of Medicine*, the Food and Drug Administration, the health insurance industry, closeted gay men, Gay Psychiatrists of New York, American Physicians for Human Rights, Senator Daniel Patrick Moynihan. Enemies were everywhere.

None of these people appreciated being called murderers. Some became more hostile as a result. Kramer's fellow board members worried that he was a loose cannon, turning potential friends into committed foes. He was vinegar in a crowd that still believed in the virtues of honey.

In its first year, the Gay Men's Health Crisis became a major social service agency, running a hot line, printing a newsletter and health recommendation brochures in four languages. GMHC had a network of buddies to help the sick, support groups, legal advisers, financial counselors and training seminars for health care professionals. Despite Kramer's regular rantings about the indifference of gay New Yorkers, a community was being built — on the coffins of the dying.

But Kramer wasn't interested in creating a gay United Way. He didn't want to serve the dying; he wanted to stop death cold. And in his book, that meant political action. Despite his fury, Kramer had a startlingly naive view of the magical qualities of politics. The son of middle-class, liberal Jewish parents in Washington, D.C., he grew up in an era when Eisenhower was everyone's grandfather and truth and justice prevailed. He'd studied at Yale and blithely accepted the myth that a Yale diploma would open all doors. It had never occurred to Kramer that the powerful might not really care what happened to anybody but their own friends, or that their power might be limited. He was convinced that if Ronald Reagan and Ed Koch would only pay attention, AIDS would evaporate.

He began on the local level, beating down the door to Mayor Koch's office. It took more than a year. Finally, on October 28, 1982, a policeman led Kramer and other members of the GMHC board into a bare, unused room in the basement of City Hall, where they sat on old straight-backed chairs for a meeting with Koch's liaison to the gay community — who'd also been liaison to the Hasidic Jewish sects. Herb Rickman arrived ninety minutes late. He promised the group virtually everything, from funds equivalent to San Francisco's AIDS budget to real involvement by the city's health commissioner.

Kramer left the meeting curiously optimistic. He'd yet to learn the cheapness of talk. It didn't take long.

"If this article doesn't scare the shit out of you we're in real trouble," he wrote in the *New York Native* in March 1983. "If this article doesn't rouse you to anger, fury, rage and action, gay men may have no future on this earth. Our continued existence depends on just how angry you get." Kramer was trying to bludgeon down the walls of denial within the gay community. He ended the article by asking for three thousand volunteers willing to get arrested at sit-ins and other acts of civil disobedience.

He heard from fifty.

The next month, when Mayor Koch made his first appearance at a function relating to AIDS, Kramer was there, outside in the pouring rain, with his volunteers. It was a symposium on the disease held at Lenox Hill Hospital, on Manhattan's East Side. Don Francis from the Centers for Disease Control had agreed to appear. Congressman Ted Weiss came up from Washington. Terrence Cardinal Cook was scheduled to give the invocation. Koch could hardly decline the invitation. "When are you going to do something about AIDS? How many people have to die?" Kramer shouted when the mayor arrived. "Hey, Ed, come out of the closet! Help your gay brothers!"

The media perked up and turned their cameras toward him. Kramer beamed.

The next morning Koch sent word that he would meet with ten representatives of the gay community. Kramer walked into the weekly morning gathering of the AIDS Network, an ad hoc organizing group, expecting to be one of them. He was late, as usual. The ten had already been chosen, and Kramer was not among them. The Gay Men's Health Crisis would send its president and its executive director. Kramer threatened to resign. Go ahead, the group answered. Gay leaders begged Kramer to calm down. He refused. The AIDS Network offered him one of its two slots. He was petulant, sure that he'd been betrayed. He stormed out.

GMHC joined the *Times*, Ronald Reagan, doctors, and most of the citizenry, gay and straight, on Kramer's shit list.

Cut off from the community he'd helped organize, Kramer wandered New York with nothing to do. One night he showed up at a party for GMHC volunteers. Uncle Charlie's, a yuppie gay bar, was filled with the energy of blaring music. Kramer barged into the DJ's booth and seized the microphone. "Tell them they made a mistake in letting me go," he yelled. "Tell them they must fight harder and not be so timid and afraid."

The volunteers didn't think they were timid. They knew they hadn't made a mistake in getting rid of Kramer. GMHC was expanding along with the epidemic and had hundreds of volunteers teaching doctors about AIDS, taking food to the sick and calming the fears of the panicked. They were doing just fine without him.

Kramer's speech at the 1983 Gay Pride Day rally was unusually subdued. "I am prouder now of gay people than ever," he declared. "Can we afford not to heal wounds and unite?" It was his final cry. No one from GMHC called to ask him to come home.

Kramer left the next month for a trip to Europe. Feeling lost and alone in Munich, he took a train to Dachau. As he wandered past the barracks and gas chambers of the concentration camp, he connected with the ghosts of the Nazi Holocaust. Nobody knew. Nobody cared. Nobody knows. Nobody cares.

He jumped on a plane to Boston, holed up in Hyannisport, on Cape Cod, and began to write a play. Larry Kramer would find some way to make people listen to him.

Robert Gallo had been too busy searching for a disease caused by HTLV to pay much attention when James Curran of the Centers for Disease Control came by the National Institutes of Health in 1981 to talk about the new immune disorder that was killing homosexuals and Haitians. But when Curran returned the following year and announced that the new ailment seemed to be attacking T cells, Gallo sat up and listened. His new retrovirus also attacked T cells. Maybe HTLV was behind this ailment.

HTLV as the cause of AIDS didn't make sense, though. In cancer, cells are immortalized; in AIDS, they die. How could the same virus kill cells in one disease and make them live forever in another? Anyway, no AIDS cases were showing up in Japan, where HTLV was endemic.

But Gallo's friend Max Essex at Harvard was sure HTLV had some connection to AIDS. He'd even found it in some tissue samples of the mounting number of the sick. And a CDC researcher named Don Francis was insisting that some retrovirus had to be involved. So Gallo decided to look into it. His lab sorted through tissue samples from patients with the new disease — looking for signs of reverse transcriptase and the presence of HTLV. It wasn't a high priority; by Gallo's own estimate, less than 10 percent of the time of his fifty associates and assistants was devoted to the task.

Then, in February 1983, Gallo received an intriguing phone call from his old friend and competitor in Paris, Luc Montagnier. The head of viral oncology at the Pasteur Institute had found something, and he wasn't sure what it might be. He and his lab staff had seen clear signs of a retrovirus in the cells of a French fashion designer with AIDS. Could Montagnier have some antibodies to Gallo's HTLV to see if that was what was growing in the designer's cells?

Gallo had news of his own. He'd found antibodies to HTLV in two gay men. Maybe he was on the verge of stopping an epidemic in its tracks.

He sent the samples Montagnier had requested off to Paris and
kept his staff looking for HTLV. They found it, but in a surprisingly
small number of AIDS patients. Even while Gallo was churning out
articles reporting his discovery of HTLV and HTLV antibodies in
AIDS patients, his laboratory assistants were complaining that they
just weren't finding his virus in most of the cases.

While Gallo continued his HTLV hunting, the French ran tests on
their tissue samples and found no trace of HTLV. In early April 1983,
Montagnier told Gallo he thought his researchers had discovered an
entirely new retrovirus. The French wrote up the results of their work
and had it hand delivered to Bethesda. Gallo had promised to arrange
for its publication in the issue of *Science* that would also carry reports
from him and from Max Essex.

When the issue appeared on May 20, the press trumpeted the
promising news: HTLV-1 might be the cause of AIDS. It was a logical
conclusion drawn from Gallo's and Essex's findings. But Montagnier
had reported the opposite, that the virus he found seemed unrelated to
the leukemia virus. Most reporters hadn't read past the abstract, which
noted that the virus seemed to be a member of the HTLV family. The
French researchers were puzzled: they had written no abstract. Gallo
had prepared it for them.

By June, Montagnier was sure he had found a new retrovirus and
that it was unrelated to Gallo's pet pathogen. Dubbed LAV, lymphadenopathy-associated virus, it seemed to be a member of the lentivirus
family, a class of virus that causes anemia in horses. He sent samples of
it to Gallo's lab. They confirmed that it was not HTLV.

But Robert Gallo didn't give up that easily. While the French were
designing a blood test and finding antibodies to LAV in patients, Gallo
was telling reporters, public health officials and other scientists that
HTLV seemed the likely cause of AIDS. In July he wrote to Montagnier
that Essex had found HTLV in half the patients he had studied, while
Montagnier had found it in only 20 percent. "Something is missing,"
Gallo wrote.

Montagnier brought him more LAV later that month, when the
two met at the first meeting of the National Cancer Institute's AIDS
task force. The French researcher showed the scientists the analysis
from his laboratory. He passed around photographs taken with an
electron microscope. But nothing Gallo was seeing or hearing would
convince him.

Montagnier is an aloof, patrician Gaul. He didn't understand that

Gallo was a scrappy, Italian street fighter. At least not until the two met again at the cancer think tank in Cold Spring Harbor on September 14, 1983. This would be that group's first meeting on HTLV, and Gallo planned to devote one session to the link between his retrovirus and AIDS. Montagnier was assigned the last slot of the session, after Gallo and Essex had presented their evidence of the link between HTLV and AIDS. Montagnier reported that since the beginning of the year, he and his team had isolated a new retrovirus in a total of eight patients, including gay men, hemophiliacs and Haitians. Their blood test for the virus still wasn't very sensitive, but it appeared to pick up 60 percent of the infections. Most important, both in its shape and its biochemistry, the new retrovirus seemed unrelated to HTLV.

Gallo went on the attack. In a series of what he calls "probing" questions — and what others at the meeting have called "sledgehammers" — Gallo suggested that the French hadn't found a retrovirus at all, that they were inept in the laboratory.

Without Gallo's imprimatur, Montagnier's findings were discounted. American scientists couldn't conceive of the possibility that a foreigner might best their country's brightest. Montagnier returned to France, stunned.

The two men continued to cooperate — to a point. Gallo's lab asked for, and received, another sample of Montagnier's virus, which an assistant in his Bethesda lab grew and determined was not HTLV. But Gallo continued to tout HTLV, writing paper after paper claiming to have isolated that and related viruses in the tissue of people with AIDS. In fact, Gallo's lab still could find HTLV in only 25 percent of the patients.

By the fall, other researchers were becoming as skeptical as the French. HTLV is "overplayed to the point where I worry that it will diminish interest in other viruses," one wrote in the *New England Journal of Medicine* in October. "There's a lot of hype associated with it."

In New York, Dr. Joseph Sonnabend, one of the city's foremost AIDS specialists, decided to see if he could find evidence of HTLV in the blood and tissue of his patients. He sent specimens off to a colleague in Nebraska. No HTLV. He sent others to a virologist in Japan. No HTLV. He tried again, sending samples to a renowned retrovirologist at Cambridge University in England. No HTLV. He submitted his findings for publication. They contradicted Gallo's party line and were rejected.

By then, the French had already applied for a European patent on their blood test for LAV. Dr. Jay Levy, a University of California virologist, had seen their work and become intrigued. In November he, too, found a new retrovirus in AIDS patients: ARV, AIDS-related virus, he called it. But he decided to save his announcement until he'd amassed further proof.

By the end of the year Gallo was pulling back from his insistence that scientists could find HTLV-1 in AIDS patients if they only looked hard enough. A mutant HTLV-1 was his newer argument, a form of the virus that wouldn't show up easily. By Christmas he was telling his superiors at NIH that he had found that mutant. Meanwhile, the French had applied for a patent on their blood test on December 5.

Montagnier didn't bother to go to the world's first major scientific gathering on AIDS. After Cold Spring Harbor, he'd decided to back off on public confrontations with Gallo. In his place, he sent Jean-Claude Chermann, a colleague who had known Gallo for two decades. Maybe he'd have more success. Chermann arrived in Park City, Utah, in February 1984 with a weight of scientific evidence. He could show that LAV selectively targeted the very type of T cells AIDS patients were missing and that the French had developed a blood test that detected antibodies to the virus in 75 percent of those infected. He even had electron-microscope photographs of the microbe, which bore little resemblance to HTLV.

Gallo began the question-and-answer session by suggesting that the French virus was a contaminant — like the contaminant that had humiliated him nine years earlier. He implied that it wasn't a retrovirus at all. When Chermann faced him down, Gallo claimed that it had to be a variant of HTLV.

Ten days after the Utah meeting, the Centers for Disease Control sent tissue samples from AIDS patients to Gallo and Montagnier. Both men claimed to have developed blood tests for their competing viruses — LAV and Gallo's HTLV variant, which he'd begun calling HTLV-3. The CDC samples set up a head-to-head competition. The tests performed equally well.

Even as Gallo prepared a series of scientific papers on his new findings, he and Montagnier began negotiating how to announce their discoveries. In early April, Gallo flew to Paris to work out the details. The CDC's Don Francis tried to play middleman, but Gallo was as suspicious of his American colleague as he was of the French. They wrangled about the classification of their viruses and came to no consensus. They did agree, however, that any declaration should be orchestrated as a joint event.

On April 23, 1984, Gallo was called back to Washington from a trip to Italy so that he could appear at a press conference called by Health and Human Services Secretary Margaret Heckler. He stood next to her as she announced to the world that the probable cause of AIDS had been found and that Robert Gallo was the American hero who'd brought hope to the dying and an answer to a dread disease.

Hours before, lawyers for the U.S. government had filed an application for a patent on Gallo's blood test for HTLV-3. Included was his sworn statement that he was the original and sole inventor, which meant that he knew of no other similar or related invention anywhere in the world.

Gallo faced the reporters packed into the conference room. "When did you make the discovery?" one asked. Gallo answered that he'd been growing large quantities of the virus for six months. It was an odd reply. There was no indication that Gallo had even discovered the virus at that time. "Is your virus the same as the ones the French have?" another queried. Gallo replied that he couldn't say yet, that he didn't have enough of their virus to make a clear comparison. Strange again, since Gallo's lab had begun growing the French LAV by December 1983.

The French watched the show in disbelief. They had been written out of the discovery entirely.

On May 4 the journal *Science* published four separate papers from Gallo's lab. The scientist claimed that he had isolated a new virus from forty-eight people with AIDS, that it was a true member of the family of retroviruses he had first discovered and that he had developed a blood test to screen for antibodies to it.

Over the years, journalists and congressional investigators have concluded that both the public and the scientific shows were monumental frauds. Gallo's lab records contain no traces of the forty-eight separate isolates he'd mentioned. His blood test came four months after the French discovery. And he had every reason to know that his HTLV-3 was, in fact, the French LAV.

It was viral plagiarism of the most egregious sort — and Gallo almost got away with it.

Larry Kramer's return to New York in January 1984 was hailed by absolutely no one. He had alienated virtually the entire gay community of New York before his departure.

As his agent read his new play, *The Normal Heart,* Kramer threw himself back into the fray, preaching the gospel of safe sex, demanding the closure of bathhouses and trying to regain his seat on the board of the Gay Men's Health Crisis. When the latter attempts failed, he wrote the group a letter, calling them "a bunch of ninnies, incompetent, cowards."

None of that was important. The important thing was the play. Kramer didn't know much about organizations, about human relations, but he knew about words, even if his first theatrical work had closed the night it opened. *The Normal Heart* would make them listen, make everyone understand. Kramer, singlehandedly, would change the course of the epidemic.

The Normal Heart was part love story, part diatribe. It was a social history of Gay America, a lecture on the price of homophobia and a cry of rage, pain and loss. The play sanctifies and immortalizes a man, Ned Weeks, who bears more than a slight resemblance to Kramer. Weeks is a writer with a disposition "as cheery as Typhoid Mary" and a talent for unbridled confrontation that alienates almost everyone. He tries to sound the alarm about the appearance of a deadly new disease and founds an organization to confront the confusion, denial and indifference. His lover — a newspaper fashion writer who lives in terror that his editors will discover that he's gay — is stricken. Weeks indefatigably battles the media, the mayor, the American Medical Association, hospitals and closeted gay men, trying to save both his lover and his community.

To no avail, of course. The organization to which Weeks gave birth disowns him for playing Cassandra shouting her way through a plague. The lover he has sought for a lifetime dies. And the conspiracy of silence continues.

"I'm a terrible leader and a useless lover," admits a battered Weeks.

But Kramer was unrepentant. "I hear you've got a big mouth," says Ned's crisp wheelchair-bound female physician.

"Is big mouth a symptom?" Weeks asks dryly.

"No," she shoots back. "A cure."

The Normal Heart wasn't successful drama, as most critics commented. It was a sermon on the mount. Too manipulative, too desperate. Kramer the would-be artist couldn't rein in Kramer the polemicist. The play envisioned a Kramer-centric epidemic and was filled with thinly veiled personal attacks, especially on Mayor Koch. Still, it made its point. On opening night in April 1985, the audience paid tribute to

Kramer with a roaring standing ovation. The *New York Times* was so mortified by the play's attack on the paper that it ran a sidebar next to its review refuting the charges. Mayor Ed Koch, who was up for reelection, called a press conference and announced increased city services for people with AIDS.

Kramer had a hit show. *The Normal Heart* ran for a year at Joseph Papp's Public Theater and was mounted in hundreds of productions from London to Los Angeles. Kramer watched himself played by Brad Davis, Joel Grey, Martin Sheen and Richard Dreyfuss.

But he did not end the epidemic. "I was naive enough to believe — or to hope — that when *The Normal Heart* opened, the following day the world would be changed," Kramer admits. He could never accept the sense of powerlessness he felt, the discovery that his voice alone could not control politics or medicine or the course of the virus.

Gallo was holding on by the skin of his teeth and the force of his bluster.

The key to shoring up his case was to prove that the new virus was a form of HTLV — *his* viral family, so to speak — and then to prevent anyone from comparing his virus to that of the French. It wasn't easy. The Centers for Disease Control had been asking for samples so they could begin doing epidemiologic work. Gallo agreed only when they promised not to use the samples to compare his virus to LAV. I'll do it myself, he said. Then he began sending memos and notes objecting to the use of "LAV" to describe the virus that he called HTLV-3. When scientists began using "LAV/HTLV-3," he objected to the precedence given the French.

The case for the new virus's membership in the HTLV family was weakened by the fact that there seemed to be no AIDS in Japan and an exploding number of cases in Africa. Gallo explained away the problem in a bizarre medical-history article in *Nature*. The virus arose in Africa, he wrote, but was transported by Portuguese sailors to the Caribbean and then to Japan. By the time it arrived in Asia, however, it had mutated into a less virulent form. The proof of his contention, he indicated, was the fact that the Japanese word for monkey, *amakawa*, came from *macaco,* Portuguese for monkey.

Except that the Japanese word for monkey is *saru.*

Meanwhile, the French were homing in on Gallo with irrefutable proof. The only sure way to compare viruses is by genetic sequencing. In December 1984 Montagnier and his colleague Simon Wain-Hobson showed up at an NIH symposium on AIDS and displayed the first gene map of LAV, which bore only marginal similarity to the HTLV family. Gallo countered with a map of his own, suggesting a striking resemblance between his virus and the HTLV family.

As scientists from around the world weighed in with their opinions, two things became clear: first, neither Gallo's virus nor Montagnier's belonged in the HTLV family, and second, Gallo's virus and Montagnier's were identical. Other viruses showed genetic similarities; these two were virtually indistinguishable.

Gallo defended himself on the first count by asserting that the French had made the same mistake about the virus's familial ties. Montagnier, who'd avoided engaging in a public debate with Gallo, exploded. "I am not interested in pursuing an endless polemic with you," he wrote Gallo on March 4, 1985, "but I wish to reestablish the scientific truth even though this implies the demonstration that you were wrong. After all, your laboratory, not mine, has spent a lot of time and money to show homology with HTLV-1 and 2. If you believe in sequence data, why don't you leave off your previous dream and admit that the AIDS virus is not an HTLV."

The second emerging truth — that the French and American viruses were identical — became an international cause célèbre. On August 6, 1985, the head of the Pasteur Institute met with officials of the Department of Health and Human Services and demanded partial credit for the discovery of what everyone knew was one virus as well as a portion of the royalties from Gallo's blood test. When the U.S. government refused to meet their demands, the Pasteur Institute filed suit, suggesting what everyone else suspected: that Gallo's HTLV-3 was the LAV that the French had sent him with the condition that it not be used for commercial purposes.

Health and Human Services attorneys responded by arguing that the virus Gallo had used to develop the American test, although genetically similar to LAV, was an independent discovery. When the Pasteur Institute insisted that they were not genetically similar but identical, the attorneys, assured by Gallo of the truth of their position, answered that claiming that the two viruses were the same was like "saying that because John Wilkes Booth and Abraham Lincoln were both people, they were identical." The dispute continued impolitely throughout 1986. The French argued that Gallo was withholding public documents. Then they offered proof that the photograph of HTLV-3 that Gallo had published in his series of articles in *Science* had actually been a photograph of LAV.

The *New York Native,* which had already declared Gallo a thief and a fraud, ran a story on the dispute headlined "Science's Greatest Living Performer." To drive the point home, Gallo's face was pasted over a photograph of Carmen Miranda in full bangles and plumes.

Finally, a group of Nobel Prize winners demanded that something be done. Science was being disgraced. Jonas Salk became an ambassador at large, shuttling between the French and the Americans to work out a solution. On Gallo's fiftieth birthday, in mid-March of 1987, he sat down with Montagnier in a hotel in Frankfurt to draw up an official chronology of the discovery of the AIDS virus that would give each man equal credit, even an equal number of lines. Montagnier and his colleagues had resisted all compromise. They knew they were right. But the political pressure was too strong to resist.

One week later, on March 31, President Ronald Reagan and Prime Minister Jacques Chirac announced a truce in the East Room of the White House. Gallo and Montagnier would henceforth be known as the codiscoverers of HIV, the human immunodeficiency virus. The proceeds from the blood test's royalties would be shared. The French agreed to drop their lawsuits.

Eight days after the first official end to the dispute was declared, scientists at Los Alamos National Laboratory in New Mexico wrote to senior NIH officials warning that Gallo's HTLV-3 was merely Montagnier's LAV by another name. The official version of the discovery of the cause of AIDS was, they asserted, a "double fraud."

With the success of *The Normal Heart,* Larry Kramer's name acquired cachet. He was no longer an outsider in his community. Gay America loves celebrities, and Kramer had become a bona fide one.

That tamed the tantrums for almost two years. Other than sending an occasional letter to the *New York Times* or the *Village Voice,* complaining about their AIDS coverage and straight America's indifference to AIDS, he threw few shrill barbs in public. Then, in January 1987, he made up for lost time by publicly blaming the Gay Men's Health Crisis for the mounting epidemic. "The Doomsday Scenario that many have feared for so long comes closer," he wrote in a marathon epistle that appeared in the *New York Native.* "Next week, 274 people will die from AIDS. Next week, 374 more will become infected with the killer virus. In four years' time, 270,000 people will have AIDS. For all the worthy Patient Services and Education that have been provided [by GMHC], the rate of infection and death continues unabated."

The letter was alternately a plea for a new direction for the organization and a rant. Like some fathers, Kramer couldn't resist berating his son for not growing up to be the man he'd envisioned. "You have become a funeral home," he charged, mocking the group for becoming a social services center. He compared GMHC's leaders to his great-uncle Herschel: an "unimaginative, whining, superior, dried-up old stuffed shirt, who was smelly and had been around too long."

How dare GMHC not be fighting for better treatment centers, public education and safe-sex training. How dare it not be at the forefront of the demand for immediate access to drugs for the dying. How dare it not smuggle in promising drugs from Mexico, not send a lobbyist to Washington, not battle with the *New York Times*.

How dare GMHC not listen to Larry Kramer.

"Since I left GMHC," he said, "your image, your sense of public relations savvy, your visibility, to put it impolitely, sucks."

Week after week, Kramer continued his relentless barrage, even while deriding his foes for attacking him rather than the real enemies. The leaders of GMHC — who were toiling to provide treatment, information and help to the mounting number of sick who were walking through their doors — finally gave in and agreed to a meeting. But they weren't willing to disband the organization and remake it according to his design. It was time for him to give up and replace the errant child. No more nursemaid to the dying. His second son would be a militant who would mobilize the gay community to topple homophobic conservatives and mealy-mouthed liberals unconcerned with the epidemic.

On a blustery spring evening, Kramer stood before a group at the Gay and Lesbian Community Center in New York and asked for a declaration of war. Looking around the room, he ordered one side of the audience to stand up. "At the rate we are going, you could be dead in less than five years," he shouted at them. "Two-thirds of this room could be dead in less than five years."

Kramer disgorged his greatest anger on the Food and Drug Administration, which he accused of withholding lifesaving medications from the dying. We need to organize, he insisted, to pick up the scattered pieces of our power and bring our enemies to their knees. It was a thrilling speech in a community that had defined itself as disempowered.

ACT UP was born.

Suddenly the kid who'd been mocked as a sissy, the man who'd never been cute enough to make it in the gay scene, had a hit play and was at the head of an army of the hippest and hottest men in the city. Finally, everyone was answering his phone calls. The *New York Times* printed his op-ed piece eviscerating the FDA and the National Institutes of Health. *Times* editor Max Frankel began a long correspondence with the very man who lost no opportunity to call his newspaper a homophobic rag. The Times-Mirror Corporation, which owns the *Los Angeles Times* and the *Washington Post,* accepted his proposal for a syndicated column. *New York Newsday* gave him a column the day Ronald Reagan made his first speech on AIDS. Kramer used it to launch what became his constant message: "There's only one word to describe [Reagan's] monumental disdain for the dead and dying: genocide."

The door to the White House opened to him, and he met with Gary Bauer, Reagan's domestic policy adviser. The assistant secretary of health agreed to an interview, as did dozens of scientists at the National Institutes of Health. It is unclear what Kramer thought he could accomplish. "Make them listen," he'd screamed for five years. They listened, but nothing much changed.

Kramer talked anywhere and everywhere. At the *Village Voice* AIDS Forum, at a New York Civil Liberties Union seminar on the U.S. Constitution, and in Boston at the Lesbian and Gay Town Meeting, where he declared, "I'm shutting up and going away." He didn't, of course, and went on to testify before the Presidential AIDS Commission, to speak at the annual black-tie dinner of the Human Rights Campaign Fund and to give interviews to every television reporter willing to listen.

He and ACT UP took to the streets. They screamed, protested, pleaded, picketed, sat-in, studied, threatened and cajoled. They hit every imaginable target, from the *Saturday Evening Post* to St. Patrick's Cathedral. AIDS funding skyrocketed, and public awareness increased. Gay men continued to die.

Kramer's response was to pump up the volume, and the vitriol. While he alternately compared himself to Cassandra and to Moses, he branded NIH, which he said stood for Not Interested in Homosexuals, an Animal House of horrors. He castigated its director of AIDS research, Dr. Anthony Fauci — the cute Italian whose nice butt ACT UP boys admired — as public enemy number one. He called Mathilde Krim, the founder of the American Foundation for AIDS Research, a "dumb incompetent, a would-be saint who should pack up her little suitcase and go back to Haifa." And he attacked Ronald Reagan,

George Bush, Cardinal O'Connor, Ed Koch, GMHC, Straight America — and most of Gay America as well.

"We are being murdered," Kramer said over and over again. There was only one solution, he insisted, turning to his roots for inspiration. "In a desperate struggle to secure their new homeland, the Jewish people in Palestine fighting to establish Israel had an organization called the Irgun. It was an underground guerrilla army, and its members were extremely disciplined and daring. They started fires. They threw bombs. They kidnapped. They assassinated. They executed their enemies. They won."

In Kramer's view of the world — which began in his Fifth Avenue apartment and ended in his five-thousand-square-foot house in the Hamptons, on Long Island — AIDS was transformed from a natural plague into a man-made disaster. "AIDS is our holocaust" became his favorite line. It was also, and not incidentally, very quotable. The metaphor was horrific and wholly unwarranted, but Kramer loved the sound of it and worked it as hard as he could. AIDS scientists were modern Mengeles. AIDS clinics were death camps. AIDS activists who didn't agree with him were henchmen of Hitler. Genocide gripped the land.

In the fall of 1989, Kramer asked for a spot on the podium at the Sixth International Conference on AIDS, the ultimate forum for an AIDS activist. He claimed the honor for himself as the founder of both ACT UP and the Gay Men's Health Crisis. The coordinating committee instead asked Vito Russo, a film historian, critic and the author of *The Celluloid Closet*. Kramer felt personally rejected and exploded. "I think you will find that it will prove a big mistake not to have honored my fervent solicitations," he wrote the physician cochairing the conference, whom he began calling San Francisco's most successful undertaker. "By snubbing me in such a fashion you have slapped in the face not only me and what I have stood for these past nine years, but every other AIDS activist. I trust that with the publication and circulation of this letter, ACT UP's everywhere will now commence their planning to join my call to action — at the conference — to let you, your committee, your conference, and the world that is watching know that, once again, an attempt has been made to silence us. You have, in effect, thrown down the gauntlet, and I intend to see that it is taken up. If you wish to view this letter as a threat, please do."

ACT UP chapters around the nation did not begin planning ways to avenge Kramer's honor. AIDS activists had not been silenced; Larry

Kramer had. When his comrades proved indifferent to his fate, Kramer upped the ante yet again. He wrote in *OutWeek* magazine:

> With this article I am calling for a MASSIVE DISRUPTION of the Sixth International AIDS Conference that is being held in San Francisco June 20–24. Every human being who wants to end the AIDS epidemic must be in San Francisco . . . either inside or outside the Moscone Convention Center or the Marriott Hotel, screaming, yelling, furiously angry, protesting at this stupid conference.
>
> HOW MANY TIMES DO YOU HAVE TO HEAR THIS BEFORE YOU BELIEVE IT! AND RISE UP AGAINST IT!
>
> THIS GOVERNMENT OF SHITHEADS WANTS US DEAD. WHY CAN'T EVERY GAY MAN AND LESBIAN GET THAT THROUGH HIS/HER HEAD? INDEED, UNCLE GEORGE WANTS ALL FAGGOTS, NIGGERS, JUNKIES, SPICS, WHORES, UNMARRIEDS, AND THEIR BABIES DEAD.
>
> HOW MUCH MORE EVIDENCE DO YOU NEED? DO YOU HAVE TO BE LINED UP IN FRONT OF A FIRING SQUAD BEFORE YOU FIGHT BACK?
>
> WE HAVE BEEN LINED UP IN FRONT OF A FIRING SQUAD, AND IT IS CALLED AIDS.
>
> WE MUST RIOT. I AM CALLING FOR A FUCKING RIOT!

Kramer's call to arms was either abhorred or ignored. No one else seemed convinced that riots would produce a cure. And Kramer didn't even appear to cheer his troops onto the battlefield. Warned that he would be arrested at the San Francisco airport and detained, the man who called for violence in the streets didn't think about taking a train.

Robert Gallo received little relief from his ordeal.

In 1987, in *And the Band Played On,* Randy Shilts published most Americans' first glimpse of the scientific dispute, seriously tarnishing Gallo's reputation. When Gallo appeared at Cambridge University, retrovirologist Alexander Karpas rose from the audience and accused him of theft. Eastern-bloc scientists claimed he had created the virus as a chemical weapon.

Gallo concluded that the mess was the fault of Don Francis of the CDC. In 1988 he sent Francis a strange letter. Addressed to Gallo himself, it affirmed that Robert Gallo was the codiscoverer of HIV. Francis was given forty-eight hours to sign and return it. He refused.

Gallo's only hope for vindication was to make the kind of discovery that would turn the dispute into a footnote. He turned his attention to developing a vaccine against HIV. Gradually, the accusations faded as Gallo either stonewalled questions or denied the truth of all allegations. In October 1989 *Newsweek* named him one of America's twenty-five leading innovators. The next month, he was granted an audience with the pope.

Then his nightmare returned, with the appearance of a special sixteen-page insert in the *Chicago Tribune* on November 19, 1989. In "The AIDS Quest," John Crewdson, one of the nation's most distinguished journalists, provided meticulous detail on Gallo's past, questioning the name of every cell culture and the date of every experiment conducted in his lab. The proof that HTLV-3 was LAV in American drag was irrefutable. Crewdson laid out a body of evidence that persuaded most readers that Robert Gallo was a liar and a cheat. The only remaining question was whether Gallo had stolen the virus or suffered yet another contamination in his lab.

Gallo answered the question himself when he tried to evade the humiliation. He suggested that one of those wily French pathogens might have slipped into his test tube by accident. But less than two weeks later, Congressman John Dingell wrote to the interim director of the National Institutes of Health and asked if he planned to investigate Gallo.

The director had little choice but to oblige. After weeks of quiet digging, in February 1990 he asked the National Academy of Sciences to assemble a blue-ribbon team to oversee the investigation, which would be run by the Office of Scientific Integrity. Throughout the late spring and summer, Gallo's laboratory notebooks were carefully scrutinized. He and key members of his lab staff were interviewed for hours in an attempt to sort out whether Gallo had stolen the viral sample sent to him by the French or mistakenly isolated a contaminant from the French samples.

Gallo acknowledged that contamination, with which he was already familiar, was a possibility. But he insisted that he had no motive for theft, that he had other strains of HIV under study during the crucial period.

John Crewdson was convinced that Gallo had been so eager to connect AIDS to HTLVs that he had wasted months chasing the wrong virus. When he saw the Nobel Prize slipping away from him, he had appropriated the French virus for himself.

Gallo became almost pathologically obsessed with Crewdson. On August 11, 1990, Gallo's wife, Mary Jane, called the police to report a break-in at their home in Bethesda. Nothing had been taken, not even the expensive jewelry sitting in plain sight on a dresser, but a purple bra was left hanging on a window latch, and desks had been ransacked. When the police asked if the Gallos had suspicions as to who might have committed the crime, Crewdson's was the name Gallo mentioned.

An informal team came to Gallo's defense. Dr. Robert Redfield, head of the AIDS program for the U.S. Army, joined Martin Delaney, the San Francisco AIDS activist; Shepherd Smith, a Republican and born-again Christian who ran Americans for a Sound AIDS Policy; and Bob Gray, a closeted gay man who had been President Eisenhower's appointments secretary, an executive at the public relations firm of Hill & Knowlton and later a member of Nancy Reagan's staff. These men believed that Gallo was an indispensable officer in the war against AIDS. At their insistence, Gallo hunkered down and stopped granting interviews.

Their spin on the story was that Gallo was the victim of an overzealous journalist trying to build his reputation by destroying the nation's most brilliant researcher. And they were remarkably successful. Most major newspapers ignored Crewdson's story. The *New York Times* mentioned it in a column on the media. The *Washington Post* tried to undermine its powerful message.

But the greatest success was in the AIDS activist community. Delaney told everyone that Gallo was so tied up in the investigation that he couldn't get any work done. We have to defend him, Delaney said; he's our brightest star, our greatest hope. Gallo himself called Larry Kramer. Things are so awful that I'm emotionally incapable of continuing my work on AIDS, Gallo told him. Kramer panicked.

Kramer and ACT UP were in the midst of divorce when Gallo called. People were still dying, so it must be ACT UP's fault, Kramer concluded. The members of the group were too young, too ill-focused, too concerned with issues that didn't interest him. Kramer lashed out at African American activists for distracting the group with useless guilt tripping. He screamed at the women members for criticizing people in the group he admired. He yelled at the men and women who'd begun to meet regularly with government scientists, accusing them of being seduced by personal connections. He threw a tantrum when a capsule history of ACT UP was written that did not mention his name.

Yet the man who hadn't hesitated to brand every other researcher in the world a murderer melted at the charm of Robert Gallo. They were an oddly compatible pair, Gallo with his hunger for scientific recognition and Kramer with his hunger for admiration and love. Kramer made Gallo feel protected from activists who were notorious for their hostility. Gallo made Kramer feel important. It was a perfect feast of egos — two men who believed they were indispensable geniuses, misunderstood and besieged by second-rate malcontents.

"Gallo is a very complicated person," Kramer says. "I don't know that we'll understand his mystery any more than we understand the mystery of Laurence Olivier. What has come out of his lab is a lot of important stuff. He's earned the right to work in a less fettered way in a time of plague. He's not an easy person. But we don't need his gifts to be imprisoned. The problem is that he has a certain difficulty relating to others. He is, in effect, his own worst enemy." The insight seemed self-revelatory.

Kramer's first public defense of Gallo appeared on the op-ed page of the *New York Times,* in an article calling for the appointment of an AIDS high command to take control of the plague. Gallo was in line for appointment, in Kramer's mind. "Dr. Gallo, who probably knows more about HIV than any other person in the world, has been hauled through the mud by critics who have accused him of everything from scientific fraud to cooking the books," he wrote.

Then, using his Holocaust analogy in a new way, he continued, "We would do well to remember that the U.S. invited a Nazi, Wernher von Braun, to come here and build our space program. The transgressions of Dr. Gallo . . . , if indeed there were any, are tiny compared to von Braun's. It is a sorry state of affairs when we must render useless our finest brains just when they are needed most."

When the *Times* did not desist from covering Gallo's continuing travails, Kramer lashed out directly at the journalist on the story. "Your one-sided hatchet job on Dr. Robert Gallo was appalling," he wrote to Phil Hilts of the *Times*'s Washington bureau. "This man knows more about the HIV viruses than any other single individual in the entire world. I don't care if he robbed Fort Knox. We can have Nuremberg trials later. After the cure is discovered . . . It is almost as if a conspiracy is afoot, to see to it that absolutely everything that could help end the AIDS plague is placed out of whack or commission.

"The Gallo story is a modern tragedy. I don't know if he did ANY-THING wrong but he has, to all intents and purposes, been rendered useless. Why aren't you writing about this tragedy, about the moral implications involved, about the sad plight in which it puts all of us, including Gallo, when an instrument of possible salvation is cruelly cut down?"

The National Institutes of Health spent ten months on a "fact-finding" inquiry into the charges against Robert Gallo. In early October 1990, bowing to pressure from its blue-ribbon panel of scientific hot shots, NIH elevated the case to a formal investigation.

Robert Gallo was flabbergasted at the turn of events. In a letter to the *Chicago Tribune,* Gallo's attorney tried to minimize the importance of the investigation, which he said had focused only "on minor issues which do not call into question either the validity of Gallo's papers or the work of his laboratory." In fact, the investigators were looking into why Gallo's HTLV-3 was a carbon copy of the French virus; Gallo's repeated denials that the French virus had been grown in his lab and the subsequent proof that it had; the backdating of published papers that seemed to have included experiments that hadn't been conducted when the papers were first delivered; and lies Gallo had seemingly told the patent office in a sworn statement.

While the investigators combed through his lab records and reanalyzed tissue samples stored in his freezer, Gallo was reeling over a new series of scandals. Two of his principal assistants were accused, and later convicted, of embezzlement and accepting illegal gratuities. Gallo himself was investigated over his collaboration with Daniel Zagury, a French vaccine researcher to whom he'd given biological materials in violation of NIH policies. Several of the Africans who'd received Zagury's vaccine had died.

Work in Gallo's lab ground to a halt so he could dedicate himself to writing a book. *The Virus Hunter* was Gallo's public defense. "To a large extent I have been the victim of nothing more sinister than my own unguarded frankness in talking to the press," he said in one of many self-rationalizing passages. In the book Gallo emerged as a fuller human being — as a man obsessed with the death of his sister from leukemia. But he answered no questions about what had happened in his lab.

Whenever Gallo did answer those questions, the story seemed to change. First he said that he had found the virus before anyone else and that the French had made a separate, and later, discovery. When the two viruses were shown to be identical, he argued that French cultures had been contaminated with his virus. When it became clear that the virus had traveled only one way across the Atlantic, he claimed that both labs had made independent discoveries, but that the patients from whom they'd drawn their samples had had sex with each other.

Finally, Gallo made one last-ditch attempt to end the whole controversy. In late May 1991, he sent a letter to *Nature* conceding that the virus he had discovered was, in fact, sent to his laboratory by the French and that it had contaminated one of his cultures. Although Gallo still maintained that he had isolated the AIDS virus in other cultures, he called for an end to "this period of controversy."

It didn't work. By the spring of 1991, the scientific world was eagerly awaiting the release of NIH's report. It was not forthcoming. In May the new NIH director, Dr. Bernadine Healy, had canceled a meeting of the blue-ribbon panel overseeing the investigation and refused to show them the draft report. The members of the panel, some of the most important men and women in American science, threatened to resign. Then NIH's lead investigator in the case, Dr. Suzanne Hadley, was ordered to turn over her files and make no further decisions in the case. Hadley, who seemed convinced of Gallo's guilt, was reined in by Healy's order.

NIH wasn't just defending American honor. The patent on the HIV test was bringing in about $2 million a year, and the split in royalties agreed upon in 1987 had been negotiated on the assumption that Gallo had not used the French discoveries to create his blood test. Gallo had ceased arguing that he'd made an independent discovery, and the French, who were hovering on the fringes of the investigation, wanted a bigger piece of the pie. The Americans wanted to keep the money for themselves.

But the pressure was mounting. In the late fall, Congressman Dingell, who chaired the House subcommittee that oversees NIH, called for a criminal investigation of Gallo. In a one-hundred-page report entitled "The Great AIDS Cover-Up," he concluded that Gallo was guilty of fraud and lying under oath.

NIH finally issued its preliminary verdict early in 1992. Investigators concluded that none of the samples from which Gallo originally claimed to have isolated the AIDS virus contained anything resembling what he found; most of them weren't even infected with HIV. The question as to whether Gallo stole the French virus was not answered, but the report concluded that falsifications and misrepresentations abounded in the work done in Gallo's lab. The blame was not laid on Gallo but on his chief virologist. Gallo got a slap on the wrist, "significant censure."

Members of the blue-ribbon panel weren't pleased at NIH's shifting the responsibility onto an underling. "I think we thought there should be two findings of misconduct," one panel member told the *Chicago Tribune*. "Or that if there was going to be only one, that they gave it to the wrong guy." The panel accused Gallo of "intellectual recklessness of a high degree." That was the last they ever heard from NIH.

While the report was still making its way into the upper echelons of the Department of Health and Human Services, where it was sent for approval, Congressman Dingell was tearing it to shreds. In a scathing critique, he accused NIH of suppressing evidence, ignoring discrepancies and waging "a campaign of public and private statements intended to clear Gallo of any apparent motive to misappropriate the Institut Pasteur virus." He dismissed the report as "a political document created for a central political purpose, namely, to support the U.S. government's position in dealing with the government of France."

Gallo's fortunes seemed to improve in November, when a panel of government attorneys overturned NIH's decision in the case of his virologist. Faced with that ruling, the Office of Research Integrity withdrew the charges against Gallo as well. But Dingell, the French and the inspector general of Health and Human Services would not let matters rest. In June 1994 the inspector general weighed in against Gallo, concluding that the French scientists were the first to discover HIV, to isolate it from patients, to describe it in print and to use it to make a diagnostic blood test. To Gallo's insistence that his samples of HTLV-3B must have been accidentally contaminated with LAV, the French virus, the inspector general responded, "The claim that 3B was contaminated by LAV comes into question since there appears to be no evidence there ever was a 3B to be contaminated."

On Monday, July 11, 1994 — more than a decade after Margaret Heckler and Robert Gallo announced the American discovery of the AIDS virus — NIH Director Harold Varmus and Maxime Schwartz, the director general of the Pasteur Institute, stood before the press in a stone mansion overlooking the NIH campus and announced what everyone already knew: HTLV-3B was LAV. The principal AIDS virus isolated by Gallo in 1984, the one most widely used in research and in the manufacture of the American blood test for AIDS, was not a new discovery but the same virus isolated by scientists at the Pasteur and sent to Gallo the year before.

Luc Montagnier was in the hallway outside the briefing room after the announcement. Robert Gallo walked by. The two did not speak.

While Gallo was suffering that final ignominy, Larry Kramer was growing happy, although happy is not a word usually associated with the acerbic and belligerent writer. His friend Gallo was looking for a new job; his days at NIH were numbered, he'd been told. Kramer's life seemed, for once, nearly perfect.

His third play, *The Destiny of Me,* had opened at the Lucille Lortel Theatre on Christopher Street, in Greenwich Village, to rave reviews. Ned Weeks, the fictional self he'd created for *The Normal Heart,* was back, now HIV positive and in the hospital undergoing experimental treatment. Two Neds appeared on the stage, the child and the adult. Their dialogue shifted back and forth between the boy growing up with an abusive father and a brother he was desperate to please, and the man looking for a miracle from a physician he'd denounced as a murderer.

On opening night, October 20, 1992, that physician, Dr. Anthony Fauci of the NIH, was in the audience with his wife. For the first time, Kramer had publicly acknowledged him as something more than an institutional straw man. Onstage, Fauci was hamstrung by red tape and apologetic for political do-nothings, but he *cared.*

When the curtain fell, Kramer approached him almost shyly. "Will you still take care of me?" he asked.

"Always," Fauci answered. "I'll always take care of you."

After the success of *The Destiny of Me,* Kramer announced his departure from activism yet again. "I've had as many farewell appearances as an aging opera star," but, he insisted, "This is it. Nobody listens to me."

That didn't stop Kramer from talking. He couldn't resist when President Bill Clinton refused to follow his prescription for a plague and NIH continued to disappoint him. Kramer focused the same old rants on new and familiar targets. In his column in *The Advocate,* a news magazine for a gay readership, he argued that everyone else had been coopted. The CDC was "the single most concentrated group of idiots in one building that this government finances." NIH continued to be "an $11-billion-a-year cesspool." And his old friend Victor Zonana, the *Los Angeles Times* reporter who had been scheduled to write Kramer's biography, had passed on the project and was "pimping for Donna Do-nothing Shalala" — Kramer's phrase for Zonana's position as her spokesman.

He missed no opportunity to criticize ACT UP or the Treatment Action Group, an invitation-only spinoff of ACT UP that concentrated solely on treatment issues. He branded the group's work "inept, useless and stupid." Its members had been Kramer's favorites for years, but they committed an unpardonable sin: they refused to invite him to join. "They do a great deal of damage," Kramer said of the group. "I don't know what's happening to them. They seem entirely bought off."

At a New York State AIDS conference in November 1993, he rose before one thousand physicians, public health workers, nurses and social workers at the heart of the epidemic and accused them of "passively colluding with intentional genocide," comparing them to Adolf Eichmann. "The difference between you and Eichmann and other Nazi desk killers who administered a system of mass killing is that you mourn for our victims and grieve for them."

He saved his most savage venom for the movie *Philadelphia,* every aspect of which he deemed intolerable. The acting was terrible, the lovers didn't seem in love and the AIDS patient's family was a total fiction. "No family exists like this in the entire world," he said, suggesting more about his own family than anyone else's. Kramer was angriest at *Philadelphia* for its absence of rancor toward American politicians. In one review he wrote, "There is not one HIV-positive person in the world who does not believe that he or she is the victim of, if not outright intentional genocide (which is what I believe), then, at least, government inaction and oversight of huge proportions. Not one."

Those who know Kramer best saw the stain of sour grapes all over his comments. He had been trying to turn *The Normal Heart* into a movie for seven years and had expected that it would be the first Hollywood movie about AIDS. Barbra Streisand had expressed interest in a film adaptation, a prospect that delighted him. But he turned on her when she put the production on the back burner during her filming of *Nuts.* Kramer declared that he would never work with her.

Nonetheless, in February 1994, when Streisand called, he flew directly to Hollywood. By March he was singing her praises in print as a brave and noble woman. When he wrote a column about taking his first capsule of AZT, he made sure gay Americans knew that Barbra was there, holding his hand. "We're going to get through this," Kramer recorded her telling him. He placed a framed photograph of himself and Streisand in a prominent spot in his New York apartment. The inscription read, "For dear Larry, We need your beautiful anger. Much love and gratitude, Barbra."

More important, Kramer fell in love. For years he'd been accused of acting out his personal frustration on scientists, politicians and other AIDS activists. When the *New York Times* printed an interview with him headlined "When a Roaring Lion Learns to Purr," even the least cynical concluded they'd been right. There was Kramer — in the newspaper he'd recently said should be tried for war crimes — with his dog, Tiger, on his lap and his boyfriend, the architect David Webster, beside him. His grimace was gone. His words seemed softer, gentler. Even those who had long complained about the master of the ad hominem attack were bemoaning the void where Kramer's anger had been.

They needn't have worried. Love might have tamed the tiger. He and David might have been busy remodeling their dream house in Connecticut. But the fifty-nine-year-old writer could not resist invective entirely. Webster was the mild-mannered one. "I don't particularly like anger or confrontation," he told the *Times*. Kramer had plenty for both of them.

"I only have so much energy, like everybody," he says. "You have to choose your targets and choose what is humanly possible. Right now, I think the best use of my time is to just keep criticizing the system and pointing out how useless it is. I spend a lot of time criticizing the NIH, harping on one point: that there has never been a cure for any major illness that has come out of NIH.

"I have nothing good to say about anything, but I'm happy. I'm in a position where I can say whatever I want, and nobody is going to shut me up."

Robert Gallo likes to sit at the picnic table in the back yard of his home in Bethesda. The trees around him are old. Their limbs are heavy. The family's black cat, Jerry, races after chipmunks. His wife, Mary Jane, brings out coffee. Gallo is one of those men who have grown into being handsome. He is utterly charming. There is no sense of stealth or deception in his protestations of innocence. He seems confounded by what he calls his persecution. John Crewdson, Congressman John Dingell, the French — "Why me?" is silently appended to every sentence.

Gallo's friends are legion. When his troubles began, former Indiana Senator Birch Bayh rushed to his rescue, trying to mediate between him and Crewdson. Frank Mankiewicz, a dean of the liberal establishment who had been press secretary for Robert Kennedy and George McGovern, offered his help. Prominent scientists were quick to support him. "He's influenced things in our lives to an incalculable degree," said Dr. Samuel Broder, until recently Gallo's boss at the National Cancer Institute. "Einstein, Freud — I'd put him on a list like that." His former NCI colleague Dr. Flossie Wong-Staal put it bluntly: "First came God, then came Gallo."

But even his closest friends aren't blind. "Sometimes his personality is not always working in the best way," said Dr. Max Essex of the Harvard School of Public Health. "Sometimes it works in a negative way. He loses his temper a lot, and he picks fights with people unnecessarily. A lot of people who don't know him have the impression he's very egotistical."

But for every devotee, Gallo has a dozen detractors. They are harder to name — people are terrified to incur his infamous wrath. Scientists dependent on federal grants won't cross him in public. Journalists and political figures know that he is quick to get even, only slightly less quick to threaten to file suit. Everyone remembers how he sent the police to John Crewdson's house. "Gallo is a uniquely disliked person," Barbara Culliton, the deputy editor of *Nature,* told *GQ* magazine. She is one of the few people who would allow her name to be attached to a negative comment about Robert Gallo.

Yet Gallo can be unexpectedly gracious and soft-spoken. His account of his travails veers from self-serving to heartbreaking. "The world changed in 1984 when I made my announcement, not in 1983 when the French said they might have found a virus," he says quietly in his back yard. "They had nothing provable. They couldn't grow it. They couldn't prove it. They couldn't test for it . . . My biggest mistake was that I should have told Heckler that we couldn't go on without the French there. But I was naive, gullible. And they have been unrelenting since 1989.

"What's the bloody motive?" he asks, as if he sincerely didn't understand why people believe he might have stolen the French discovery. "The patent? They told me to do it. I didn't know what a patent was.

Even if I deliberately stole the virus, they should give me a medal. Look what I've done for humanity."

Imagine what it's like, he says, leaning forward across the picnic table. Day after day, year after year. "One time there was a piece in the paper saying they were going to charge me with mail fraud. My mother saw it on TV. Imagine how that felt?"

Gallo's friends have told him to get out, to quit NIH and forget AIDS research. "They all tell me, 'You've got two Laskers, you found the first human retrovirus, the second human retrovirus, and IL-2. Sit back and smoke cigars. You have everything to lose and nothing to gain.' They were right. This is a high-pressure field with lots of craziness and visibility. The fatter the head, the bigger the reward. This kind of culture linked with the media does great harm."

But Gallo relishes the battle. He might be charming, but he is instinctively competitive. He admits he's not averse to elbowing a friend on the basketball court. He'll never quit; it isn't in his DNA. He even seems to revel in the continual reweaving of the conspiracies that he believes have been mounted to destroy him. He talks again and again about the seven break-ins at his home. "Who would have done that? Who is out to get me?" These days Crewdson is no longer his prime suspect. He points the finger alternately at the French and Congressman Dingell's investigators.

"Me, why me?" he asks endlessly. "Why are they doing this to me?"

John Crewdson provides the obvious answer. "What Gallo can't see, in his own mind, is that everything that's happening to him now is his own fault. So he casts around for a villain. But he doesn't see that it's him. What's really happening to him is because of Gallo. He's done all this to himself."

By the fall of 1994, Gallo had become so controversial that his boss at NIH warned him to give no more interviews. "In this field, the right thing to do is to keep quiet and stay out of the media," he says during an interview.

But he seems incapable of such discretion. His bitterness toward Don Francis is still palpable. In the HBO movie of *And the Band Played On*, Gallo's character played the villain to Francis's hero. "Imagine," Gallo says, "Francis thought he was going to set up a retrovirology lab at the CDC. That would be like the blind leading the blind. He's a mediocre nothing." He refers to Dr. David Ho, director of the Aaron Diamond Institute, the only private AIDS research lab in the country, as "Dr. Diamond Head. He's not much of a scientist, but he knows how to play the political game." And of Dr. Anthony Fauci, he says, he "likes to hog the spotlight. He always has to be in center stage."

One of the few people about whom he has anything positive to say is Larry Kramer. "He's been very supportive to me," he says. "I admire him. He's a fighter. He's like me. He doesn't fear *them*."

The heaviness in Gallo's voice belies his next words. "That frees us."

TWO

Evidence to
the Contrary

With Robert Gallo at her side, Margaret Heckler stood behind a podium in the Hubert H. Humphrey Building in Washington, D.C. Lights flooded her face, cameras rolled, reporters clutched their notebooks expectantly.

"Today we add another miracle to the long honor roll of American medicine and science," announced Heckler, the secretary of the Department of Health and Human Services. "Today's discovery represents the triumph of science over a dreaded disease. Those who have disparaged this scientific search — those who have said we weren't doing enough — have not understood how sound, solid, significant medical research proceeds."

It was April 23, 1984. Nearly two thousand Americans were dead of AIDS. More than one hundred new cases were being reported every week.

For the first time since young men began showing up at their doctors' offices with strange cancers, the government was offering a shred of hope to the dying: the cause of the disease, a type of virus called a retrovirus, had been isolated. An end to the nightmare was in sight. Within six months a blood test would be available, Heckler proclaimed. Within two years a vaccine would be ready for testing.

Gallo looked grave and proud. The director of tumor cell biology at the National Cancer Institute had been called home from Europe to receive credit for the path-breaking discovery. For two years researchers around the globe had been searching frantically for the cause of the baffling immune disorder — looking for viruses in the tissue of the sick, investigating the immune-suppressive qualities of the recreational drugs they used, testing the impact of semen in their bloodstreams. Heckler beamed at Gallo, the winner of the race, the man who would become the nation's greatest weapon in the scientific war against AIDS.

She never mentioned that a year earlier, a team at the Pasteur Institute in Paris had isolated the very retrovirus Gallo was now claiming to have discovered, or that the French had twice sent samples of their virus to Gallo before he allegedly discovered it. (She had planned to, Gallo insists, but was unable to deliver her full remarks because of a sore throat.) She never mentioned that Gallo's research had not gone through standard scientific review or that his discovery had been validated by absolutely no one.

Scientists listened to Heckler's press conference with relief, but also with more than a little bemusement. In science, after all, advances are usually announced by their discoverers in specialized research journals, not by politicians posing before banks of television cameras. Researchers offer proof, not pronouncements.

Some scientists were more bewildered than bemused. Heckler's explanation seemed too pat. How could young, healthy men be dying from a virus scientists could barely find in their bodies? Why was this virus selectively targeting gay men? They sat back and withheld their applause, waiting for the evidence.

Eleven years and more than a quarter of a million deaths later, they are still waiting — and there is still no vaccine.

In the decade since Heckler's surprise announcement, the international war against AIDS has become a desperate battle against the virus whose discovery she proclaimed, the human immunodeficiency virus. In the most intensive disease hunt in human history, scientists have cross-sectioned and spliced HIV. They have cultured, activated and mapped it. They have figured out how it reproduces. They can draw a picture of it. Some have even built a six-foot-tall model of it. But they are missing one important piece of the puzzle.

"We do not yet know *how* HIV causes AIDS," Dr. John Coffin of Tufts University, a member of the international committee that named the virus, told the delegates to the Sixth International Conference on AIDS in 1990. That situation has not changed.

Nevertheless, virtually every physician and researcher on the face of the planet assumes that HIV is the cause of AIDS. The evidence seems to be overwhelming: the one thing all AIDS patients seem to have in common is the presence of HIV in their bodies. Junkies spread it by sharing needles, hemophiliacs get it through blood products and gay men pass it along through semen. Semen and blood are excellent transmitters of viruses. If basic researchers haven't unlocked the key to the virus's deadly functioning, it is because unraveling a complex virus is hardly a simple task.

But that unraveling continues to elude the efforts of hundreds of scientists, and troubling anomalies in the model of AIDS have complicated their efforts. A new virus, unrelated to HIV, has been discovered that seems to cause Kaposi's sarcoma. A significant number of people infected with HIV are living and thriving with no signs of illness.

Gradually, then — inevitably, in fact — a small but persistent band of skeptics has begun to wonder aloud at the validity of the trinity of AIDS dogma: that AIDS does not occur in the absence of HIV, that HIV alone causes AIDS, and that everyone infected will inevitably fall ill and die.

Most of the dissidents are easy to dismiss. They are members of that eclectic collection of writers, activists, quacks and conspiracy theorists who jump on almost any bandwagon, sometimes to publicize their own pet causes, sometimes to satisfy an emotional need to be contrary. There is Joan McKenna, a Berkeley-based "alternative healer," who aggressively promoted the hypothesis that AIDS was merely syphilis in disguise. She was joined by Dr. Stephen Caiazza, a young East Coast physician who was so sure McKenna was right that he repeatedly injected himself with syphilis bacteria, trying to develop AIDS.

John Lauritsen, a market researcher — trained at Harvard, as he invariably points out — insists that AIDS is the result of the abuse of poppers, an inhaled form of butyl nitrite popular in the gay recreational-drug scene. (He's the kind of writer who practices the exclamation-point-and-bold-print style of journalism, declaiming such things as "Science has plunged into whoredom.")

Chuck Ortleb, the editor of the *New York Native,* the first paper in the country to pay attention to AIDS, now uses his weekly as a bully pulpit from which to preach that AIDS does not exist. It is, he is convinced, part of a larger problem of immune-system destruction that includes chronic fatigue syndrome and a rising number of cancers. The culprit: a ubiquitous form of human herpes virus. Ortleb believes that many scientists and federal officials know that something is systematically ravaging the immune systems of Americans but are involved in cover-ups at the highest level. Behind the coverup, he suspects, are elements both from the government and from right-wing groups.

But enough of the HIV dissidents have real credentials — Nobel

Prizes and memberships in the prestigious National Academy of Sciences, positions at leading laboratories and universities, established medical practices in major cities — that make them impossible to ignore.

Dr. Joseph Sonnabend, for example, a South African whose Greenwich Village practice catered to gay New Yorkers long before anyone ever heard of AIDS, was one of the first physicians in the nation to treat the growing number of infected. He knew that the young men he was suddenly seeing with cancers typical of the elderly, or with pneumonias most common among malnourished Third World children, had been unhealthy for years. He had already treated them for hepatitis A and B, for syphilis, gonorrhea and herpes. He refused to believe that their medical histories were irrelevant to their increasingly serious illnesses. Sonnabend doesn't dismiss HIV out of hand, but he is skeptical of arguments that the virus alone explains the destruction around him.

The most recent thorn in the side of the AIDS establishment is Dr. Kary Mullis, the 1993 Nobel laureate in chemistry who won the award for developing the first technique for rapidly multiplying and mass-producing targeted segments of DNA. It is this technique that allows researchers to find HIV even when it is carefully hidden in the human body. "Human beings are full of retroviruses," Mullis says. "We don't know if it is hundreds or thousands or hundreds of thousands. We've only recently started to look for them. But they've never killed anybody before. People have been living with retroviruses for millions of years."

But the most persistent critic of the HIV research crowd is Dr. Peter Duesberg, a microbiologist at the University of California at Berkeley, a researcher Robert Gallo himself once extolled as "a man of extraordinary energy, unusual honesty, enormous sense of humor and a rare critical sense." Everyone involved in cancer research knows Duesberg is a stubborn polemicist, but his scientific accomplishments in retrovirology are too important for his critique to be dismissed out of hand. The problem is that Duesberg refuses to grant HIV any role whatsoever in the new medical phenomenon. "A harmless passenger virus," he says of it, one of the many microbes that cause human beings trouble only when their immune systems are already devastated. That devastation is the result of drug use, he insists, despite all evidence to the contrary.

Duesberg has been joined by several hundred scientists and writers attracted by his arguments and his credentials and by the chance to sling some mud at the medical establishment. They are senior researchers in the United Kingdom and Spain and brash physicians from Australia and the United States. The group became hard to ignore when Luc Montagnier, chief of AIDS research at the Pasteur Institute, the man Margaret Heckler was too ill to mention as the discoverer of HIV, declared that HIV alone might not cause AIDS. He seemed to agree with Duesberg that HIV was a pussycat, but added that it could become a raging tiger when triggered by other infections.

How can these scientists — reputable men highly regarded in their fields, at least until recently — be so skeptical about what virtually the entire world accepts as truth?

For one thing, the dissenters say, the numbers just aren't adding up. For years after Heckler's announcement, the Centers for Disease Control projected the number of people expected to turn up with HIV infection. It was more than a sophisticated guess. Epidemiologists know from years of experience how a new virus spreads in the human population: quickly, geometrically. They can draw a curve of early explosive growth, then a gradual tapering off. But the predictions for HIV were consistently wrong, and the CDC was repeatedly forced to revise and dramatically lower its estimates.

HIV has not spread at anywhere near the rate that would be expected of a newly introduced sexually transmitted disease. It is dawdling. In fact, HIV tests of military recruits and blood donors suggest that HIV infections were no more common among the general population in 1992 than they were in 1985. Why isn't HIV following well-established epidemiological patterns? No one has provided an answer.

Then there's the fact that people infected with HIV just don't seem to be dying at anywhere near the expected rate. Of course not, said Dr. Steven Jonas, a professor of preventive medicine at the State University of New York at Stony Brook. "There's no historical precedent for [a disease] spreading uniformly throughout the population and killing everybody that gets infected. Look at the Black Death that hit western Europe around 1365. Most people focus on the fact that it killed a third of the population of western Europe. What they don't consider is that two-thirds of the population didn't die." Why should AIDS be different? Nobody has provided an explanation.

The dissidents point up other nagging problems with the HIV hypothesis:

- Transfusions with HIV-tainted blood are supposed to be the surest way to become infected, yet not all hemophiliacs transfused with blood-clotting concentrate from contaminated blood wind up testing positive. For example, of forty-eight Scottish hemophiliacs who received clotting factor from the same batch of HIV-infected blood, only sixteen ever tested positive for HIV antibodies. Why? Nobody knows.
- HIV isn't found in very many of the T cells it purportedly kills. Scientists can find the virus in only one in ten thousand T cells early in infection, and only one in forty in late-stage AIDS cases. How do all the rest of the T cells get massacred?
- A few HIV-positive people suddenly test HIV negative without any treatment — although AIDS experts contend that the body cannot kill HIV by itself. In 1994, for example, Tulane University researchers reported on five hemophiliacs infected in the late 1970s and early 1980s who no longer have any signs of the virus in their bodies.
- Only 4.5 percent of the prostitutes in New York City who are not intravenous drug users are infected with HIV, although they have had thousands of sexual contacts, many undoubtedly with infected men, without using condoms. Yet prostitutes have always been spreaders of sexually transmitted diseases. Why is AIDS different?
- Most of the spouses of those who were infected — including Arthur Ashe's wife, Jeanne Marie, Magic Johnson's wife, Earleatha, and Rock Hudson's lover, Marc Christian — have no sign of HIV in their bodies, although they had regular sexual contact with their partners, without using condoms, for years.
- The New York City Department of Health has identified six HIV-positive men who were regular sperm donors between 1978 and 1985. Although the virus is transmitted more easily through artificial insemination than through vaginal intercourse, only one of the 176 women who received sperm is believed to have been infected through insemination, and none of the children born to these women has tested positive.
- Mice that have never been exposed to HIV can still produce antibodies to the virus. Since the "AIDS test" is for antibodies rather than the virus itself, can we be sure that all those who are antibody positive are actually infected?
- AIDS is still not spreading very far beyond the groups in which it first arose. More than 96 percent of all AIDS cases can still be

attributed to homosexual sex, blood transfusions, intravenous drug abuse or sex with an IV drug user or hemophiliac.

- People seem to be getting AIDS in the absence of HIV. Kaposi's sarcoma and *Pneumocystis carinii* pneumonia, the diseases most common to AIDS patients, are cropping up in individuals without any trace of the virus or other immune disorders. The Centers for Disease Control have recorded the cases of more than three dozen gay men with Kaposi's sarcoma — and without HIV.
- HIV infection doesn't seem to be universally fatal. Despite all the dire predictions, between 5 and 10 percent of the Americans infected fifteen years ago show no sign of illness, no evidence of damage to their immune systems. Why? Nobody knows.

Most researchers insist that such apparent contradictions are to be expected in the early stages of research into a new disease. They say new techniques have already enabled scientists to find HIV hiding in bodies in which it escaped detection by earlier methods. New tests are able to measure the type and concentration of virus, and new research has shown that some strains of HIV are more virulent — and more infectious — than others.

All of what they say is true, but none of it even begins to fill the cracks in the hypothesis that HIV alone causes AIDS.

The dissidents' refusal to accept the gospel of HIV has provoked one of the nastiest spats in modern science. Nonscientists assume that learned M.D.s and Ph.D.s have high-minded debates, trading theories and data in civilized discourse. They publish statistics and refutations of statistics in arcane journals. In the spirit of Copernicus and Einstein, they seek the truth.

In this case, they have mostly slung mud.

The real argument is reduced to a few pithy statements and retorts: AIDS follows HIV, mainstream researchers say. Correlation doesn't prove causation, critics respond. But 99 out of 100 AIDS researchers agree that the virus is sufficient to cause the disease. "This isn't an election," dissidents remind them.

Then the gloves come off. Dr. Robin Weiss, a British AIDS researcher, and Dr. Harold Jaffe of the CDC call Duesberg a flat-earther who is "bogged down in molecular minutiae and miasmal theories of disease." Duesberg responds in kind, accusing his critics of creating a "totalitarian science environment. If you don't agree with the government, with the official theory, with the Gallos, you get locked out. And most scientists just go along like good soldiers and do as they're told."

Dissidents insist that the HIV-as-the-sole-cause-of-AIDS crowd has no choice but to call them names because leading proponents are so enmeshed in their dogma — professionally, emotionally and financially — that they cannot allow any honest discourse. In fact, officials at the Centers for Disease Control and the National Institutes of Health actually cut off discussion of the very possibility that HIV alone might not be guilty of producing AIDS by accusing the inquirer of trying to undermine the campaign for safe sex. Journalists are cautioned away from the story: Duesberg is crazy, mainstream scientists charge; he's a screeching homophobe. If reporters push, the scientists refuse to cooperate, accusing them of endangering public health.

The paranoia is hardly one-sided. Duesberg is convinced that the HIV theorists are part of a conspiracy of retrovirologists who have allegedly "seized the reins of political power within the NIH-funded establishment. Their colleagues will not buck the system for fear of losing access to research grants. They are bolstered by the pharmaceutical industry, which is growing fat off antivirals that not only do not kill HIV — which is harmless anyway — but are, themselves, toxic."

Dr. Charles Thomas, a former professor at Harvard, founder of the Group for the Scientific Reappraisal of the HIV/AIDS Hypothesis and president of the Helicon Foundation, goes even further. AIDS, he says, is part of a wider conspiracy of "scary science," which includes claims that nuclear power is dangerous, that pesticides cause cancer, that pollution causes acid rain — and that HIV causes AIDS. A political libertarian, Thomas believes that concern over these alleged disasters is a plot by scientists, university professors and the media to increase the size of government and to bolster funding for science.

If there were no more infectious diseases, Thomas reasons, the budget of the Centers for Disease Control would be in jeopardy. So the CDC and its friends had to create public panic over swine flu, hantavirus and HIV. "The reason that the whole shabby sore of HIV is being held in place is there's so much money riding on it. The federal government is spending about $4 billion on just this single subject, and all that $4 billion is predicated on the idea that HIV causes these diseases. If HIV doesn't cause these diseases, then that money is being wasted . . . and the people who are the recipients of that money don't want it to stop."

Few of the other heretics are quite so extreme. They believe that the problem is more subtle: they accuse the establishment researchers of just being human.

Americans tend to place science on a pedestal as perhaps the only objective force in society. Every schoolchild is taught to revere the scientific method as the paragon of rigor, the unbridled quest for truth. That view presupposes that scientists have no specialties that guide, and bias, their research; that they have no pet theories they fervently believe in; that they have no friends they wish to promote, no funders to appease, no university committees or deans to impress, no prizes to which they aspire. In the end, the HIV critics remind us that scientists are as human as factory workers or used-car salesmen. A retrovirologist wants to believe he can make a crucial contribution, and so is predisposed to retrovirological explanations for disease. A bacteriologist who finds a new bug wants it to be important to humanity. Working researchers need grants to pursue their work, to win promotions and pay raises. And everyone dreams of a Nobel Prize.

It does not make for a perfect scientific world. Then again, there never has been one. The greatest scientific advances have always been made by researchers pushing against the walls of dogma, and dogmatists inevitably push back. Many of the men and women we think of today as great scientists — from Galileo to Darwin — began as dissidents. It wasn't so long ago that Robert Gallo himself was mocked for believing that retroviruses could cause sickness in humans.

The official version of AIDS:

In the beginning there is HIV, a retrovirus that incorporates its genes into the chromosomes of host cells and turns them into factories for their own reproduction. HIV hits the bloodstream with a burst of fury, looking for its favorite cells, macrophages or T cells, both essential parts of the body's immune system. HIV attacks the T cells but, initially, does not destroy them, using them instead to mass-reproduce.

Most newly infected people aren't aware that HIV is inside their bodies. Just after infection, some suffer from rashes, from swollen glands or mild fevers, as if hit with a case of the flu or a touch of mononucleosis. But the symptoms disappear quickly as the body's defenses rally, pushing the virus into hiding inside lymph nodes. Scientists used to believe that the virus then lies relatively dormant either in the lymph nodes or in specific types of blood cells, often for years. More recently, however, they've concluded that the virus replicates constantly within the lymph nodes, although its activity remains virtually invisible in the blood. During this period, the presence of HIV can be detected indirectly — by measuring whether the body is producing antibodies to fight it — or directly, by employing sophisticated medical technology.

Gradually, however, the lymph nodes break down and the virus escapes. The newly freed cells mass-produce viral particles that spread through the lymphatic tissue and charge through the bloodstream, attaching themselves to previously uninfected cells.

With other bugs, even that would not necessarily spell disaster. Healthy bodies harbor dozens of viruses and other microorganisms that never cause any noticeable harm. But in the case of HIV, most scientists believe that the body's defenses just aren't sufficient to the monumental task of keeping at bay the millions of new viral particles produced each day. Most researchers think that the immune system gradually collapses under the onslaught. Others suggest that a more virulent form of the constantly mutating virus emerges and decimates the immune system.

But all agree that as HIV enters the final and most lethal stage of its relationship to the human body, nearly all defenses — to it and to a wide array of diseases — collapse. Bacteria, other viruses and bugs that wouldn't hurt a soul under normal circumstances suddenly run riot. When that begins to happen, an HIV-infected person comes down with one of the dozens of illnesses that qualify him for a diagnosis of AIDS. In the absence of any drug that kills HIV without killing the body that nourishes it, scientists see just one inevitable result of HIV infection: death.

If this were a murder case, all the evidence would be deemed circumstantial. Nobody can see HIV destroying T cells, so nobody is sure how it does its dirty work. When Gallo announced his discovery of a new retrovirus that could infect T cells and macrophages — the very immune cells depleted in AIDS patients — scientists expected to find that HIV was somehow sneaking through the body undetected by the immune system, killing off T cells and macrophages, thus devastating the body's defenses from the inside.

After more than a decade of hypothesizing and investigating, however, almost everyone agrees that HIV does not swarm through the body undetected, that the immune system mobilizes to fight off infection and manages to win, at least for a while. What happens, then, to reverse the outcome of the battle and to cause the immune system to collapse? Does it just burn out from the struggle? Does the virus trigger an autoimmune reaction, as in lupus or Crohn's disease, whereby the body's defenses turn against themselves? Does HIV cause T cells to commit suicide en masse? Does it somehow force uninfected cells to clump together with infected ones, paralyzing their ability to defend the body? Does a more deadly mutant virus emerge? There are five or six decent hypotheses. There is no consensus around any one.

Even this uncertainty doesn't bother the more reasonable critics of HIV orthodoxy very much. In science, after all, there often is no smoking gun. Sometimes circumstantial evidence is the best you can expect. But where HIV is concerned, they point out, even the circumstantial is riddled with holes.

Robert Koch was a German scientist who had a peculiar obsession with proof. Born in 1843, three years after his teacher, Friedrich Gustav Jacob Henle, made the stunning assertion that living organisms too small to see with the naked eye could cause disease, Koch become one of the first disciples of the new science of bacteriology, and he advanced it considerably. He discovered both the organism that causes tuberculosis and the organism that causes cholera — eventually winning the Nobel Prize for his work.

It is hard to imagine today how astounding those discoveries were at the time. When scientists first began studying the world through a microscope, they found it teeming with microorganisms. There was no way to watch them operate in living beings, so how could they tell which were harmless and which were lethal?

Koch, who had served as a field surgeon in the Franco-Prussian War, became an ace detective. He developed all kinds of new investigative techniques, along with what were to become the basic rules for definitive proof that a given germ causes a given disease: (1) You have to find the germ in every case of the disease; (2) you have to be able to isolate it from the body and from other germs; (3) you have to reproduce the original disease in a healthy animal by inoculating it with the isolated microbe; (4) then the same germ must be retrieved from the newly infected host.

Koch wasn't inflexible. He understood that some cases wouldn't fit neatly into his set of rules. In those cases, however, he cautioned that a simple association should never be confused with causation. In other words, just because everyone in your neighborhood with measles also has blond hair doesn't mean that blond hair causes measles. That is now the first lesson in Science 101, but in Koch's day it was a revolutionary concept.

Koch, whose principles are still taught to every student of epidemiology, isn't very popular with the HIV crowd these days: their virus fails his test. HIV can be isolated from the body and from other germs, but only with difficulty, because most of those infected don't have much virus that can be found in the bloodstream.

HIV fails the other tests outright. First, the virus cannot be found in every case of AIDS. In 3 percent of diagnosed AIDS cases, no HIV antibodies have been discovered. Are these people HIV negative or are their bodies producing no antibodies to the virus? And while no one has tried injecting HIV into a healthy human being, scientists have stuck all kinds of mice and rats and monkeys and chimpanzees — and none of them got anything resembling human AIDS. None of this disproves the HIV hypothesis, as dozens of scientists point out each time Duesberg lectures them on Koch's postulates as if they were first-year medical students. HIV's failure of Koch's test can be easily explained:

- The virus or its antibodies are not found in all cases of AIDS because the tests for it are not yet sensitive enough.
- Koch's second rule doesn't apply to viruses because they cannot be grown in pure culture — thus they cannot by definition be isolated from all other germs. That failure to follow the letter of Koch's laws, they explain, has not created controversy over the causes of other viral diseases, like influenza and polio. Koch himself abandoned his second rule when confronted with asymptomatic cholera carriers and Typhoid Mary.
- Something in animals other than humans may prevent the development of AIDS. Koch himself acknowledged that his third rule presented difficulties in proving the causes of tuberculosis and cholera.
- The development of AIDS in people infected through transfusions of contaminated blood or clotting-factor concentrates is sufficient to satisfy Koch's final rule.

But most mainstream AIDS researchers won't get into the Koch argument, insisting that his postulates are hopelessly out-of-date, since they were designed around bacterial infections. They cannot be applied to viruses, which are a borderline life form with no metabolic structure and no ability to reproduce independently. For those scientists, the bottom line is that in almost every case of the condition called AIDS — a cluster of diseases frequently accompanied by weight loss, incontinence and dementia — they can find antibodies to HIV. The virus seems to be the only thing that the sick — gay men in New York, truck drivers in Uganda, prostitutes in Thailand and abandoned children in Romania — have in common. That's just too much of a coincidence to pass up.

Robert Root-Bernstein isn't overly concerned with Robert Koch or his postulates, either. He's less interested in theoretical paradigms and would-be microbiological anomalies than in the number of people who are HIV positive but don't have AIDS and the number of people with an affliction that looks suspiciously like AIDS but who aren't HIV positive. The young physiology professor hasn't created quite the ruckus among establishment scientists that Duesberg has; he has never been part of that establishment. His faculty position is at Michigan State, not Harvard or Berkeley. The only credential that stops his opponents from dismissing Root-Bernstein as a crackpot is his MacArthur Foundation "genius" grant.

For seven years Root-Bernstein has been asking an embarrassing question: If HIV is the sole cause of AIDS and inevitably causes the fatal disease, how come so many of the HIV infected aren't getting sick? The establishment has a quick answer: They eventually will. It just takes time.

How much time? asks the mild-mannered professor.

The response keeps changing.

When HIV was first discovered, scientists at the CDC suggested that most of the infected would begin to fall ill within twelve to eighteen months of infection. They didn't. So the CDC did what it has done again and again: it raised the projected incubation time. In 1986 they set it at two years. In 1987 they upped it to three. In 1988 it grew to five, in 1989 to ten and by early 1992 from ten to fifteen. The CDC didn't have much choice.

Epidemiologists there were working from blood samples drawn in the late 1970s from 6,875 sexually active gay and bisexual men in San Francisco. Scientists had never heard of AIDS or HIV when they froze the blood. They were concerned about hepatitis B, which had been infecting the livers of gay men disproportionately. In 1985, when the HIV antibody test was licensed, all that six-year-old blood from the nation's highest-risk AIDS group suddenly became critically important. It was a laboratory for the study of the progress of HIV infection.

Sure enough, 67.3 percent of the samples turned out to be HIV positive. Researchers followed 489 of the infected men to see how long it took them to get sick. Only 8 percent developed full-blown AIDS within four years of infection, but then the percentage began rising dramatically. Within six years, 20 percent were sick; within eight, 37 percent; and within ten years, just above half. The odd thing was that the rate then began to level off. A year later it had risen only to 54 percent. Even after fifteen years it still had not reached 80 percent.

These figures, Root-Bernstein argues, suggest that HIV alone is a poor explanation for AIDS. But it gets more complicated: almost all the frozen blood samples were from men who also had hepatitis B, syphilis, gonorrhea or herpes. Their immune systems were already on overload from the massive assault — which makes them terrible predictors of how HIV would operate in healthier blood. Even the CDC admits that the San Francisco group is "a nonrepresentative sample." Nonetheless, it has been the basis for the ever-rising CDC estimates of the median incubation period for HIV.

"Look," says Root-Bernstein, "if they keep going at this rate, we're going to have people who live to ninety who were infected with the virus at fifteen, and they will still be arguing that HIV causes AIDS and that AIDS is an inevitably fatal disease."

Root-Bernstein has never suggested that HIV has no role whatsoever in AIDS, but he is firmly convinced that AIDS is more complex than the work of a lone assassin. Like Sonnabend, he argues that AIDS is the result of repeated insults to the immune system — by a whole host of microbes, by recreational and prescription drug use, by promiscuity, exposure to semen, transfusions and malnutrition. In his view, then, it is hardly a surprise that AIDS has remained relatively confined to populations in which the immune system is battered by repeated blows.

Look at gay men in urban America, Root-Bernstein argues in his book, *Rethinking AIDS: The Tragic Cost of Premature Consensus*. He is referring particularly to the gay men who lived in the fast lane of drugs and anonymous sex in bathhouses and parks — the very men most likely to have AIDS. They were walking paradigms of how to overload your immune system. Hepatitis, cytomegalovirus, syphilis, gonorrhea, chlamydia, gay bowel syndrome, anal fissures and papilloma virus ran rampant in the community. Added to these assaults were antibiotics used to control the infections, steroids to create more manly physiques, poppers and cocaine to keep the party going.

The immune systems of these men were so overburdened that it was often difficult to distinguish the HIV-positive men from the HIV-negative. Two researchers at St. Mary's Hospital in London tried. In 1982, before HIV was discovered, they took blood from 170 symptom-free gay men. Four years later, after the development of the HIV test, 48 of them turned out positive. But the uninfected men were just as likely to have abnormal immunological tests as the infected. When other researchers followed up on the same patients three years later, they concluded that "in symptomless infection, HIV does not appear to cause more impairment [of immune function] than that seen in their uninfected peers."

Even Robert Gallo confirmed that pattern in a 1987 study of one hundred healthy homosexual men in Trinidad. The median T cell count of the HIV-negative men was 560, almost half the normal figure. Yet some of the infected men had normal T cell counts.

The other groups considered at high risk for AIDS also suffer from the same pattern of immune devastation. One hundred intravenous drug users in Atlanta and Chicago studied by Emory University researchers all showed immune suppression, although only 12 percent were HIV positive. The health of the nation's addicts is so abysmal that the CDC acknowledges that it "cannot discern . . . to what extent the upward trend in death rates for drug abuse reflects trends in illicit drug use independent of the HIV epidemic."

Transfusion recipients are in the same boat. Transfusions suppress the immune system in proportion to the amount of blood given, and the typical transfusion patient who develops AIDS received between 16 and 21 units. Furthermore, particularly before blood screening was instituted in the mid-1980s, the blood supply was not safe from hepatitis viruses, cytomegalovirus and Epstein-Barr virus. Recipients of blood were assaulted, then, with many of the same microbes devastating the immune systems of gay men.

And the nation's hemophiliacs, routinely infused with blood-clotting factors, suffered from chronic immune suppression. In the fall of 1983 and the spring of 1984, the T cells of twelve hemophiliacs and six nonhemophiliacs were measured. The hemophiliacs had an average of 475 T cells per cubic milliliter, the others an average of 1,157 cells. In retrospective studies, none in either group tested positive for HIV. "I can't see anything different in the death patterns of hemophiliacs now from four years ago," Dr. David Aronson, of the Division of Blood and Blood Products at the National Center for Drugs and Biologics, said to a reporter in 1983.

More telling is that even HIV-negative members of these groups suffer from some of the same infections considered to be the clearest signs of AIDS. Kaposi's sarcoma — a form of cancer that before AIDS had been found only in elderly men — has been turning up in young gay men who indisputably do not have HIV. Physicians in New York recently reported on five elderly patients with *Pneumocystis carinii* pneumonia (PCP) — and no HIV.

"Maybe I'm seeing anomalies, but everyone in science knows that the anomalies are keys," Root-Bernstein says. "They are nature's way of telling you that something is wrong with your dogma. Look at Copernicus, Galileo, Einstein. Anomalies line their paths. If we insist that HIV is the sole cause of AIDS, then if we have people who aren't infected developing the same symptoms as AIDS patients, we are forced to conclude that we have a second epidemic, or a third, or a fourth."

Most American adults have a small scar on their upper arm or thigh from a smallpox vaccination. Smallpox, once a deadly scourge that killed millions, has been virtually wiped out by vaccination, an ingenious medical technique which introduces a minuscule amount of weakened or dead disease-causing microbes into the body. The body responds by producing antibodies, natural antidotes that kill off the invading pathogen. The theory behind vaccination is that once you have antibodies to a given disease, you are practically immune to it.

The theory has been proven in practice, not just with smallpox but with typhoid and diphtheria, polio and cholera. So why is it such devastating news when a person tests positive for HIV, which means that there are antibodies to HIV in his blood?

Shyh-Ching Lo, the virologist in charge of AIDS programs for the Armed Forces Institute of Pathology, doesn't believe it should be. The presence of antibodies to HIV, far from being a sign of doom, is proof that the body is coping with the virus, Lo contends. That proof makes him wonder how it is that HIV particles manage suddenly to whip the antibodies — which is the implication behind the theory of HIV. "There is no good explanation for why and how the virus breaks out of the antibody protection," Lo says. "I'm not saying that HIV plays no role in AIDS — the data show a clear correlation with disease — but AIDS is much more complicated than HIV."

With no grants or establishment support, Lo went looking for a more convincing explanation on his own. In 1986 he announced that he had found it: a previously unknown variety of an organism called a mycoplasma, which, together with HIV, caused AIDS. For nearly three years his theory was ignored. His research was turned down for publication nearly a dozen times before the *Journal of Tropical Medicine*, which is available in only a few hospital libraries and on no major electronic databases, agreed to print his findings. His grant applications were rejected. Even the presentations he made at professional meetings got him nowhere; his colleagues just didn't show up.

Lo's revolutionary finding was dismissed in part because it was based on a complicated new technique that he had devised for identifying mycoplasmas, which are extremely difficult to find because they have no cell walls. Given the stakes, no one was willing to give Lo the benefit of the doubt. The fact that he wasn't affiliated with a prestigious research center, wasn't part of the NIH-funded AIDS research establishment, certainly didn't help his case. Then, in December 1989, an official at the National Institute of Allergy and Infectious Diseases (NIAID) decided that Lo's work merited a closer look. The agency flew a dozen specialists to San Antonio to examine his data. Those experts in AIDS and other infectious diseases expected, they admitted, to demolish the unknown researcher.

Lo presented his findings. He had detected an organism he was convinced was a mycoplasma in cells taken from AIDS patients. He couldn't find the organism in cells of healthy individuals. When he injected the organism into four silver leaf monkeys, three quickly developed low-grade fevers. All four lost weight and died within seven to nine months of infection. When they were autopsied, there was his mycoplasma — in their brains, their livers and their spleens. Lo also reported finding the mycoplasma in the damaged tissue of six HIV-negative humans who had died of unspecified causes after suffering from suspiciously AIDS-like symptoms.

Robert Koch would have been proud of him.

Lo did not argue that his mycoplasma — *Mycoplasma incognitus* — caused AIDS. "This might be a key cofactor that promotes disease in HIV-infected individuals" was his modest assertion. "It might be an opportunistic infection that takes advantage of immune compromise. Or it might be the primary cause of the disease, with HIV perhaps helping it along. All I know is that it is there and that it changes the properties of HIV. But it is too early to know how or what that means."

The scientists quizzed Lo for two days. They knew that tiny bacteria-like mycoplasmas have a nasty tendency to contaminate their lab experiments and that they can cause immune suppression and debilitating chronic disease in animals. But in human beings mycoplasmas are known to cause only nonlethal diseases — mild pneumonias and some genital infections.

"When I showed the mycoplasmas from my pathology studies, they didn't believe they existed," Lo recalls. "When I showed them that the organism existed and proved it was a mycoplasma, they said my cultures were contaminated."

Two days later, Lo had turned the scientists' skepticism into interest. "The documentation was absolutely solid," said Joseph Tully, the head of mycoplasma programs for NIAID. The participants formally recommended further study of the link between the mycoplasma and AIDS, and experiments with drugs that could kill the new microbe.

One year later, NIAID had funded no such research. When asked why, a spokesperson for Dr. Anthony Fauci, NIAID's director, said Fauci would "not talk about mycoplasma or any other AIDS cofactor." By 1994, NIAID was spending some money on Lo's lead: $1.3 million out of a total AIDS research budget of more than $500 million.

Fifteen minutes wouldn't be enough, Luc Montagnier knew. The announcement was too important, too controversial. If the organizers of the Sixth International Conference on AIDS wouldn't give him, the discoverer of HIV, more time, he would find another way.

It was June 1990, and the conference was scheduled to open in San Francisco in a week. Montagnier planned to announce that he had been wrong for almost seven years. He was about to explode a bomb in the midst of a multi-billion-dollar international research establishment built on the bedrock truth he had helped create. HIV, he was about to argue, was a benign virus that becomes dangerous only in the presence of a second organism. His candidate: a mycoplasma. In culture, he said, HIV is harmless and passive. When you add the mycoplasma he'd isolated, it becomes a killer.

Montagnier had published that opinion three months earlier in the French journal *Research in Virology*, suggesting that T cells burst when infected simultaneously with HIV and his mycoplasma. But in San Francisco he planned to go further, to tell scientists about a simple experiment he had conducted. Montagnier had added tetracycline, which kills bacteria but not viruses, to white-blood-cell cultures in which both HIV and the new mycoplasma were growing. Almost immediately, in the face of this common antibiotic, the sort that people get every day to help them battle such common ailments as pneumonia and acne, the T cells stopped bursting.

Montagnier made his announcement at a special session of the conference, sponsored by the American Medical Association, which agreed to give him more than fifteen minutes. As he spoke, Shyh-Ching Lo sat in the audience, enjoying his moment of vindication. Montagnier, the great man of AIDS, had hit upon exactly the same microbe as Lo had. The two had not shared their data. They didn't know each other. Separately they had made the same discovery. But Lo seemed to be the only person in the room who was excited. Of the twelve thousand people at the conference, only two hundred came to hear Montagnier's talk. By the time he had finished, almost half of those had walked out.

Montagnier was used to skeptical responses and outright dismissals, especially on this side of the Atlantic. Few American scientists had taken his discovery of the AIDS virus seriously until a year later, when Robert Gallo claimed to have discovered it too. But this time Montagnier came with his HIV credentials. He had hoped for a better reception.

After the presentation, Dr. Jay Levy, a University of California virologist who was also an independent discoverer of HIV, approached Montagnier and accused him of mistaking a simple contamination of his lab for a major new discovery. Here the exchange grew heated.

Levy: "I've looked in twenty patients and I can't find your mycoplasma."

Montagnier: "They're very hard to find."

Levy: "We know how to look." With that, he turned his back and walked away.

Most of the people who controlled the course of AIDS research dismissed Montagnier's presentation as cavalierly as Levy did. "It's just a hypothesis," said Peter Drotman, a CDC spokesman. "We don't believe it. HIV is not a benign infection." The small number of dissenters who had hoped that Montagnier's support would be a turning point in their struggle were horrified. "There was Montagnier," said Peter Duesberg, "the Jesus of HIV, and they threw him out of the Temple."

What is AIDS? According to the federal government, it is not a disease but a twenty-six-page single-spaced collection of diseases, conditions under which the diseases must occur, test parameters and guidelines.

The only thing that holds this mind-numbing definition together is HIV. If you have a certain type of pneumonia and HIV, you have AIDS. If you have that type of pneumonia and don't test positive for HIV, you are just a poor slob who has been around too many people spewing pneumonia germs. The same holds true for cancers and viruses and fungi, and bacterial infections that usually occur only in turkeys. If you have any of them without HIV, you're a freak. If you have them along with HIV, you're an AIDS patient.

If HIV is not the sole cause of AIDS, then the years of desperate searching for a way to kill a virus in already infected people — a feat medical science has never accomplished with any virus — might have been spent more productively on other courses of research.

For scientists, that's the worst possible news. In hotel lobbies and bars outside medical conferences and in off-the-record conversations, dozens of AIDS researchers admit they are disturbed by the persistent failure of the most monumental medical research effort in the nation's history to yield clear proof that HIV alone kills. Yet in public, and for the record, few will express these doubts. They have learned all too well the lessons of Sonnabend, Duesberg, and Lo.

Sonnabend was one of the founders of AIDS research, delving into the mysteries of the new syndrome at St. Luke's Hospital in New York before most Americans had heard that a new plague was seeping into the population. Sonnabend never received any of the multi-million-dollar grants that fueled research at major universities and attracted medical residents and young scientists to one of the few fields of bio-medical research in which the pot of money was actually increasing; he simply tried to keep the dying alive.

When the first gay men in New York were trying to figure out how to stave off the infections that were killing their friends, they consulted Sonnabend. When Dr. James Curran, the head of the first CDC task force on the new disease, needed advice on how to proceed, he consulted Sonnabend. When Dr. Mathilde Krim, the Israeli cancer researcher, wanted a colleague to help guide the work of her new AIDS foundation, which became the American Foundation for AIDS Research, she consulted Sonnabend.

A full year before HIV was discovered, and declared to be sexually transmittable, Sonnabend and his patient Michael Callen developed the concept of safe sex and described its practice in a pamphlet, published as "How to Have Sex in an Epidemic." That advice was adopted worldwide. Searching through the literature in 1982 for some clue about how to deal with the pneumonia that was killing his patients, Sonnabend hit on the idea of using the sulfa drug Bactrim or aerosolized pentamidine — standard procedures with organ transplant patients and other severely immune-compromised individuals — not only to treat the disease but to prevent it. That approach is now routine medical practice.

In 1983 Sonnabend became the editor of the first medical journal devoted to AIDS. His inaugural article, "The Etiology of AIDS," hypothesized a "multifactorial model of disease." He suggested that there is no single pathogen causing AIDS and wrote that "the disease arises as a result of a cumulative process." Although scientists both at the CDC and at NIH had come to believe that an infectious agent was to blame, Sonnabend continued to propose a more complex view in meetings, medical journals and in the press. Even after Gallo and Heckler's press conference, Sonnabend refused to fall in line behind the theory that a single infectious agent was causing AIDS. He couldn't ignore the fact that nearly everyone coming down with the syndrome had some prior immune problem.

So the ax fell. Sonnabend was fired as editor of the research journal he created and ousted from the editorial board. He became a pariah in the field he had helped to invent. With one exception: patients continued to flock to the physician believed to have the best diagnostic eye — and the best track record for preventing AIDS-related complications — in New York.

Peter Duesberg fared even worse, becoming, in his own words, "the enemy within" for persisting in his view that HIV is a benign virus. When National Public Radio attempted to stage a debate between Duesberg and a supporter of the HIV hypothesis, producers could find no one willing to confront him. "Critiquing a dubious theory would take time away from more productive efforts," Dr. Anthony Fauci of NIH told NPR producers. John Maddox, the editor of *Nature,* became so exasperated at Duesberg's refusal to back away from his theory that drug abuse leads to AIDS that he banned the California researcher from the magazine. "Has Duesberg a Right of Reply?" Maddox asked in a headline in 1993. "Duesberg has forfeited the right to expect answers by his rhetorical technique," Maddox wrote, explaining that the scientist continued to posit unanswerable questions and then interpret silence as proof of a lie.

For twenty-two years, Duesberg had been listened to, praised and funded for his work. After all, he had discovered a viral gene that might cause cancer and been rewarded with membership in the National Academy of Sciences, long before Robert Gallo was so honored. He was the first person to draw a genetic map of a retrovirus. From 1985 to 1990, he'd enjoyed a luxury few scientists could imagine: a prestigious, no-strings-attached research award from NIH called an Outstanding Investigator Grant.

By the time the grant came up for renewal, Duesberg had ceased to be an insider; his views on AIDS had made him anathema in his own world. On October 26, 1990, he received an unequivocal response to his renewal request: "Despite the applicant's eminent track record, the relatively low past productivity, the logically and functionally flawed rationale, and the poor prospect of the proposed study for advancing knowledge in important areas, greatly weakens the overall merit of this application." Application denied.

Establishment AIDS researchers say that Duesberg was defunded because he wasn't producing anything more than confusion. Duesberg contends that the review committee was "penalizing me for developing concepts contrary to those of the committee members." Although those members would not comment on the review, saying that it would be illegal to do so, their names and credentials are relevant. Two of the ten members of the committee — Dr. Dani Bolognesi and Dr. Flossie Wong-Staal — are among the nation's important HIV researchers, and both have close ties to Robert Gallo. Three others claim never to have seen Duesberg's application. A fourth says that he gave his opinion by telephone, a recommendation for renewal.

Today Duesberg's phone rings constantly, but the calls are from other HIV dissidents and members of the alternative press who support them. Duesberg is rarely invited to speak at major universities or research centers. His laboratory is virtually empty; few graduate students are interested in a mentor who has been branded a quack. Rather than teaching advanced courses in microbiology, he has been assigned to supervise undergraduate labs.

And the list of casualties of HIV orthodoxy goes on.

Robert Root-Bernstein complains that he has been branded a homophobe for suggesting that few heterosexuals who don't abuse drugs will fall sick with AIDS. He has been fired as a columnist for *The Sciences* and was attacked by Robert Gallo, in his book *Virus Hunter,* for "peddling sophism." Root-Bernstein takes comfort from history. After all, he says, Galileo died while under house arrest, but was ultimately vindicated. He even received an apology — more than 350 years belated — from the Vatican. Darwin was despised and is still blamed for everything from the fall of religion to the promiscuity of America's young.

Once he began suggesting that HIV alone has never been proven to cause AIDS — and that some of the AIDS research budget should be spent on alternate hypotheses — Kary Mullis became a scientific outcast. But instead of attacking his science, his deriders took aim at his personal life. They had plenty of material. When he was awarded the Nobel Prize, he quipped that it would be "a great way to pick up babes." He lives on the beach near San Diego, he says, so he can surf regularly. His first published scientific paper described his view of the universe while on LSD.

"The Nobel Prize gives you a kind of immunity, so this stuff doesn't bother me a bit," he says. "I've got my money from the Swedes, so I'm fixed. I'm a free agent. There's nobody on the planet that can fuck with me, and I can say precisely what I think. I don't mind that they say I'm making an ass out of myself. Unlike them, I know I'm an ass."

And Montagnier, who discovered HIV and thus has a special stake in its importance, has been lectured to as if he were an incompetent graduate student who didn't know his way around a lab.

"Who are these people who are so much wiser, so much smarter than someone like Luc Montagnier?" asks Dr. Harry Rubin, the dean of American retrovirology. "He became an outlaw as soon as he started saying that HIV might not be the only cause of AIDS. The minute someone suggests that the orthodoxy might be wrong, the establishment starts to call him crazy or a quack. One week you're a great scientist; the next week you're a jerk. Science has become the new church of America and is closing off all room for creative, productive dissent."

Given the consequences, it is hardly surprising that scientists skeptical about the current theory of AIDS have hesitated to speak out. "I'd bet my professional reputation that something more than HIV is involved in this disease," said one federally funded AIDS researcher. "But I wouldn't bet my grants."

Human beings construct paradigms to create order out of chaos. Any attacks on those paradigms threatens order, so paradigm shifts are invariably slow. Yet to some extent, such a shift has already begun within AIDS research. By 1990 leading AIDS scientists were talking about the same kind of cofactors suggested by Sonnabend and Root-

Bernstein, about genetic factors that protect some of the infected from illness and about weaker strains of HIV that might not be fatal. They have little choice. The number of infected individuals not getting sick is growing, and even mainstream researchers now estimate that as many as 10 percent will probably never fall sick.

This shift is rarely acknowledged openly; it is too scary. There is a multi-billion-dollar research establishment at stake, and dozens of senior scientists would suffer considerable embarrassment. Most of all, there is the dread of discovering that time, money and human lives have been squandered. "What epidemiologist or federal official wants to admit that the entire thrust of research and education might be misguided?" asks Robin Haueter, an AIDS activist in New York. "What person with AIDS wants to consider the horrendous thought that we have wasted all these years of research, that an end might not be anywhere in sight?"

THREE

Magic Bullets and Bottom Lines

We Americans no longer harbor any illusions about our politicians. Too many have betrayed us, revealing the bitter triumph of self-interest even among those professedly dedicated to public service. We understand charitable organizations — even churches — to be corrupt, and we accept that corporations and their officers are even worse.

Yet we bow before doctors and scientists, deferring to their seeming omniscience; we assume their altruism, despite the lavish salaries they earn. In our naive, hopeful thinking, these white-smocked men and women are warriors against the unknown, and they will always slay the opposition, if they are simply given enough time, money and trust. In honor of their oath, they will do us no harm. In service to their conscience, they will do us great favors. They will point the government onto the right and righteous path, paving the way to more effective drugs and more affordable access to them.

The search for a cure for AIDS has revealed this image to be a fantasy. The odyssey and the scientists involved have been guided by the same force that has driven research into every other public health concern, from heart disease to cancer: the bottom line.

Basic science is becoming a dying institution, a dinosaur in a scientific world geared toward the production of salable products. Pharmaceutical companies drive American biomedical research, and they inevitably ask the following questions: Is the market big enough — are enough people suffering from a particular disease to make drug production worthwhile? Can we produce and test a drug cheaply enough to sell at the standard 400 to 500 percent profit? Will our research be good enough to pass muster with the Food and Drug Administration before the disease runs its course? What is the possibility of a lawsuit if we fudge a bit and push a drug onto a fast track? (A polite way of asking: Will the patients taking our drug die anyway, or are they likely to linger long enough to sue?)

When AIDS began to demonstrate its profit-making potential, drug companies from New Jersey to Switzerland dusted off compounds long discarded as treatments for cancer and leprosy and tested their effectiveness against HIV. A hundred compounds seemed to kill the relatively vulnerable virus in test tubes and petri dishes. Most of them would have killed patients, too, if they were injected into their veins.

In an ideal scientific world, the few promising compounds that seemed nonlethal would have been submitted to disinterested government scientists for study. The most exciting would have entered the official testing network — the AIDS Clinical Trials Group — where objective researchers would screen the drugs thoroughly for safety and efficacy.

A logical, civilized process. A model of cooperation between the public and private sectors whereby drug companies would provide the medications and scientists would test them at federal expense.

A fantasy.

Government scientists demand millions of pills to conduct their research, so drugs of promise belonging to cash-poor manufacturers languish untested. Well-financed companies hire university scientists as consultants, then give them honoraria, free trips to conferences around the world, research grants, cocktail parties and dinners at elegant restaurants. These same scientists dominate the federal research network. They decide which drugs get tested, perform the tests and, ultimately, recommend approval or disapproval of drugs. Not surprisingly, drugs owned by the companies for which they consult get priority for testing and receive faster FDA approval, even though there is minimal proof of the drugs' effectiveness. Treatment strategies involving no medication — thus promising no profit — receive short shrift.

Activists terrified by the mounting death toll have demanded more — more money, more testing, more approvals, more drugs. They have become the strange bedfellows of multinational corporations seeking federal research funds to defray the cost of drug development and the acceleration of the drug approval process. Then, the activists have become the enemies of those same corporations when they begin to sell their federally financed drugs at astronomical prices.

Meanwhile, fifteen years have passed, and people living with AIDS have wound up with only four drugs to help fight the destruction of their immune systems.

First there was AZT, which was approved with less than a year's research that was demonstrably flawed. Then ddI won approval, before the first full human trial had been completed. Next came ddC, despite such shaky evidence of its efficacy that it was recommended for use only with AZT. Finally, in June 1994 d4T was added to the arsenal — without any evidence that it prolonged survival, or was safe.

Americans have long clung to the belief that science can do anything. But after a decade of research and clinical trials that cost more than $6 billion in federal funds alone, what people with AIDS get, statistically speaking, from these drugs is:

- Between three and eight weeks of added life
- A two- to six-month delay in the onset of full-blown AIDS
- Some minor decrease in the number of opportunistic infections over the course of HIV infection and AIDS
- Serious side effects that at best make patients feel terrible and at worst can kill them.

That is what has been called victory in the battle for treatments and a cure for AIDS.

Dr. Margaret Fischl was thirty-two years old, one year out of residency and an obscure assistant professor at a minor medical school in Miami. A hard-working, serious young woman, she had been a good student at the University of Miami and looked to be on course for an unexceptional career in academic medicine. Her previous research was hardly on the frontiers of medical science. The one study she had published was titled "An index predicting relapse and possible need for hospitalization in patients with acute bronchial asthma."

Then came the young men whose bodies disintegrated before her eyes, refusing to respond to the most aggressive treatment medicine could devise. Fischl did something out of the ordinary, something that would mark her for the rest of her life: she paid attention.

Still a resident in general medicine, she enlisted in the struggle against a disease that still had no name. She became a one-woman crusade in her hospital, her university and the Florida legislature for funds to educate the public about the new disease, to try to prevent an epidemic and to build a treatment program to cope with it.

When the scientific establishment woke up to the looming epidemic, Fischl moved to join its ranks. "A lot of famous people, much more famous than her, got into the act," said her boss, Dr. Robert Rubin, vice provost at the University of Miami. "These were international experts in virology, in vaccine development, in immunology and genetics. Margaret was thrown right into the center. She is not a basic scientist. She is not going to win a Nobel in virology. She is a clinical scientist. Suddenly she was competing with people twice her age and ten times her experience." Her grant requests were turned down because she had no experience in gene cloning or retrovirology. She lived with constant stress, "the intellectual stress of being told, 'You're not a real scientist,'" Rubin said.

Nonetheless, eight years later Fischl flew to San Francisco, to appear before the delegates to the Sixth International Conference on AIDS. Activists with bleached hair and leather jackets had flooded the streets chanting, "One billion dollars, one lousy drug." At the time, AZT was the only approved anti-HIV drug, and young men who'd been told they were dying weren't impressed with scientific productivity.

Fischl was nervous. Terrified of being attacked by the activists, she'd been escorted onto the speaking platform by burly security guards. Seated next to her were virologists and immunologists from three continents. She was there as their equal, one of the most powerful members of the AIDS research establishment in the United States. It was a moment of honor and glory — made possible for Margaret Fischl, and the world, by Burroughs Wellcome.

AIDS is more than a disease; it's a scientific opportunity. Young physicians and researchers dreaming of the Nobel gold, or at least tenure and advancement, jump on the AIDS bandwagon. Government bureaucrats compete to make sure their agencies get a share of the $1.3 billion the federal government is doling out annually for AIDS research. Private laboratories line up at the government trough for their share of the kibble. Pharmaceutical companies scramble to strike their own mother lode in the form of a chemical compound that will prove deadly to the AIDS virus and not to the sick. Given the more than 40 million people worldwide facing a killer disease with no cure, such a drug would have seismic implications for the bottom line.

It didn't start out that way — which left Dr. Samuel Broder in a bind. In 1984 the director of the National Cancer Institute was appointed clinical director of its special task force on AIDS. His mission was to find drugs to fight the virus his colleague, Robert Gallo, claimed to have discovered. Broder had a small lab with a small staff and faced a monumental task. Science hadn't even conquered viruses, as anyone who's suffered with the flu or German measles well knows. HIV was worse, a retrovirus cleverly designed by nature to evade human defenses. Retroviruses insert their genes into the genetic material of cells and commandeer them. No one had ever found a way to remove retroviruses from those cells without killing healthy cells as well.

Broder strived to change that. He needed help, and the logical place to turn was to the nation's pharmaceutical companies. Despite the potential for profit, the enthusiasm was hardly deafening, because drug development is an awesomely expensive gamble. Most companies estimate that it costs $100 million to $200 million to bring a drug to market. In the early days of AIDS, the pessimism around the development of antivirals, and the fear of working with a lethal virus, meant that few companies were willing to wager that much.

Broder drummed up support wherever he could, offering the services of his lab at NCI in Bethesda to screen compounds that seemed promising. The one company he was most intent on enlisting was the giant British pharmaceutical firm Burroughs Wellcome, which had experience with the class of drugs Broder thought might work. It also had deep pockets — from the sale of over-the-counter drugs such as Sudafed, Empirin and Actifed — technical know-how and an enviable warehouse of chemical compounds looking for diseases to fight.

Burroughs Wellcome officials were less than enthusiastic when Broder flew to their American headquarters in North Carolina in October 1984. But he spoke eloquently about potential profits. No one knew how many people worldwide were infected with HIV, or what percentage of the infected were likely to fall ill, but the best guess was between six and eight million infections, increasing exponentially.

The pitch worked. When Broder left, Wellcome's researchers pulled some old compounds out of its stockroom and shipped them off to Bethesda, where NCI researchers added them to the growing number of drugs arriving from four dozen drug companies. Among Wellcome's compounds was a herring and salmon sperm extract developed by a Detroit researcher, Jerome Horowitz, in 1964 as a possible cancer treatment. His concoction, AZT, had never made it into human testing. It had been so ineffective against cancer cells, and so toxic, that Horowitz didn't even take out a patent.

In February 1985, however, that drug showed some activity against HIV in Broder's test tubes. It was quickly anointed the most promising drug in the batch, as the possible treatment, if not the cure, that patients and the U.S. Congress were demanding of the NIH scientists spending their tax money. Within four months, Wellcome asked the Food and Drug Administration for permission to begin testing AZT on human beings. Permission was granted within the week — unprecedented speed. In less than a month, on July 3, 1985, a Boston furniture salesman took the first tablets in the phase I study required to prove the safety of any new medication. He was gradually joined by ten more patients at the National Cancer Institute and eight at Duke University.

The drug didn't kill anyone. Nor did it seem to make anyone terribly sick — the two requisite conclusions for a phase I study. That's when Fischl got into the act. Burroughs Wellcome needed a group of researchers and their patients, at various sites around the country, to run the critical phase II study to see if a drug actually worked. Fischl was selected as a codirector, a position that would put her on the fast track for more research grants and for publication in the *New England Journal of Medicine*. The other codirector was Douglas Richman, a renowned virologist.

How did a newcomer, a total unknown, get the lead billing on such a crucial study? Fischl won't say. She refers all such questions to Burroughs Wellcome. "Most of the sites were picked based on [the local researchers'] reputations with antiviral work," Wellcome's spokeswoman said. Margaret Fischl had published no antiviral work.

Fischl, Richman and their colleagues selected 269 men and 13 women with AIDS to be their guinea pigs. The patients were more than willing. Word of the new miracle drug had already electrified the nascent AIDS grapevine. Some patients lied or tried to bribe their way into the study. Others exploited political connections to gain a coveted place. A few offered to purchase bootleg AZT from Burroughs Wellcome employees.

Almost from the beginning, there were signs that the drug was trouble. Two months into the trial, which began in February 1986, dozens of the 145 patients on AZT, rather than the placebo against which it was being tested, developed anemia. Their bodies just weren't producing enough red blood cells, and they suddenly needed transfusions. Researchers panicked, said Robert Yarchoan, an NCI scientist working with the study's investigators. The new drug was killing healthy bone-marrow cells at an alarming rate. Physicians who had referred their patients threatened to pull them from the study. The pressure was mounting to end it altogether, but Fischl was resolute. "She was convinced AZT was working," Yarchoan says. "She was convinced it was worth the risk." Fischl resisted the pressure — and prevailed.

None of the subjects died of anemia. But by the middle of September, nineteen of the placebo patients had died, joined by only one patient receiving AZT. Researchers had planned to keep the trial running through December, a total of eleven months. Instead, they shut it down after seven. How could they allow patients to keep taking placebos when the benefits of AZT seemed so apparent?

Members of the media were called in and told that a "promising" drug had been discovered. The effect was galvanic on the thousands dying horribly in and out of AIDS wards and on the corporate fortunes of Burroughs Wellcome, which had the exclusive right to produce AZT for seventeen years. The company's profits began to skyrocket, doubling in the following two years, to almost $200 million.

On January 16, 1987, the Anti-Infective Drugs Advisory Committee of the Food and Drug Administration met in a conference room at the FDA's aging Parklawn Building to make a decision that would affect AIDS patients throughout the world. Burroughs Wellcome sent a team of nine; billions were at stake. Fischl, who had celebrated her thirty-seventh birthday a few days earlier, was there. This was her study, her reputation, her future. Dr. Itzhak Brook, the committee chairman, and his colleagues were given one day to decide whether AZT should be approved for the market.

No one was under any illusions about the bind in which the committee found itself: AIDS activists and politicians were screaming for the federal research effort to produce something, and AZT was all those researchers had. But some members of the committee staff objected to the hurry-up atmosphere. "We're all under tremendous pressure, and there's no question that politics is a much greater part of AIDS drug development than approval and availability of drugs in less publicly visible diseases," said Ellen Cooper, the FDA medical investigator who had analyzed the AZT study data.

Despite the media hype, Cooper didn't like what she had seen in the research data. She worried about approving a drug on the basis of a single trial that was stopped before its completion, a trial that had fewer than three hundred subjects, most of whom had taken AZT for less than six months. She hated the idea of approving any drug without knowing anything about its long-term effects.

Cooper was also concerned about judging the effectiveness of the drug when so many of the subjects were being treated with a host of other medications. That kind of contamination would have discredited most drug trials. How could the FDA be sure that AZT was the drug responsible for patients' survival? Approval, she concluded, would be a "significant and potentially dangerous departure from our normal toxicology requirements."

When the reviewers sorted through the data, they had encountered one puzzle after another. After the study was terminated, in September, the patients on placebos were switched to AZT. Even so, in the following three months, thirteen more people from the original placebo group died, and there were seven deaths among those who had been on AZT from the beginning. Suddenly the survival rate between the two groups didn't look so dramatic — not 19 to 1, but 4 to 1.

"I was struck by the fact that AZT does not stop deaths," Dr. Stanley Lemon of the University of North Carolina Medical School told the packed meeting room. "Even those who were switched to AZT still kept dying. There are so many unknowns that it is hard to exactly know the truth. We do not really know what will happen a year from the beginning. The data is just too premature and the statistics are not really well done. The drug may actually be detrimental. We do not know."

But the FDA committee members kept harking back to the 19-to-1 ratio from the early part of the study. The final vote was 10 to 1 in favor of approval, with Itzhak Brook the only dissenter.

Dr. Joseph Sonnabend waited months for Fischl and her team to publish the final results of their study. He was eager to add a new weapon to his meager arsenal of drugs to help the growing number of sick, but he wasn't willing to join AZT's promoters without studying the results carefully. Government press releases didn't impress him; data did.

A medical researcher trained in infectious diseases at the University of Witwatersrand in Johannesburg and the Royal College of Physicians of Edinburgh, Sonnabend had done research on antiviral treatments and the immune system at the International Institute for Medical Research in London in the 1960s, before the field had entered the scientific mainstream. He wound up in New York in the 1970s and put his expertise in sexually transmitted diseases to work in the gay community.

When Sonnabend finally read the AZT study report, he had questions, but none more troubling than this: Why had so many placebo patients died? "I was suspicious of the study from the beginning because the mortality rate was simply unacceptable," Sonnabend says. "My patients were simply not dying in those sort of numbers that rapidly."

He reviewed the data and tried to figure out what had happened. He couldn't, because Fischl hadn't provided any detailed information about what had actually killed the placebo patients. AIDS, after all, does not kill; it allows other infections to do so. Even what little information he could glean was inconsistent. The causes of death provided to the FDA did not match those in the article on the research Fischl had written for the *New England Journal of Medicine*. "Sloppy research," Sonnabend concluded.

He pressed on. As he puzzled through the death reports, Sonnabend began to worry that the patients on placebos might have died because they were neglected. Had the physicians caring for them been inept at warding off and treating these infections, he asked publicly, or were they unwittingly treating placebo patients differently from those on AZT?

That was theoretically impossible, he knew. To avoid such differences in treatment, controlled scientific experiments are almost always double-blind: neither the physician nor the participant knows which patients are on the drug being tested and which are on a placebo. And Fischl's *New England Journal* article was specific: this had been a double-blind study.

Except, as every patient in the study knew, and FDA scientists acknowledged, it was not. The study's participants were members of a community that was already savvy about the ways of science — and intent on receiving AZT. From the first, they could distinguish between the two types of pills they were given: they tasted different. Many realized they could send their pills to commercial laboratories for analysis and discover whether they were on AZT or the placebo. Some who weren't getting AZT persuaded those who were to share it. Their agenda, after all, wasn't scientific purity, it was survival.

The patients' wasn't the only side of the blind that was broken. The side effects of high doses of AZT are so extreme that researchers knew who was on AZT just by how frequently the participants needed blood transfusions. (Which was another thing that bothered Sonnabend: Could the short-term benefits attributed to AZT actually have been the result of transfusions of fresh blood?) And beyond the transfusions, the standard lab tests — in which the action of AZT on the blood was clearly visible — would have told researchers instantly who was on the drug and who was taking a placebo. In other drug tests, such information is erased by lab workers to keep clinicians from seeing it. In the testing of AZT, it was not. It didn't need to be, Fischl argued, insisting — despite a wealth of evidence to the contrary — that the blind had never been compromised.

Dr. Samuel Broder, the NCI director, defended the integrity of the study in a different way. Special precautions to preserve double-blinding were not necessary, he said, because researchers could be trusted not to be biased. In fact, Broder objected to Sonnabend's entire line of reasoning. "That's an accusation of fraud, not bad scientific design," he said.

Despite Broder's defensive response, scientific fraud is hardly unknown, especially among ambitious young researchers working in the high-pressure, high-stakes environment of competitive universities. Few scientists can forget the case of Dr. John Darsee, a rising star at Harvard who had turned out nearly one hundred research papers before he turned thirty-three. His brilliant career was cut short when lab mates caught him forging test results. Dr. Robert Slutsky, another superstar-to-be, managed to produce one research paper every ten days between 1983 and 1984. Investigators discovered that he had pulled off that miracle of productivity by fabricating data — inventing results from animal and patient studies he never executed.

Darsee and Slutsky were hardly unique, so Broder's protestation of any inference of fraud on the part of Margaret Fischl rang a little hollow. In fact, Sonnabend insists he never accused Fischl or her colleagues of fraud. He simply asked why, if unblinding presented no significant problem, Fischl, as author of the study, claimed to have overseen a double-blind study. "Double-blinding exists for a very clear reason: to ensure that no unconscious bias can creep into the way we treat patients. If there were not a need for it, it would not exist," he said. "What I am saying is that the study doesn't tell us what we need to know. It was technically substandard. For all we know from that study, AZT may even be better than they claimed. But it may be worse."

In October 1987, a year after Fischl's study ended, Dr. Gordon Dickinson, then her research collaborator at the University of Miami and now head of the AIDS program at the Veterans Administration Medical Center in Miami, presented the results of his own study of patients receiving long-term AZT treatment. During their first six months on the drug, patients gained weight and experienced increases in their T cells — one of the building blocks of the immune system. But after that, he reported, they began losing both weight and T cells and developing serious infections. "I'm pessimistic about AZT," he told the local press.

Fischl did not dispute the finding but took sharp exception to Dickinson's analysis. She tersely reminded reporters that she, not Dickinson, was the chief AIDS researcher at the University of Miami. "We absolutely recommend continued therapy despite falls in T cells and infections," she said without clarifying who else was included in the "we" or why continued therapy would be justified in the face of such negative markers.

By then, Fischl's career was skyrocketing. As AZT became one of the most tested drugs in history, her résumé grew with references to her authorship or coauthorship of dozens of key studies. She became a star at the University of Miami, a franchise player whose research brought in more than $10 million a year in federal and private grant money, half of which went directly into university coffers. She was elected the sole U.S. representative to the International AIDS Society, which coordinates the global effort against the disease. She became one of only ten members of the executive committee of the AIDS Clinical Trials Group and the chair of its HIV Research Agenda Committee. The ACTG directed the then $70-million-a-year government AIDS research effort and for years channeled most of its research dollars into further study of AZT: AZT in early HIV infection, AZT for children, AZT for health care workers pricked with needles filled with HIV-infected fluids, AZT for pregnant women and AZT in combination with other antivirals. Drug companies usually do some post-licensing testing, but the ACTG spent 80 percent of its federal funds on AZT.

It's not that there were no other drugs worth testing. A congressional committee, patient groups and even the Institute of Medicine have criticized the ACTG for its overemphasis on AZT at the expense of work on treatments for the cancers and the fungal, viral and microbacterial infections that actually kill people with AIDS. Activists, journalists and politicians have gone further, asking why the research network did so. Was Burroughs Wellcome exercising too much influence over the group? If scientists like Fischl owe their prominence to the very corporations whose drugs they test, can they possibly be objective? If pharmaceutical companies wield that much power over the careers of researchers, can the American public trust anything these scientists say?

Such uncomfortable questions were asked not just about Fischl and her fellow AIDS researchers or about Burroughs Wellcome, but about the entire American scientific community, raising chilling concerns about the state of the nation's science. Such concern surfaced even before AIDS raised the stakes, both for researchers and for pharmaceutical companies. After World War II, biomedical researchers grew increasingly dependent on federal funds to equip their laboratories and finance their work. Universities didn't pay the freight, even for researchers with faculty positions. In fact, universities skimmed hefty percentages — more than half, in some cases — off the top of research grants as "overhead." But in recent years government largess hasn't kept pace with the cost of research. Only one of every five grant applications to the National Institutes of Health now receives funding. Where can researchers turn to pay their lab bills?

Industrial support is the only option, an option most scientists long rejected as selling out to Mammon. The potential problems are glaring: How will basic research be funded when it produces no profit? Will scientists continue to pursue the research they believe is important or will they select new projects on the basis of corporate fundability, thus the potential for corporate profit? Will their acceptance of funds dilute researchers' objectivity? Will they be willing to risk giving pharmaceutical companies bad news about their drugs, even if it means jeopardizing future grants? Will the relationship between corporations and researchers create an atmosphere of secrecy, dampening the free exchange of information essential to scientific progress? Can science be trusted to police itself?

These are serious questions about who sets the scientific agenda of the nation and how honestly it is followed, but they have been dismissed by much of the scientific community, which protests the insult to its integrity and insists that clear institutional safeguards are in place.

Several chilling incidents cast doubt on those assurances. In 1987 Dr. Erdem Cantekin of the University of Pittsburgh accused his colleague, Dr. Charles Bluestone, of grossly exaggerating the effectiveness of antibiotics in treating middle ear infections in children. Bluestone had established a center to study that ailment at Pittsburgh's Children's Hospital in 1980 and had attracted hefty grants from the National Institutes of Health. He had also accepted millions of dollars in honoraria, research funding and speaking fees from the pharmaceutical companies whose products he was endorsing as treatments. Nonetheless, a university committee cleared Bluestone of charges of impropriety because it concluded that his findings had been supported by other studies — an odd finding, since an international research group had contradicted him. The person who wound up being punished was Cantekin. A university committee suggested that his tenure be revoked, and his office was moved to a windowless cubicle above a supermarket.

In 1988 a congressional investigation revealed that more than a dozen researchers who'd run a large study of a new drug that dissolved blood clots had owned stock in the company that produced the medication. Not surprisingly, the researchers concluded that the new drug, t-PA, tissue plasminogen activator, was superior to a competitive product. They failed to mention that both drugs performed equally well by some measures and that the other medication sold for one-tenth the price of t-PA.

The chairman of the congressional subcommittee investigating the case, Ted Weiss of New York, stated that it was "an unequivocal conflict of interest" for any scientist doing federally funded research to have a financial stake in its outcome.

Yet such conflicts were neither illegal nor uncommon. "Seeking a profit from your research is the ordinary, expected thing," said Leonard Minsky, executive director of the National Association of Universities in the Public Interest.

AIDS research has not gone unscathed by the exposure of conflicts of interest. Syed Zaki Salahuddin, a key researcher in Robert Gallo's lab, pleaded guilty in 1990 to accepting illegal gratuities from a company that supplied goods and services to Gallo's laboratory. It was worse than that: Salahuddin's wife, Firoza, was one of four original directors of the company in question, a piece of information Salahuddin omitted from the financial disclosure statements he submitted regularly to the National Cancer Institute.

Two years later, Gallo's lab was embarrassed anew when his principal deputy, Prem Sarin, was found guilty of embezzling $25,000 that had been sent to the lab by a German pharmaceutical company to pay for an assistant to screen a potential AIDS drug. Prem took the money as a personal consulting fee and used the lab during working hours to perform the tests the German company requested.

Some financial relationship between researchers and private companies — usually somewhat less sleazy than Salahuddin's and Prem's — is standard procedure. In December 1989 Dr. Martin Hirsch, the former chairman of the AIDS Clinical Trials Group, acknowledged at a federal hearing that almost all the federally funded AIDS researchers were receiving money from the pharmaceutical companies whose products they were testing.

Many researchers are paid to conduct drug trials for pharmaceutical companies. Some serve on the companies' advisory boards, and most accept at least occasional speaking fees from them. FDA committee hearings open with disclosures of conflicts of interest. It is not unusual for four or five committee members or their invited guests — the big names in AIDS research — to admit to financial relationships with the companies whose drugs they are evaluating.

By the late 1980s, the situation was beginning to appear, if not become, out of control. Hoping to preempt conflict-of-interest legislation brewing in Congress, the National Institutes of Health unveiled, in January 1989, a new regulation prohibiting federally funded researchers from having a financial stake in any company "that would be affected by the outcome of the research or that produces a product or equipment being evaluated in the research project."

The scientific establishment was not pleased. "The proposed guidelines are inoperable, are an affront to the personal integrity of the vast majority of scientists, are an invasion into the private lives of multitudes of individuals," a prominent cancer researcher wrote in a typically indignant letter to the federal agency. Of the seven hundred responses NIH received to its proposal, more than six hundred were hostile.

In the face of that opposition, Secretary of Health and Human Services Louis Sullivan backed off and quietly canceled the new regulation. A congressional committee responded by holding hearings on scientific conflicts of interest and concluded that neither the nation's universities nor NIH was adequately monitoring and controlling conflicts of interest. The committee proposed banning federally funded scientists from conducting research on drugs owned by companies to which they had financial ties.

The scientific community mobilized to ward off legislation, promising that universities would deal with scientific misconduct and conflicts of interest more vigorously. The AIDS Clinical Trials Group, which had no policy on conflicts of interest or even on disclosure of financial relationships, took action of its own. During the group's 1994 reorganization, its staff and executive committee proposed a straightforward disclosure policy. Scientists wouldn't be barred from maintaining financial relationships with drug companies but would be required to inform the research network if they owned company stock or received consulting fees or honoraria.

"Wake up and smell the roses," said Dr. Charles van der Horst of the University of North Carolina, a member of the ACTG executive committee, to his fellow researchers at their meeting in July 1994. "It is not kosher to have stock or patents or an equity in a company and push their drug. Save that for the rubber-chicken circuit. We will not let you do it anymore at the ACTG."

A howl of protest rose from the ranks. "People are incredibly uptight about conflict of interest, and I really don't understand it," said van der Horst. "It's not like we're asking for tax forms, the exact amount of stock they own or the exact amount of money they get for presentations. But when we're looking at a large protocol or an application to run a committee, we need to know if the principal investigator has stock in the company. We need to look at a conflict-of-interest statement along with a curriculum vitae."

Margaret Fischl herself does not oppose prohibitions on ownership of stock or other interests in companies. "This is not relevant to me," she explained. "We are not salaried through pharmaceutical companies. I do not own stock in pharmaceutical companies . . . I have never gotten a 'kickback' from Burroughs Wellcome, if that is the terminology."

But owning no stock and receiving no "kickbacks" doesn't guarantee that Fischl and her colleagues are not influenced by the pharmaceutical industry. "It's not that we think that scientists are greedy bastards," said Diana Zuckerman, who worked on conflict-of-interest issues for former Congressman Ted Weiss. "It's that we have to ask if close working relationships with scientists and officials at drug companies, if becoming friendly with folks there, does not bias what a scientist decides to study or thinks, whether he knows it or not.

"Money is only one way that people are influenced. There is the pressure to publish that is facilitated when a drug company gives you a grant; the tremendous desire to say something new works; the prestige that bringing in grants and consultancy fees earns you within your university."

Fischl thinks that's nonsense: research cannot be influenced that easily. "It's not just the pharmaceutical company, you're also working with the FDA. They are involved with designing the study from the beginning."

But questions of subtle influence still remain. Fischl, for example, might not have received a salary or consulting fees from Burroughs Wellcome, but she made "advertorials" for AZT — television spots explaining the virtues of the drug, bought and paid for by Burroughs Wellcome. For years, her picture appeared in AZT ads in magazines distributed to physicians. The company paid her for the first study of AZT, and she built her entire career around that product. "These people fly you around the country to speak at conferences," says Dr. Joseph Sonnabend. "They promote you and your research. You get a bit of fame and glory. Maybe being on the emotional take is ultimately more insidious than being on the dollar take."

On August 17, 1989, newspapers around the world trumpeted a dramatic new finding: early treatment with AZT can stave off AIDS. "Today we are witnessing a turning point in the battle to change AIDS from a fatal disease to a treatable one," announced Louis Sullivan of HHS.

The news electrified Wall Street. Burroughs Wellcome's stock surged by 33 percent in a single week. The *Wall Street Journal* estimated that annual sales of AZT, the most expensive drug ever put on the market, would reach $1.2 billion by 1992 — half of that pure profit.

At that moment, 1.4 million Americans were assumed to be infected with the AIDS virus. "Eventually all of them may need to take AZT so they don't get sick," said Dr. Anthony Fauci, whose federal agency sponsored the two studies on which the finding was based.

Press releases announced that the major study, of which Fischl was a second author, was based on 3,200 HIV-positive Americans who had not yet progressed to full-blown AIDS. Over a two-year period, half had been given AZT and half a placebo. The authors concluded that "HIV-positive patients are twice as likely to get AIDS if they don't take AZT."

Once the data became available, however, the news seemed less exciting. The research, it turned out, was based not on 3,200 subjects but on less than half that number, 1,338; the remainder had either dropped out of the study or been enrolled too late to be counted. The average subject was followed for one year. While only 25 of the 910 participants on AZT progressed to AIDS, only 33 of the 428 placebo takers joined them — 7.6 percent got sick while taking a placebo, 3.6 percent got sick on AZT. That looked impressive, but statisticians didn't share the enthusiasm. Some researchers say that considering the small number of subjects in each group who got sick, the statistical difference between them was not great. It could have been a random occurrence.

Fischl does not accept that argument. "A two- to threefold difference is not attributable to chance." She called the findings "a quantum leap."

Other scientists were skeptical. Three months after the announcement, a group of European AZT researchers openly challenged the study's conclusions in an article in *Science*. The Europeans claimed that the Americans had withheld the raw data from them for three months. When the data finally arrived, they wrote, it did not support the results the Americans had announced. Quite the opposite: the Europeans argued that AZT had been recommended for wider use for political, not scientific, reasons.

Meanwhile, members of the Veterans Administration's AIDS research team were also looking over the new AZT data. They were two years into their own three-year study of the effects of AZT on patients infected with the AIDS virus but not yet sick. If there was clear proof that AZT delayed the onset of AIDS, how could the VA ethically continue a study in which half the patients were given placebos?

VA researchers took an early look at their own data, then met with representatives from the National Institutes of Health and the Food and Drug Administration. There was something wrong: their results contradicted Fischl's conclusions. The VA's scientists found no meaningful difference in the progression to AIDS between AZT patients and placebo patients. They decided to continue their study.

A few months later — at about the same time that Fischl was delivering her paper in San Francisco encouraging the use of AZT for one million Americans infected with HIV but not yet sick — the National Cancer Institute announced that almost half the people who had taken AZT for three years could expect to develop an aggressive form of lymphoma, a deadly cancer of the lymphatic system.

AZT's supporters rushed to the defense of the drug. "I cannot fathom why AZT would be causing lymphoma," Fischl said in San Francisco. "It's just that people are living longer" with depressed immune systems, predisposing them to cancer.

Paul Volberding, head of the AIDS program at San Francisco General Hospital and one of Fischl's coauthors in the AZT studies, agreed. "Whatever is going on, it's certainly not as simple as 'AZT causes lymphomas.'"

But no one could be sure, because no one had compared the lymphoma rates of AIDS patients who took AZT with the lymphoma rates of those who had refused to take the drug.

Whether AZT was harmful or not — and whether or not it was as effective as Fischl and her colleagues claimed — was not the only question. Even researchers convinced of the value of the drug worried that by spending so much time and money studying AZT, federally funded AIDS scientists were bypassing other drugs and other avenues of research. As of August 1989, the government was supporting twice as many drug trials — and spending four times as much money — on AZT than on all other potential AIDS treatments. Of the six new anti-HIV studies announced for 1990, four involved the use of AZT in combination with other drugs. In that year nearly 80 percent of the patients enrolled in federally sponsored AIDS drug trials were in studies related to AZT. That percentage hadn't changed in 1994.

Dozens of promising drugs and therapies have been left by the wayside as limited funds have been channeled into deciphering how AZT and its cousin compounds work. Many of the drugs that have been ignored are owned by small corporations that do not have the money to wine and dine scientists and federal officials — which Burroughs Wellcome does regularly. They are unwilling, or unable, to give large grants to community-based AIDS service organizations and to court activists with grants — all of which Burroughs Wellcome does regularly.

In fact, many of the promising treatments are not owned by drug companies at all, and can't be. They are unpatentable products — food or chemical derivatives or natural products based on foods. If they have been tested at all, they have been relegated to the Office of Alternative Medicine, which has a budget of $3.5 million for all diseases, compared to the ACTG budget of $111 million for AIDS drug research alone. Some treatments are immune-stimulating procedures that might involve no drugs at all.

Scientists in the ACTG banked all their hopes and their funds on killing the virus. But HIV disease turned out to be more complicated than the simplistic Pac-Man model of a virus racing through the body infecting and killing cells. With HIV the internal logic of the immune system goes haywire. No one is sure why or how. Immunologists still don't know, and they were virtually locked out of AIDS research when the funding was channeled to virologists. Only after fifteen years of epidemic were the first trials geared toward rebuilding the immune system, rather than murdering the virus, approved by NIH. But funding for immunology is still a pittance, even though no one yet knows whether an immune system gone astray can be put back on track, whether its suicidal instincts can be changed and whether its disease-fighting "memory" can be replenished.

Furthermore, all the emphasis on AZT and its cousins has left relatively little money for research into treatments for the diseases that actually kill people with advanced HIV infection, especially the less common ones like microsporidiosis or progressive multifocal leuk-oencephalopathy. The money and prestige, after all, are in anti-HIV drugs.

The problem was that the ACTG stormed in to find a cure for AIDS without understanding how HIV does its dirty work, or why some infected people fall ill immediately while others remain healthy, even after fifteen years. Without basic research conducted by geneticists, immunologists and microbiologists, there can be no answers to these questions. Without those answers a cure — even an effective treatment — is a remote possibility. In the critical moment of the epidemic, just after the discovery of HIV, only two researchers at the molecular biology laboratory at Cambridge University — the lab with the world's highest concentration of Nobel laureates per floor — were working on AIDS. From the start, research into AIDS was driven by the initiative of pharmaceutical companies. The cart was put before the horse, often by a deadly distance.

A pall fell over the AIDS research establishment in July 1993 when five chronic hepatitis patients died during the testing of fialuridine — FIAU — a member of a family of drugs called nucleoside analogues, which includes AZT, ddI, ddC and d4T. Scientists were caught off guard: FIAU had reportedly been proven safe in animal studies and early human trials. Fifteen patients had begun taking the medication in the spring. One week they were fine. Two weeks later, many were on the verge of death. Seven required liver transplants.

Dozens of researchers scurried to figure out what had happened. FIAU had seemed a near miracle when it was first tested in 1989 and 1990. Scientists had turned to the drug hoping it might fight HIV. It did not, but it seemed to kill the hepatitis B virus. Until then, the only treatment for chronic hepatitis B was a medication administered by injection and known to cause severe side effects. FIAU, a liquid preparation taken orally, promised to be just as effective with none of the drawbacks.

Dr. Jay Hoofnagle, director of the division of digestive diseases and nutrition at the National Institute of Diabetes and Digestive and Kidney Diseases, mounted a small safety trial of the drug in April 1992. Twenty-four patients were treated with liquid FIAU — flavored to taste like Grand Marnier — for one month; the hepatitis B virus disappeared in nine of them. Except for those taking the highest doses of the medication, the patients seemed to tolerate FIAU well.

The only major complaints were of nausea and vomiting, which Hoofnagle took as a good sign. Before hepatitis is flushed out of the body, it tends to flare up and cause nausea. At worst, he assumed the side effects were the routine ailments of hepatitis sufferers. The only problem he attributed solely to FIAU was tingling and pain in some patients' feet, a condition called peripheral neuropathy. That had been anticipated and was even listed as a possible side effect on the patient consent forms — neuropathy is a classic side effect of nucleoside analogues.

Hoofnagle moved ahead with a six-month trial to test the drug's effectiveness. Beginning in March 1993, ten of the patients from the earlier trial were treated for one month, then new patients were gradually added to the research group.

Everything went well until early June, when three patients from the new group complained of severe nausea and vomiting. Supervising physicians directed them to stop taking the drug, assuming the symptoms would disappear quickly. They did not. One woman became so ill that she was flown to NIH from North Carolina. Hoofnagle still wasn't alarmed, because he suspected that the virus was simply flaring. But when he checked the woman's blood work, there was no sign of hepatitis in her body. What was poisoning her liver?

On the morning of June 25 another patient, a Virginia man who had also been complaining of nausea, was taken to the emergency room of a hospital in Fredericksburg and diagnosed as having lactic acidosis. Hoofnagle panicked: acidosis results from a potentially fatal buildup of waste materials in cells. The symptoms are not characteristic of hepatitis B. Something was terribly wrong.

The next day, Hoofnagle contacted all the patients, directing them to stop taking FIAU and to come in to Bethesda for testing. He discovered that five more patients — including two who had been on the drug for only five days — had lactic acidosis. The group was a nightmare of liver failure, kidney abnormalities, pancreatitis and neuropathy. On July 4 Hoofnagle's sickest patients, among them the Virginia man and the North Carolina woman, received liver transplants. The man died the next day. The woman died in late August.

In hindsight, the warning signs that something dangerous was happening should have been clear. Two years before that final, fatal study, a Yale University pharmacologist had sounded them, in the journal *Molecular Pharmacology*. Yung-Chi Cheng had found that some nucleosides — including AZT and its related compounds — could cause severe liver malfunctions. Hoofnagle did not see Cheng's work until the weekend after his patients started dying. He insisted that he had thoroughly searched the literature on potential toxicity before beginning his studies but had somehow overlooked the Yale team's results.

More chilling was the fact that serious problems had arisen — and been discounted — in every FIAU study that had been done:

- Of the twelve AIDS patients in a 1988 FIAU experiment at the University of California at San Diego, directed by ACTG researcher Dr. Douglas Richman, at least five experienced sudden increases in liver enzymes. One might have died as a result of the drug.
- Of the forty-three AIDS patients in a 1990 trial at the San Diego campus, at NIH and at the University of Washington — where the researcher was AIDS expert Dr. Lawrence Corey — at least five had high liver enzyme levels. Three deaths might have been caused by the drug.
- Of the twenty-four patients in the 1991 NIH pilot study, eight had elevated liver enzymes. One death might have resulted from the drug.

Even early animal studies of FIAU — conducted with woodchucks — had suggested severe liver toxicity.

In fact, the drug's manufacturer, Eli Lilly, knew there might be trouble with FIAU even before Hoofnagle's final trial began. Lilly had mounted its own study of the drug's impact on normal volunteers, the first time that healthy people were given the drug. Liver enzyme levels soared and severe liver abnormalities developed, reactions that the company could not blame on the volunteers' health or other medications. Lilly did not notify Hoofnagle of the results. The company failed to inform NIH and the FDA for weeks. They simply waited and hoped for the best.

The FIAU fiasco sent shock waves through the AIDS research establishment. Given the speed with which AIDS drugs were being released, they knew that if FIAU had shown promise against HIV, it would surely have been in the bodies of thousands of patients before anyone could have recognized its toxicity.

Their concerns weren't entirely theoretical. Physicians began asking whether disaster had really been averted. Could any of those thousands of patients they'd put on AZT, ddI and ddC have suffered fates similar to the FIAU trial participants, fates ignored by researchers who had confused their symptoms, and their deaths, with causes other than the drugs — with the seemingly inevitable onset of AIDS? There was no way to be sure, because no one tracks all the ailments AIDS patients suffer during the course of their disease. No one routinely performs autopsies on them. Researchers and clinicians report "incidents" only when they believe the symptoms might be related to drugs. The FIAU case made clear how hesitant researchers were to reach that conclusion.

Suddenly everyone began paying attention to the few physicians who had been warning of AZT-related liver damage for years — well before FIAU provoked concern. Dr. Allen Arieff saw his first cases of unexplained lactic acidosis in AIDS patients in 1990, when he was a visiting professor at Mount Sinai School of Medicine in New York. Two patients there had died of the rare condition, and Arieff couldn't figure out why.

When he returned home to California, Arieff, haunted by the deaths, began looking for more. By the summer of 1991, he'd found seven. When he mentioned their cases at a scientific meeting, a dozen or more scientists spoke up with similar experiences. Joel Freiman, an FDA epidemiologist, had discovered the problem on paper, in the lists of "adverse reaction" reports on AZT filed with his agency. Researchers at NIH had turned up three other cases of unexplained fatty liver. While Arieff was talking to his colleagues about their cases, Freiman had documented fourteen more.

No one thought to warn patients taking AZT.

The cases were published in medical journals, but no one wanted to consider the possibility that AZT might be destroying livers. In June 1993, however, just before the FIAU patients began to die, the FDA asked Burroughs Wellcome to send out a warning letter to the nation's infectious disease specialists. They complied. But like Cheng's article and the warning from Arieff, that signal too was ignored by the medical community.

After an FDA task force convened to investigate the disaster issued its report in November 1993, the agency's commissioner, David

Kessler, admitted that the data warning of FIAU's toxicity were apparent from the beginning. The problem, he said, was overoptimism, which led researchers and Eli Lilly to systematically misinterpret every patient problem and complaint as unrelated to the drug. The FIAU debacle sent up a dozen warning flares, not just about undue optimism, but also about the quality of the research done by scientists running clinical trials in America.

Right in the middle of the unfolding FIAU scandal, a bomb exploded that made those flares seem dim by comparison. The preliminary results of the Anglo-French Concorde trial, the longest and largest study of the effects of AZT on asymptomatic HIV-positive people, had been released in April 1993. The study had followed 1,749 HIV-positive people given AZT either early in their infection or only after they developed AIDS. After three years, the survival rate was 92 percent in the early treatment group and 94 percent in the deferred-treatment group. The rate of progression to AIDS was an identical 18 percent in both. So the study concluded that early intervention with AZT, the standard of care in American medicine, was irrelevant.

The results contradicted the studies done by the AIDS Clinical Trials Group, which had made AZT a household word. The American researchers did not accept the European challenge to their work graciously. After the French and British scientists presented their results at a closed meeting at NIH, the director of the Division of AIDS issued a terse press release: "At this time we see no basis for changing the current recommendation to initiate antiretroviral therapy for HIV-infected persons whose CD4 + T cell count falls below 500 per microliter of blood."

Dr. Paul Volberding, the researcher at San Francisco General Hospital who was Fischl's coinvestigator on most of the early American AZT studies, said, "[The Concorde investigators] conducted the study as well as I've seen any done. The issue is, how do we interpret the data? One approach is to say there is no benefit to early AZT therapy. Another approach is to say there is a benefit, but it is a transient one." When Fischl was asked how she planned to incorporate the Concorde results into her practice, she said she would continue giving AZT to her patients "from when they have 800 or less CD4 cells." It was clear that she rejected the Concorde findings.

Two months after the release of the preliminary Concorde data — and just as the FIAU patients were beginning to fall sick — the AIDS establishment flew to Berlin for its annual gathering. In the halls and bars, U.S. scientists were on the defensive. Their honor, and competence, had been impugned by a bunch of Europeans. They responded by nitpicking at the Europeans' research design and statistical competence. They even groused about the announcement being made in a letter to *The Lancet* without full presentation of the data — a strange criticism from a group that regularly announced its results in press releases.

Dr. Maxime Seligman, a French AZT expert who codirected Concorde, responded to the Americans' complaints and their insistence on continuing early intervention with AZT: "One shouldn't be too dogmatic or simplistic. Obviously, you should give a drug as early as possible. That is classic medicine. But that is for a reliable drug. I wouldn't give AZT [early] based on the data we have here."

The Americans' protestations against the Concorde results rang hollow because they had broken a cardinal rule of research by terminating their studies before they could see the long-term impact of the drug. Fischl's trial had ended six months earlier than planned. Volberding's major study, which compared asymptomatic patients who did and did not take AZT, was canceled after an average follow-up of eleven months. In fact, the only American study that ran its full length — three years — was conducted by researchers from the Veterans Administration. It had produced the same results as Concorde.

Activists, many of whom had thrown themselves into the politics of AIDS still clinging to a naive image of science as benevolent and omniscient, responded to the American scientists with cynicism and even fury. After all, scientists had staked only their careers on AZT. AIDS patients had staked their lives on it.

Beyond the embarrassment, a stark new reality emerged from the Concorde study. The basic technique that the Americans had been using to gauge the effectiveness of drugs, the CD4 cell count, was shown to be useless. Traditionally, drug trials test new medications against clinical endpoints: the onset of specific diseases or symptoms, or death. But with a disease that progresses so slowly, and over such a long period of time, the use of clinical endpoints means that trials would go on for years. Neither AIDS patients nor their physicians were willing to wait, so they turned to so-called surrogate markers, biological indicators of the progress of a disease which can be substituted for clinical endpoints.

Surrogates are tricky, because what seems a clear indication of disease progression in treating a patient might be meaningless in judging a drug. For years, for example, cardiologists prescribed drugs to heart attack survivors to control irregular heartbeats. They knew from experience that irregular heartbeats in those patients increased the probability of a second heart attack, so it seemed logical to try to prevent them. Things didn't turn out according to their plan. When they finally studied the impact of giving patients such medications, they discovered that the drugs were actually tripling the death rate.

AIDS researchers didn't learn that lesson. Knowing that a drop in CD4 counts — the number of a critical white blood cell — suggests disease progression, they selected that measure to test the effectiveness of drugs. Medications that raised CD4 counts were deemed worthy of testing; those that did not were discarded. But the researchers never verified that artificially stimulating CD4 cells with chemicals would slow the progress of the disease or prolong life.

The Concorde study showed that it does not. AZT increased the CD4 cells of the patients given early treatment, but that rise did not correlate with sustained life. No one knew why. Some researchers speculated that the stimulated CD4 cells just didn't work very well. Others suggested that AZT might force CD4 cells out of reservoirs like the lymphatic tissue, and that the rise might be dangerous.

Everyone agreed that the news was ominous. Suddenly more than seven years and billions of dollars of research were open to question — along with the competence of the entire AIDS research establishment. The value of almost all of the drugs AIDS patients were taking was also called into question, because they had been approved on the basis of their ability to increase CD4 cells. Even more distressing was the thought of all the drugs that had been discarded as ineffective because they had not raised the counts. How would researchers proceed without a valid surrogate marker?

Berlin offered American AIDS researchers yet another humiliation — and another warning of the dangers of their approach to science. It again involved Margaret Fischl. She was running an ACTG trial testing whether AZT, its cousin ddC or a combination of the two was more effective in treating AIDS patients. The press release sent out in advance of her report at Berlin made the results clear: "The researchers observed no significant differences between any of the three treatment regimens." But in Berlin Fischl rose and touted the merits of the combination therapy, at least for one select group of patients. Activists jeered and openly challenged her for dancing the "combo mambo." Statisticians in the room shook their heads in dismay.

The line between analysis and massaging the data to bolster a hypothesis is often a fine one in science. Most clinical research designers are careful to avoid the type of "subset analysis" — searching through every conceivable category of patient until you find a group that illustrates the desired results — in which Fischl was engaging. If scientists "look at subgroup after subgroup after subgroup, by the laws of probability one in twenty of these comparisons is going to come up bingo even when nothing is going on at all," said David Sackett of McMaster University in Hamilton, Ontario.

"Fischl was a classic case," said Thomas Fleming, a biostatistician from Seattle who sits on numerous committees that monitor clinical trials. "But it appears in all clinical areas that are new to clinical trials. Everybody thinks their disease is different, the exception. We are seemingly unwilling to learn from history, from other disease settings."

Why was Margaret Fischl in particular so immune to this lesson? Perhaps because her AZT research was her sole claim to fame; to allow it to be debunked would be to sink back into anonymity. Her colleagues argue that the problem is more complex, that she was still scarred from those early days when fellow physicians snored through her presentations on AIDS, when she was a junior faculty member and the head of her medical school dismissed her predictions of a looming epidemic as alarmist. When she later became a name-brand AIDS researcher, the phone in her office began ringing constantly with patients begging to see her. Before long, she found herself in charge of dozens of nurses, physicians, lab technicians and office workers handling the care of thousands of patients.

This status and admiration were inevitably mixed with difficulty: the politics of getting federal grants; the delicate diplomacy of dealing with colleagues jealous of the sudden prominence of a young upstart; the messy confrontations with patients and activists diverting their anger over an epidemic into fury at her. And rather than learn to extract the bits of legitimate criticism from this constant onslaught, Fischl seemed to withdraw. It appeared to be the reflex of a particularly private person. "Everyone was driving her crazy," said Robert Rubin, the vice provost of the University of Miami. "Something snapped in her psyche." She wouldn't allow her office to hand out her complete résumé, wouldn't grant interviews and would literally break into a trot — or hide in her hotel room during a fundraising event — to avoid a reporter. She rarely discussed her private life: many of the people who worked closely with her didn't know if she was married or single. Her superiors insist that this was not a sign of aloofness, but rather fragility. "Sometimes she sits down and cries," said Rubin. "If the public could see that, they would be less critical."

Some might. Not the ones who tethered so many of their hopes to AZT and the integrity of her research. Certainly not the ones who bet their lives on it.

After the AIDS researchers returned home from Berlin, the news only got worse when the most exciting and hopeful research study in years was added to the growing list of discredited scientific work.

In February 1993, the country had been electrified by the announcement from Massachusetts General Hospital that the "Achilles' heel of HIV" had been discovered. Yung-Kang Chow, a Harvard Medical School student, had developed a new approach to killing HIV with a combination of AZT, ddI and a new type of antiviral called Nevirapine. It was, in essence, a triple punch that would circumvent HIV's wily ability to mutate quickly into resistance to any one drug.

Mass. General and Harvard cranked up their press machines and sent out a twelve-page press release suggesting that a cure for AIDS was at hand. Neither the *New York Times* nor network television news could resist a packaged handout from Harvard — even if it came with no proof. Not only was some hope being offered to the dying, but the inventor was the perfect romantic American hero — dubbed Dr. Hope by one New York paper. Chow was a thirty-one-year-old Taiwanese in his first year of medical school. One night, while poring over grant applications at the dinner table, he was struck by the bold possibility of forcing HIV to mutate itself into oblivion.

With what seemed like a virtual cure being hyped by the mainstream media, AIDS research centers were inundated with calls. The excitement was so great that the AIDS Clinical Trials Group, which had been planning a small trial using Chow's approach, expanded the number of sites from ten to sixteen, doubled the number of patients in the trials and pushed hard to get them up and running without delay.

To many researchers, however, the news seemed too good to be true. It was. Soon after the Berlin conference, researchers from England and the United States reported that they were unable to duplicate Chow's results. Chow's mentor, Dr. Martin Hirsch, one of the nation's most prestigious AIDS researchers, admitted that his protégé had committed a critical error that invalidated his work. Yet the ACTG trial was not canceled. Its investigators insisted that Chow's concept was valid, even if his work was not.

It was the summer of 1994. While her colleagues in AIDS research were off in Japan for the annual gathering of the clan — the Tenth International Conference on AIDS — Dr. Deborah Cotton was cooped up in her cubbyhole office at Massachusetts General Hospital. She had too many sick patients to fly off to yet another conference. She barely had time to repack her bags and kiss her husband and three kids between meetings of the FDA's Anti-Viral Drug Advisory Committee, the National Task Force on AIDS Drug Development, the AIDS Clinical Trials Group, the Institute of Medicine and the sundry think tanks that regularly demanded her expertise.

It seemed that her life had become a continual round of meetings organized to reconsider every truth AIDS researchers had built, month by month, corpse by corpse, for a decade. She had just returned from the eighteenth meeting of ACTG researchers in Washington, D.C., a grim series of mediocre research proposals and even more mediocre research. No new treatment seemed to be on even the most distant horizon. To make matters worse, the ACTG had its back against the proverbial wall. After seven years of spending one-quarter of the federal AIDS research budget on drug testing, the group was under attack from activists, politicians and other scientists asking how the ACTG could expect to come up with effective drugs if its researchers still didn't understand how HIV caused disease.

"The focus on drugs and vaccines made sense a decade ago, but it is time to acknowledge that our best hunches have not paid off and are not likely to do so," wrote Dr. Bernard Fields, a prominent Harvard virologist, in a proposal for a rethinking and revamping of AIDS research published in May. Fields listed, in painfully clear prose, the central questions that were still unanswered: How does HIV spread throughout the body? Why do some infected people remain healthy for years while others die quickly? What part of the immune system is most effective in fighting HIV? How does the virus destroy the immune system? Can HIV be eliminated from the body after infection? With no effective treatment on the horizon, Fields declared, it was time to answer these questions, "time to turn to basic science."

Activists were more blunt in their criticism. "With better basic research five years ago, we'd have more answers today," said Greg

Gonsalves of the Treatment Action Group, a spinoff of ACT UP. "It's hard to make the case that money was not wasted."

Senior scientists affiliated with the ACTG insisted that they had little choice but to gamble everything on the possibility of hitting the medical equivalent of a grand slam, of finding a magic bullet without unraveling the disease — and leaving the intricacies to post-cure curiosity seekers. "When Congress was pumping money in, they were asking, 'How many patients do you have on clinical trials? What, only five hundred? You should have a thousand,'" recalls Dr. Anthony Fauci. "I would dutifully say, 'Mr. Chairman, the number doesn't make any difference — you gotta ask the right questions.'"

But they did not. They lost the gamble and were poised on the edge of a scientific black hole. Dr. William Paul, the new head of NIH's Office of AIDS Research, had already announced his intention to shift money out of clinical drug trials into basic science. It seemed a logical move, since there were few new drugs waiting to be tested. Paul had been warned about the heat he would take, so he hired a New York publicist to handle the incoming flak.

It was not an easy time, and Cotton didn't expect it to get any easier in the near future. "I don't want to see the ACTG disbanded," she said. "We are better than we were, but we need total honesty about how modest our achievements are to date."

Having survived the fourteen-hour-a-day, five-day ACTG meetings, Cotton was getting ready for her next round of meetings, a series of conferences on new surrogate markers. AIDS researchers were still embarrassed by the failure of CD4s and the other indicators they had adopted and used for a decade. Many were still talking about CD4s as if they were meaningful guides to a drug's worth. Most knew that if they didn't find a new tool, they would be left studying drugs the old way — the long way — by waiting for patients to fall ill and die.

The latest miracle marker — the surrogate du jour — was a test researchers had used for years to measure the amount of virus in a patient's blood. It sounded logical that reducing the amount of virus, the so-called viral load, would help infected people live longer — but then it had also sounded logical that raising the number of CD4 cells would prolong life. Logic, while essential to creating hypotheses, should never be confused with proof. The experience with CD4 cells taught that drugs can provide seeming benefits that mask reality, and that beneficial drugs often don't leave the footprint that scientists expect.

Viral-load testing was an enticing possibility as a surrogate marker, but it was also an exciting new toy. Scientists wanted to play with it. Biotechnology companies wanted to sell it. But there still was no proof that it was a meaningful measurement in judging a drug. And proof wasn't easy to develop. The only way to validate a surrogate marker is to mount a large and lengthy clinical trial to compare it to disease progression. That would bring drug approval to a standstill for years.

Donna Freeman of the FDA summed up all the conundrums when she quoted Lewis Carroll at a meeting on surrogate markers:

"Alice: Which way should I go?

"Cat: That depends on where you are going.

"Alice: I don't know where I'm going.

"Cat: Then it doesn't matter which way you go!"

Cotton was also getting ready for a meeting of the FDA's Anti-Viral Drug Advisory Committee that promised to be one of those contentious sessions that lead nowhere. After years of demanding that the testing and approval of AIDS drugs be speeded up, activists had split over the FDA's relaxed and revved up approval process. For years, companies had delivered data showing that their drugs increased the number of CD4 cells by ten or twenty — less than a normal day's variation — for a few weeks. If the drugs did anything more, no one knew what it might be; the studies had been too brief, too small, too sloppy.

The Treatment Action Group, a collection of the nation's most knowledgeable research activists, was demanding that the FDA force pharmaceutical companies to prove the worth of their drugs before approval. Cotton was both frustrated and amused. For years she'd been criticized as the hard-ass on FDA advisory committees for voting against the fast approval of drugs and for questioning the use of unproven surrogate markers. After ddI was approved, against her advice, she had spoken out sharply. "The public may think that this was a decision based on science," she had said. "It is not. It is a decision based on scientific hunch and a policy decision that we need another drug other than AZT. The message to other pharmaceutical companies is: 'Don't spend too much time crossing t's and dotting i's and making sure you have good data from clinical trials. Instead, go early and often for approval.'"

Her warning had been prophetic, but seated in her office during the depressing summer of 1994 she was not gloating. "Too many years of Catholic school," she said with a shy laugh.

Too many years of AIDS was more like it. "It's not an easy time to be in this field," she said quietly. "Now the FDA will approve any-thing, and the ACTG is driving for accelerated approval. I got more flak from my colleagues than from the activists when I opposed ddI and ddC. Everything about early approval is good except that it is bordering on magical thinking. It's a quick fix, as if this were a war and we could just stop it.

"Now everything is unraveling. We thought it would be five years and we'd have an answer. Instead, we're back to questioning whether to use CD4 cells as a marker. The FIAU disaster hangs over us. If FIAU had worked in HIV, there would be people beating down doors for liver transplants now.

"It's humiliating. I don't know whether I'm underusing drugs or overusing drugs. My patients are all dying anyway. But having these drugs makes doctors feel better. Now they never have to say they have nothing left. They love it. They love the art of medicine. They don't care if they don't have the data to back it up. I do."

As 1995 began, the news grew even more grim for American AIDS researchers and the patients who depended on them. The triumph of the year before had been the highly touted discovery that giving AZT to HIV-positive pregnant women could cut by two-thirds the possibility of transmitting the virus to their fetuses. But in February 1995, Johns Hopkins University researchers announced that giving women vitamin A, which costs two cents a day, might be just as effective.

Then the first in-depth study of the effectiveness of AZT as a treatment for children was ended early — not to announce the overwhelming virtues of the drug, as had happened with the adult trials, but because researchers realized that the drug was a disaster. AZT was not delaying progression to disease; it was causing bleeding and bio-chemical abnormalities. Dr. Anthony Fauci, who had excitedly recommended the use of AZT in adults months before any studies were completed, said, "We don't know what to recommend because you cannot make a recommendation based on a study that is not finished."

Researchers from Columbia University, a husband-and-wife team, discovered a new virus that caused Kaposi's sarcoma. Federally funded researchers had been searching in vain for a cure for KS for a decade and had been unable to find any other pathogen associated with the disease. They were upstaged by two unknown scientists working without any federal support.

Dr. William Paul, the new director of the Office of AIDS Research at NIH, was so disgusted with the mess that he created a committee of outside advisers to reassess the war on AIDS. No one was convinced that they could accomplish very much. "There are a lot of people who are part of the system and who are not going to want to see the system change," said Dr. David Baltimore, a Nobel laureate and professor of biology at Massachusetts Institute of Technology. Nonetheless, the committee was given a year to complete its task. In that time, twenty thousand Americans were expected to die of AIDS.

For Margaret Fischl, the news was even worse. In October 1993, the virologist who performed the dozens of tests that validated her research ran into trouble with the hospital whose laboratory he ran. Dr. Lionel Resnick had used that facility to fulfill his contracts with Fischl, with other universities, and with drug and insurance firms. But he had instructed his clients to send payments to his private company, Vironc, which had a mailing address that turned out to be his home. Investigators estimated that he had siphoned off more than $1 million for work performed at the hospital lab. Resnick insisted that there had been a misunderstanding and agreed to repay the hospital.

The matter was handled quietly until February 1995, when the *Miami Herald* got hold of the story. Suddenly Fischl was being questioned by university officials, federal prosecutors and the FBI about her relationship with Resnick and his company. She declared both her innocence and her puzzlement that suspicion had fallen on her, although she had hired Resnick and personally authorized the payment to him of more than $400,000. She staunchly defended her colleague.

Despite Fischl's protestations, her superiors at the University of Miami and officials at NIH began investigating Resnick's work, and Fischl's along with it. Fischl was annoyed. "I'm very concerned for the effort to stop AIDS," she said. "I personally find all this very stressful."

FOUR

Riding the AIDS
Gravy Train

AIDS isn't just a disease. It's a booming industry that bolsters the stock prices of multinational drug companies; it buys prestige, or at least BMWs, for young physicians who would normally still be struggling with student loans; it fuels the expansion of the biotechnology industry; it provides jobs for bereavement counselors and benefits coordinators, AIDS spokesmen and activists; and it spawns thousands of new businesses to service the needs of the dying and the fears of the healthy.

Even in the midst of recessions, there are few cutbacks in the industry that is AIDS. No layoffs are expected for those who make their living off the imminent demise of 40 million citizens of the planet.

By the fall of 1994, these advertisements were appearing in popular magazines:

"Terminally ill . . . there are options." Call Page & Associates for information on their services for the "special needs of the gay terminally ill."

"Traveling with HIV? . . . You can vacation in Key West with confidence that all your medical needs can be taken care of here. Call us for a free brochure. ImmuneCare of Key West."

"If You Suffer From A Terminal Illness, Living Well Is The Best Revenge. But it takes money . . . Sell your life insurance policy and improve the quality of your life."

"If you are HIV positive or have AIDS, take the time now to make a Lasting Impression." For $19.95, you can leave letters or cards to be sent to loved ones on specified dates after your death.

The *Wall Street Journal* was carrying the nation's most complete coverage of the latest medical advances, along with the impact, real or projected, on stock prices of the relevant corporations. Stock market analysts specializing in AIDS offered tips on the potential of the AIDS-related hospice industry, the fortunes to be made in home health care and the risks of biotechnology startup companies. Investment counselors advised both the dying and those seeking to make a profit off them.

POZ magazine — a glossy monthly for the nation's growing HIV-positive population — made its debut in April 1994, offering an editorial message of hope and dozens of pages of advertising for the despairing. Covering himself with a brief disclosure, its publisher, Sean Strub, received hefty consulting fees from Johnson & Johnson and lobbied ceaselessly for the approval of its HIV home testing kit.

Burroughs Wellcome, the first pharmaceutical company to gain approval for an anti-HIV drug, already had estimated profits of $1 billion from AZT alone. Its income from the most popular preventive medication for AIDS-related pneumonia could not be calculated. Because it is not an American company, Burroughs Wellcome is not required to release the type of information necessary to gauge precisely what AIDS means to its bottom line.

Physicians who joined the war against AIDS had overflowing practices, yet some dismissed long-time patients if they lost their medical insurance when they became too sick to work. Many continued to prescribe aerosolized pentamidine to prevent *Pneumocystis carinii* pneumonia, although the drug Bactrim was more effective. Pentamidine demanded a monthly office visit and $150 or more a pop. Bactrim took a simple prescription and $8 a month. Doctors ordered record numbers of blood tests, claiming that constant vigilance is the price of survival. Patients suspected something more than their survival was the guiding force.

Home health care companies mushroomed to service victims of a chronic disease that makes the infectious environment of a hospital dangerous to their health. They regularly paid physicians "referral" fees to keep the clients coming.

For laboratories, condom manufacturers, latex producers and every brand of huckster — from the guy in Florida who created the National AIDS Information Center to provide the names of "certified AIDS-free physicians" to the leaders of courses in miracles — AIDS has been a bonanza.

On Wall Street and in the bars and backrooms where the deal

makers gather, everyone knows that one man's suffering can become another man's salvation. The market niche is too lucrative not to exploit. In a nation where health and profits are viewed as complementary, the AIDS Industrial Complex was inevitable.

Pharmaceutical companies have been the biggest winners, but they are hardly alone in capitalizing on the demand for an elusive magic bullet. True charlatans — the purveyors of pond scum and bottles of what were labeled CD4 cells — surfaced before HIV had a name, and the demand created a bull market. They thumped on thymus glands and channeled the power of crystals through copper helmets (the treatment was free, but the crystals cost $300 each). They lured the desperate across the border into Mexican clinics that served up a concoction mixed with cranberry juice. It was a real deal: only $2,500 for a complete remission.

The mythical cure of 1986 was reticulose, advertised as a lipoprotein–nucleic acid complex by a Miami Beach company with its international headquarters up the back stairs of an art supply store on a seedy outdoor mall. Available in Tijuana at the same clinic where Steve McQueen received laetrile treatments before he died of cancer, the reticulose cure cost $6,000 for the three-week regimen — although the company's owner assured callers that it took just nine days to get rid of Kaposi's sarcoma.

The following year it was the secret "highly virucidal" potion offered in Costa Rica by Maurice Minuto of Long Island, New York. He wasn't doing it for the money, he insisted. His only motivation was "a little piece of paper called the Nobel Prize."

The great advance of 1989 was peddled for $3,000 to $5,000 by a used medical equipment salesman in Fort Lauderdale: an intravenous drip of a mysterious fluid administered to patients in a concrete-block building without air conditioning or running water in Port-au-Prince, Haiti. The miracle was, in fact, a treatment developed for equine encephalitis.

In 1992 there was the African herbal remedy promoted by Afrique Hope — at $20,000 plus travel expenses to Ghana. A 50 percent discount went to the first six to sign up.

The following year Basil Wainwright's $7,800 "ozone generator" promised to stimulate the immune system by blowing ozone into the rectum. Wainwright didn't give up even after he was jailed in Florida for mail fraud, conspiracy and trafficking in an adulterated medical device. He continued his sales pitch with media interviews from his jail cell in Fort Lauderdale. He was quickly supplanted, however, by a Clearwater, Florida, company offering intravenous infusions of salt water that had been charged with electricity, a procedure invented in Logan, Utah. Patients were treated for $15,000 and the price of a trip to Providenciales, in the Turks and Caicos Islands.

By 1995, the great advance being offered was Chinese chi cong therapy, which was promoted by a Taiwanese restaurateur in Manhattan. He didn't make much headway; his therapy demanded two years of celibacy. But AIDS patients always found a choice in the "alternative" scene. Chi cong's competitor was *uña de gato*, cat's claw, a plant rumored to be displacing even coca as Peru's cash crop.

The number of treatments accompanied by testimonials and pseudoscientific proof has been so mind-numbing that it is almost impossible to separate the quacksters from the "alternative healers," practitioners of medical treatments that have some basis in science and that are amenable to being proven or disproven. Freon enemas, a Mexican offering, are clearly in the former category. But what can a person with AIDS make of nutritional supplements and hyperbaric treatments, the oxygen therapy that cures the bends, which offers at least some slim scientific rationale?

Not much, consumer fraud zealots say. The zealots themselves are hardly neutral. They make handsome profits off their writings and speaking tours condemning all treatments and medications not stamped with FDA and American Medical Association seals of approval, including chiropractic adjustments and acupuncture. Their favorite targets are vitamin companies and health food stores, the $4 billion industry that plays to America's obsession with the illusion of health-in-a-bottle. In 1989 volunteers from the Consumer Health Education Council called forty-one health food stores and asked for their expert on nutrition. Talking vaguely about a brother with AIDS and his wife who still had sex with him, the callers asked for products to improve both his health and her chances of avoiding infection. All forty-one stores suggested some solution, from vitamins to geraniums, immune boosters, homeopathic salts, Bach flower remedies and herbal baths. Thirty said they carried products that cured AIDS.

Inside Edition took a hidden camera into four New York City health food stores. The manager of a General Nutrition Center recommended amino acids for AIDS, saying that they "helped block the chemical inhibiting the growth of the virus" without being toxic like AZT. Alacer Corporation of Irvine, California, sold E-mergen-C, a multivitamin and mineral drink with a note on the package claiming that HIV "can be successfully inhibited in its action with approximately 12 grams of vitamin C daily." Futurebiotics of Brattleboro, Vermont, pushed Maximum Immune Support as providing a broad spectrum of immune defenders. And Natural Organics promoted an Immunizer Pak Program, providing "a powerful blend of ancient herbs gathered from the far corners of the world to bring you a potent and effective immune booster formula."

The lies were so egregious that New York City passed a law declaring claims of a product's benefit to the immune system deceptive advertising unless the product was clearly labeled with information on its effects against HIV. Regulators could barely keep up with the abusers, who repackaged vitamins and minerals as immune boosters and jacked up their prices accordingly.

Physicians and nutritionists agree that vitamins and minerals might improve the health of people with AIDS, but their advice bears little relationship to the formulas being sold as elixirs.

But the hype works. In the years prior to the emergence of AIDS, many Americans swore off junk food and opted for nutritional purity, convincing themselves that youth and energy could be purchased wherever the vegetables were organic. Gay Americans especially, obsessed with youth and anatomical perfection, became gluttons at the nation's health food trough. AIDS gave them dire motivation to pig out as never before. Their vulnerability became gullibility. A study in St. Louis found that people with AIDS were spending an average of $356 a year on vitamins, minerals, herbs and other unproven treatments, and some as much as $9,000 annually.

There were scams within scams, as the members of the nutrition crowd devised new ways to avoid proving the worth of their products. International White Cross, a Texas company selling a product called Immune + PLUS, anticipated trouble with the Federal Trade Commission when it distributed literature hinting that its mixture of wonders would cure AIDS. "At the conclusion of the original study, 26 of 28 patients showed significant improvement, and no patient remained in the AIDS category," the sales pitch asserted on the basis of an extremely questionable study done by an extremely questionable physician.

The company devised an ingenious strategy to avoid trouble. It found a small tribe of Native Americans, the Hopland Band of Pomo Indians, strategically located a hundred miles north of San Francisco, and gave them exclusive marketing rights to the product. "Amazing Results Improve Immune System," the Hopland Band's advertisements said. "180 Day Test Shows Immune System Reactivated," read materials the Pomos handed out at the Native American AIDS conference in Tulsa, Oklahoma, in November 1990. They invited gay men from San Francisco and Native Americans from across the West to drop by the reservation and watch a video on Immune + PLUS, which sold for $297 a month plus tax, shipping and handling. No credit cards accepted.

When federal officials moved against International White Cross and the Hopland Band, the tribal chairman, Donald Ray, agreed to cooperate but reminded the deputy attorney general of California that the tribe had sovereign immunity. Then he wrote a line that could not have been better if written by a captain in the PC police: the product "has basic ingredients which have been part and parcel of Native American health care and culture for over 500 years."

The communities most affected by AIDS are peculiarly, particularly vulnerable to the quacks who have always tended to crawl out from under their rocks when disaster offers an opportunity. People with AIDS aren't like any other desperate group; they're already the nation's outsiders, pariahs accustomed to alternative ways of living, receptive to anti-establishment messages, eager to dissent.

From the first days of the epidemic, the gay community prickled with conspiracy theory. The belief that the government, the medical community and all other subunits of the much-touted establishment were indifferent to, if not responsible for, the epidemic was almost universally accepted. While the black community was awash in speculation that HIV was genetically engineered to murder Africans, gay leaders and spokesmen opted for a more sophisticated theory: the virus itself wasn't part of a plot, but the government's refusal to stop the epidemic was. Larry Kramer said it over and over again: AIDS is intentional genocide. AIDS is intentional genocide. AIDS is intentional genocide.

It was natural, then, for AIDS patients to turn to medical practitioners outside the mainstream who advertised themselves as the caring alternative to establishment indifference. They might have been leeches, but they made sure that they were gay-friendly ones, and they crafted their message to dovetail perfectly with the language of gay activists. They touted the importance of people with AIDS having a choice, borrowing a phrase coined by activists in their battle with the

Food and Drug Administration over access to experimental drugs. They reminded potential customers that scientists don't have all the answers — an argument that AIDS treatment activists had used to gain entree to meetings and workshops.

Tom Howard, the recruiter for the Turks and Caicos salt-water cure, cannily insisted he wasn't trying to make money and that he was being persecuted by authorities who had no vision and no incentive to find breakthroughs. He accused the health research industry of being in cahoots with greedy pharmaceutical companies — voicing a belief ten years of AIDS had confirmed in the minds of AIDS patients.

The modern snake-oil salesmen sermonize on the ridiculing of Louis Pasteur for his suggestion that disease might be caused by bugs too tiny to see. A community that has experienced decades of persecution feels the bond — and is reeled in. They and their families have become so convinced that even the failure of quack treatments can't derail their enthusiasm.

"Rage, rage, I live in constant, absolute rage," said Dotty Hollingsworth, whose twenty-nine-year-old son, Michael, had a seizure in the Miami airport on his return trip from the Port-au-Prince clinic where he'd been infused with the equine encephalitis treatment. He died less than two months later. "I don't know if it was a scam or not," she said. "I don't think so. He was probably just too far gone. But I do know that what medicine offered him was a scam. I live in rage at the doctors, at the Food and Drug Administration, at the medical establishment."

Not everyone offering up a treatment for AIDS is a nut or a scamster. Take Dr. Jonas Salk, the inventor of the first polio vaccine and the most puzzling hypester-cum-humanitarian of the epidemic.

Salk is a certifiable hero. In a world in which presidents and statesmen rarely make the Most Admired list, even schoolchildren whose news intake is limited to the antics of Michael Jackson and the cast of *Beverly Hills 90210* know his name. Although the polio vaccine he developed fell out of use in 1961 when it was superseded by the Sabin oral vaccine, Salk is still honored for his contribution to ending a scourge that had killed or maimed Americans for fifty years.

By the time AIDS became medicine's newest obsession, Salk had disappeared from the scientific scene. Working out of his institute on a bluff by the sea in La Jolla, California, he'd become a kind of philosopher, jotting down notes and ideas in dozens of notebooks, waking up in the middle of the night to capture his thoughts. He'd even published dense philosophical tracts with such titles as "Anatomy of Reality: Merging of Intuition and Reason."

But like so many who've basked in the limelight only to wind up an entry in a history book, Salk couldn't resist another challenge. The lure of AIDS was strikingly similar to the lure of polio.

In 1987 Jonas Salk proposed creating a vaccine that would turn HIV infection into a nonlethal condition. So-called therapeutic vaccines weren't unheard of. Unlike vaccines that are given to prevent infection, therapeutic vaccines are given to the infected to boost the body's natural immune response and prevent, or minimize, illness. Before the invention of antibiotics, they were used with limited success against syphilis and tuberculosis, and they are still used to help those infected with rabies to avoid illness — although few were convinced that the rabies model had much application in the case of HIV infection.

When Salk jumped into the fray, Daniel Zagury, a French scientist collaborating with Robert Gallo, had been working on a therapeutic vaccine for AIDS for more than a year and had already inoculated volunteers with his preparation. But Salk emerged from scientific retirement to proclaim the concept as his unique insight. To finance his venture he formed a new company, Immune Response Corporation, which traded on his name and the allure of enormous profits from a vaccine.

Few scientists paid much attention. Salk was considered to be over the hill, unschooled in modern techniques of gene splicing and genetic manipulation. His polio vaccine was pedestrian compared to what would be necessary to switch off HIV.

But at the Fourth International Conference on AIDS in Stockholm in 1988, the silver-haired scientist, then seventy-three years old, announced that he had solved the problem of AIDS vaccine development, at least conceptually. Although other scientists were designing vaccines using synthetic fragments of HIV to stimulate the body's immune response, Salk declared their efforts misguided and proposed using whole, live but inactivated HIV. Not surprisingly, it was the same approach he'd used for polio.

The audience was startled. Few scientists were convinced that a therapeutic AIDS vaccine was possible, and using live virus as its basis was not only arcane — the rantings of an old codger who hadn't moved into the modern world — but dangerous. The inactivation of the polio virus in Salk vaccines had never been entirely successful: one bad batch of vaccine had caused 204 cases of polio and 11 deaths — which was why the Salk vaccine became outmoded with the introduction of Sabin's alternative.

Salk was not deterred by the skepticism of other scientists, by the fear of accidentally reinfecting patients or even by the objections of the Food and Drug Administration, which considered an HIV vaccine made with live virus to be dangerous. Salk circumvented the FDA by mounting his trials in California, where state law permitted local researchers to test new AIDS therapies manufactured in the state without federal approval.

Everyone knew that Salk had secret trials under way at the University of Southern California medical school. Everyone had heard that he had tested his vaccine in chimpanzees, with no evidence of safety problems. Salk and his Immune Response colleagues weren't saying much more, but many scientists and activists heard that he had also vaccinated twenty-two male volunteers.

Despite the company's silence, Salk's name attracted more than $20 million in private investments. Colgate-Palmolive bought in, for a 12 percent share. France's largest vaccine producer anted up $7.5 million in exchange for marketing rights to the hypothetical vaccine in Europe, Africa and Latin America.

On the eve of the Fifth International Conference on AIDS in Montreal in 1989 — the moment Salk annually chose for his announcements — the vaccinologist admitted to the *Wall Street Journal* that developing a vaccine for AIDS would be more difficult than devising one for influenza, or even polio. "AIDS is like a cross between latent infection, cancer and autoimmune disease," he said. "If we haven't solved those three, it would be surprising if we solved this right away."

But when he sauntered to the conference podium, Salk announced that his approach to vaccine development had succeeded: he had saved two chimpanzees. They'd cleared HIV from their bodies after being vaccinated. When they were exposed to the virus again, they resisted infection. The preparation also seemed safe for human use. Salk wouldn't say much about whether the vaccine would work in humans. Asked point-blank if patients should regard his findings as a breakthrough, he responded, "I wouldn't put it in those terms." But no one could talk about anything but those two chimps.

Salk's timing was flawless. Just months after the conference, Immune Response began talking about a public offering of its stock. The company had twenty-nine employees, no marketable product, no sales and no earnings. But it had a hot potential product: an AIDS vaccine with almost limitless possibility for sales. An estimated 15 million people were infected worldwide at that time, and that number was expected to double by the year 2000.

It also had the hottest name in the vaccine business. "That's the kind of sizzle investors long to buy," Gordon Ramseier, the chief executive officer of Immunetech Pharmaceuticals, told the *Wall Street Journal*. When the company's name was posted on the NASDAQ board in May 1990, investors paid an average of $7 a share for the chance to own a piece of a vaccine that the world's leading AIDS researchers had already denounced.

The price went straight down from there. After all, Salk had no product, and he wasn't releasing the results of any studies. Even the announcement by Roger Cardinal Mahoney, the archbishop of Los Angeles, that he had asked nuns and priests over the age of sixty-five to volunteer to be injected with the Salk vaccine — and that Cardinal O'Connor of New York might sign up — made no impact on brokers. By the end of 1990 the miracle stock closed at 2⁷/₈.

Then, again on the eve of an international AIDS conference — this one in Florence, Italy, in 1991 — Salk reemerged, piggybacking on the work of Dr. Robert Redfield of Walter Reed Army Institute of Research. Redfield had tested a therapeutic vaccine on thirty infected volunteers and reported in the *New England Journal of Medicine* that the vaccine seemed to stabilize the immune systems of patients who responded to it for up to twenty-seven months.

The vaccine tested by Redfield, who had been talking about the potential for a therapeutic vaccine as early as 1986, bore no similarity to Salk's. In fact, it utilized the very protein coating of HIV that Salk was discarding. But Immune Response had issued a press release trumpeting Redfield's work: "The published results indicate that vaccination against HIV can boost immunity to the virus in already-infected patients. This finding supports the approach first proposed by Dr. Jonas Salk in 1987, that HIV-infected patients may be aided by treatment with a therapeutic vaccine." In interviews, Salk seemed to take credit for Redfield's advance. "I am very pleased about this," he said. "It's always nice to see someone else pick up an idea and provide some verification that there is some merit to this."

In Florence, the sometimes doddering scientist, who had had a love-hate relationship with the media since he began a nasty dispute with Albert Sabin, the inventor of the polio vaccine that consigned

Salk's to the dustbin, staged a full-court press event to announce that he would inject himself with his HIV preparation. He did not mention that he was following the example of Sabin, who'd tried out his own vaccine before giving it to others, and of Daniel Zagury, who was his own first volunteer for an AIDS vaccine. "I want to answer the implicit question, Would you take it yourself?" Salk said. "Since actions speak louder than words, that's the obvious thing to do."

That week, ABC News selected an AIDS researcher as its Person of the Week. That researcher was Jonas Salk.

Two weeks later, capitalizing on the publicity, Immune Response announced that it expected to begin vaccinating volunteers by the end of the year and invited investors to participate in its golden future. "We don't say this vaccine will eliminate the HIV infection," CEO James Glavin said. "But it does give you something to fight the infection. We may be able to prevent someone who is HIV-infected from progressing into getting AIDS conditions."

Glavin admitted that the company's finances were a disaster: Immune Response had lost almost a million dollars in the second quarter of 1991 and income had dropped. But, once again, the lure of a new Salk vaccine — a second miracle from the American scientist who'd been passed over for the Nobel Prize the first time around — was too strong to be deflated by reality. Mark J. Simon, a biotechnology stock analyst, issued an "aggressive buy" recommendation, calling Immune Response "the best AIDS play in America today."

The stock price shot up to 19½ and kept on going — to 22½, to 62¾, rising 29 percent in one day even though no data on the efficacy of the vaccine would be available for more than a year. When the basketball star Earvin "Magic" Johnson announced that he was infected with HIV, Immune Response's stock rose $3.50 a share in heavy trading. It ended 1991 at 39¼ — a gain of 1,265 percent in a single year. The business weekly *Barron's* called it "the year's most astounding stock."

By the spring of 1992 the bottom was beginning to fall out. The clinical trials that had so excited investors — the trials the company had announced would begin by the end of 1991 — had been delayed. "Product liability" concerns were the only reason offered. The stock price fell to 28½.

Four months later Salk was back on the podium at the international AIDS conference — the eighth, in Amsterdam. This time he announced that he had solved the problem of AIDS vaccine development, at least conceptually — again. Again he declared current approaches to vaccine therapy misguided, even harmful. Again he unveiled a new strategy. Vaccines for smallpox, flu and polio stimulate the body's production of antibodies to the infectious agent, triggering the humoral arm of the immune system. Forget stimulating antibodies, said Salk. Suppress them instead, and try for a delayed-type hypersensitivity, or cellular immunity, the kind of immune reaction provoked when an allergic person is exposed to poison ivy. The strategy does not demand a new type of vaccine, Salk said, just that minuscule amounts of it be administered.

For the audience, it was déjà vu all over again.

Salk's concept was, as before, not original. He was piggybacking again, this time on the work of Dr. Gene Shearer and Dr. Mario Clerici of the National Cancer Institute, who had studied HIV-negative health care workers who'd been stuck with HIV-infected needles, and HIV-negative children of infected mothers. Shearer had reported finding HIV-specific cellular responses in those individuals, but no HIV antibodies. He suggested that exposure to minuscule amounts of HIV might elicit precisely the type of immune response necessary to protect people from infection.

What Salk showed as proof was shaky data from a preliminary vaccine trial. Four years earlier, he had vaccinated twenty-two HIV-infected men, and twelve of them produced no antibodies to HIV, which seemed like a failure at the time. In Holland, however, Salk reinterpreted that apparent failure, converting it into evidence of success. The twelve showed classic delayed-type hypersensitive responses, he said, and were doing better than the ten who had produced antibodies.

While many scientists agreed that cellular immunity was important, other vaccine researchers were quick to point out that both types of immune response, cellular and humoral, were necessary. Dr. Dan Hoth, the chief of AIDS drug development at NIH, wouldn't even go into a full explanation of his disagreement, dismissing Salk's latest presentation as "a maximum amount of speculation from a minimum amount of data."

As usual, Salk was not dissuaded. In August 1992 he announced a full, double-blind, placebo-controlled test of his vaccine to determine once and for all if it would work. The trials would conclude by the end of the year, and the data would be released in January. The only sticking point was the type of proof he was prepared to offer.

Salk knew it would take more than a few short months to prove that his vaccine worked. People infected with HIV simply don't fall ill that quickly, with or without a vaccine. Instead, he said that he would use surrogate markers, blood tests to measure the body's immune response.

Salk's plan ignored the refusal of the Food and Drug Administration to accept such tests as proof of a vaccine's value. If the agency stuck to that position, Salk would have to mount a study with thousands, not hundreds, of volunteers, lasting years rather than months.

Stock analysts trying to forecast Immune Response's fiscal health reassured investors that the FDA would bow to political pressure and approve Salk's vaccine on the basis of surrogate markers. One analyst pegged the probability at 65 percent. Another, Brandon Fradd, himself a doctor, was an open booster, calling the Salk approach "a breakthrough in HIV therapy." However, he acknowledged that "as a scientist and physician, I would be the first to say there's not much efficacy data," but he assured his clients that the FDA would accept Salk's approach if Salk produced significant proof that the vaccine had clinical benefits.

On August 13, 1992, Salk presented data he'd collected in an early safety trial of the vaccine, a study of its impact on sixty HIV-positive, asymptomatic patients. It was a rehash of the results he'd presented to an underwhelmed audience at the Amsterdam meeting. Those results hadn't received the attention they deserved in the investment community, one stock analyst said, because Dr. Anthony Fauci, the head of AIDS research at NIH, had reminded every reporter who would listen that there was not a shred of evidence that any of the ten to twelve AIDS vaccines, including Salk's, worked.

But in August Salk tried again, announcing that his vaccine seemed to stimulate both humoral and cellular responses. It didn't make much more of an impression the second time around. After all, Salk himself had argued against stimulating the humoral response.

Immune Response's stock fell to 21¾. Less than a year later, two weeks before the 1993 meeting of the international AIDS research establishment — this one in Berlin — rumors flew across Wall Street that Salk had proof that his vaccine worked and that he could prevent HIV infection from turning lethal. At Immune Response's annual meeting, corporate officers released just enough information to titillate investors and nudge their stock price upward: the grand old man's team would present the results of two studies on June 9, at the Ninth International Conference on AIDS.

"There will be no public discussion of the data prior to that date," insisted Bronwyn LaMelle, Immune Response's investor relations officer.

The company would not say any more about Salk's research results, but brokers specializing in biotechnology stock could talk of little else. Mark Simon, the biotechnology stock analyst, was still bullish, although he admitted he had no inside information. Brandon Fradd followed suit, arguing that the company wouldn't have waited until the Berlin meeting to disclose bad results. He was so enthusiastic about the stock that he speculated the company might file for FDA approval of the vaccine by the end of the year.

The stock's price rose 3 ⅝ in a single day and more than 1,276,300 shares were traded — against an average daily volume of just 321,600. The giddy ride lasted for more than a week, as the price of the stock rose 50 percent from May 21 to June 1, when it ended at 27¼.

In Berlin, reporters eagerly awaited the third day of the conference, when Dr. Alexandra Levine of the University of Southern California would present the results of three studies by the Salk team. Stock analysts flew in from New York and grabbed the front rows in the lecture hall so they could report back to their offices, slide by slide, by cellular telephone. The world's leading AIDS researchers packed into a large hall in the International Congress Center.

Levine first presented the results of a study of twenty-three gay men who had received eight doses of the vaccine over a three-year period. None had experienced any difficulty beyond some pain at the injection site or temporary fever and rash — side effects typical of most vaccines. Twelve of the twenty-three showed delayed hypersensitivity reactions, a positive response to a skin test that measured some aspects of cellular immune functioning. Those twelve, Levine said, had fewer opportunistic infections, fewer deaths and higher CD4 counts than the placebo group. Her conclusion: there is a strong correlation between delayed hypersensitivity reaction and a stunted progression of HIV.

The second study was designed to test for the optimum dose of the vaccine. Forty infected patients, all with minimal deterioration of their immune systems, were given either a placebo or one of four doses of Salk's vaccine. The results: patients receiving moderate to high doses produced both humoral and cellular immune responses.

To the uninitiated, it sounded like a breakthrough. But none of that material was new or particularly surprising. In fact, no one was sure what Levine's results really meant, since no one knew how to measure humoral or cellular immune responses. The surrogate markers Salk was using had never been validated; there was no evidence that they correlated with a slowing of the disease process.

Finally Levine presented the most recent study, a trial of 103 asymptomatic patients. Flashing slide after slide, she showed that the treated group had increased humoral and cellular responses and that they had gained more weight than the untreated. Most important, she said that the amount of virus in their blood increased only 10 percent over the course of a year, while the amount of virus in the blood of untreated patients increased almost 50 percent — at least by one measure. That finding might have been startling and exciting, since the amount of virus generally increases as the immune system is ravaged. But by other measures — ones she mentioned only in passing — there was no difference in the viral burden of the two groups and no difference in their CD4 counts.

As the audience filed out of the hall, the world's leading AIDS researchers produced instant analysis. "I'm less than enthusiastic," said Dr. David Ho, the virologist who runs the Aaron Diamond Research Institute in New York. Dr. Max Essex of Harvard declared that the results would have been given no attention at all if not for the aura surrounding Salk's name. Dr. Anthony Fauci said, "Let's not explode this into 'We have the answer.' You cannot make any conclusion that this is clinically useful."

Dr. Robin Weiss, a respected British scientist, was more blunt: "It was a dog-and-pony show."

Major vaccine researchers couldn't be more specific in their criticism because Levine hadn't provided detailed data on the individual patients, the kind of data essential to interpreting the trends she presented. They reserved most of their remarks for the surrogate markers Levine said had proved the value of the vaccine. "We simply don't know what these markers mean," said Dr. Dani Bolognesi, the Duke University vaccine expert. "They haven't been validated . . . Those are small changes, and small changes that we don't know what they mean doesn't give you real confidence that this is beneficial."

Salk would not be derailed. Eschewing the afternoon press conference organized for the day's presenters, he held his own briefing at the posh Berlin Excelsior Hotel, even providing a bus for reporters to make the twenty-five-minute trip there. With cameras rolling, a public relations firm providing drinks and snacks, and satellite transmission to financial analysts worldwide, the diminutive researcher, dressed in a modest brown suit, stepped up to the microphone. "We've been ex-plorers," Salk declared. "We're like Columbus going to India and finding America and saying, 'That's not where I was headed.' The science has now begun to reveal that there is a logic to the magic" of a vaccine for those already infected. While the results weren't conclu-sive, he declared, "It's the first whiff of spring, you might say."

Reporters asked Salk for more specifics on his studies; he refused to provide them. Then their queries were shoved aside with questions phoned in from stock analysts overseas. The reporters were reeling as they filed out of the bizarre press briefing that was more like an inves-tor relations reception than a meeting with journalists. Almost no one had even caught the off-handed dismissal of Immune Response's ear-lier announcement that the FDA would approve the vaccine by the end of 1993 or early 1994. "No timetable," Salk's spokesmen had sud-denly declared.

"What am I supposed to tell my desk?" reporters asked one an-other. "It's so embarrassing. He's Jonas Salk and he keeps doing this."

Standing at the curb waiting for a taxi, Bob Massa of the *Village Voice* muttered, "Report it as a circus designed to manipulate his stock prices. There certainly wasn't anything scientific about what was going on in there."

Wall Street, for once, agreed. The next day, Immune Response's stock dropped 26 percent, to $16.

For thirty years, Jonas Salk was locked in battle with his scientific archrival, Dr. Albert Sabin. Salk might have produced the first vaccine that ended the long, terrifying polio summers that had gripped the nation for most of the century. But Albert Sabin produced the vaccine that lasted. In fact, by the late 1960s, it was almost impossible to find Salk's vaccine on the shelves of American pharmacies.

The three-decade rivalry between the two scientists was an epic in the annals of modern medical backbiting. "Albert Sabin was out for me from the very beginning," Salk said in 1991. "In 1960, he said to me, just like that, that he was out to kill the killed vaccine." Sabin was no more complimentary. "It was pure kitchen chemistry," Sabin said of Salk's vaccine. "Salk didn't discover anything."

Scientists have tended to side with Sabin. After his vaccine dis-covery, Sabin went on to become the president of the Weizmann In-stitute of Science in Israel. He was awarded the Feltinelli Prize of the Accademia dei Lincei of Rome, the Lasker Clinical Science Award and the Presidential Medal of Freedom, America's highest civilian honor. Salk, on the other hand, became a celebrity after the first dose of his vaccine was injected into a Virginia student on April 26, 1954. He received carloads of congratulatory telegrams and hundreds of requests for appearances. Marlon Brando portrayed him on the silver screen. But he was never elected to membership in the prestigious National Academy of Sciences. He was never awarded a Nobel Prize — thanks to his competition with Sabin, most scientists assume. While the public saw Salk as "a demigod, to many in the scientific community he seemed a demagogue," explained Allan Brandt of Harvard.

In the summer of 1992, the two men had their final skirmish when Sabin published a paper in the *Proceedings of the National Academy of Sciences* in which he argued that an AIDS vaccine was inherently impossible. The dispute remains unresolved — and neither of the old rivals will be around to gloat over its conclusion. Albert Sabin died on March 3, 1993, at the age of eighty-six. The following year Salk enjoyed a moment of triumph when his vaccine trial results were finally published. Even the very scientists who had mocked the old man began to overlook the hype and study the data. Not great, they declared. But not bad, either. In January 1995, the Food and Drug Administration gave Salk approval to administer his preparation to hundreds of volunteers to test its value. It was the first vaccine to receive such approval.

Salk, however, was deprived even of the possibility that those glimmers of glory would become final vindication. He died on June 23, 1995, at the age of eighty.

Salk wasn't the only over-the-hill brand-name scientist to get caught up in AIDS. He was joined by Dr. Henry Heimlich, the Cornell University–trained physician best known for his maneuver to relieve choking. That's not the only thing that bears his name. As a young chest surgeon, he devised the Heimlich Operation, a primitive way to reconstruct the esophagus; the Heimlich Chest Drainage Valve, first made from a rubber dime-store toy; and the Heimlich Micro Trach, which provides portable oxygen for patients with debilitating lung disease.

Heimlich is anything but modest about his achievements. "I have never had a failure," he says. "It may take a while for the others to see what I see. But eventually, they do. Like I always say, 'If your peers understand what you've done, you are not being creative.'"

Heimlich's creative contribution to AIDS research is the notion of giving patients malaria. It's cheap. It is readily available. And, Heimlich insists, it will produce immune substances that might help patients overcome HIV. His cure involves inoculating patients with malaria parasites, allowing them to suffer ten to fourteen fevers — which could spike up to 106 degrees — for three weeks to a month, then administering anti-malaria medication. The fevers would disappear along with the HIV. No real danger to the patients, Heimlich insisted, because he planned to use the most benign strain of the protozoan.

The idea of using malaria to treat other diseases wasn't an original one. The controversial Austrian neuropsychiatrist Julian Wagner von Jauregg won a Nobel Prize in 1927 for using malaria to treat syphilis of the brain. In 1981 Dr. Leonard Greentree, a physician in Ohio, published a paper on malaria therapy as a potential cure for cancer. Heimlich had sought out Greentree for support, both medical and financial, in using malaria against HIV. It was not forthcoming. Greentree wanted controlled studies of the treatment in animals first, then humans. Heimlich, however, is philosophically opposed to animal research.

Heimlich went out on his own. He even asked the Centers for Disease Control for samples of malaria-infected blood. When the CDC balked, Heimlich's foundation moved overseas.

AIDS specialists were more than a little skeptical of the notion of purposely infecting HIV-positive people with plasmodium, the protozoan that causes the severe anemia, spiking fevers, convulsions and renal failure characteristic of malaria. "Heimlich's life-saving maneuver for people who aspirate food doesn't qualify one as an HIV expert," said Dr. Anthony Fauci, branding the malaria therapy as "dangerous and scientifically unsound." When Heimlich began talking about experimenting on human beings, twenty scientists and physicians petitioned the federal government to investigate his so-called induced malaria therapy.

Heimlich wasn't fazed by the attack. "[That petition] is an annoying and painful thing," he told the *Los Angeles Times*. "But this happens. It's very common in my life. Some people think if they attack a famous person, they can become as famous . . . It's happened before," he said. "It's politics. Or it's financial. Or one scientist knows another. Or somebody is working on a vaccine for Lyme disease or for AIDS or what-have-you and they're afraid we'll get their funding."

Anyway, Heimlich didn't need to worry. He already had the money in hand to do the work he'd proposed — thanks in large measure to Joanne Carson, who'd opened her Bel-Air home and her guest list to Heimlich in the spring of 1993. He wowed guests like Jon Voigt, Patti Davis and Bruce Davison with stories of a 1990 study in Zaire that purportedly found that a group of children with both malaria and

AIDS were doing fine, even after two years. None of the stars thought to ask Heimlich what happened to them after that period of time. One reporter did. "You're wondering? What about me?" he said. "Nobody tried harder than we did [to find out]."

All Heimlich said he needed to put an end to the plague by 1994 was $591,800 — a modest sum considering the millions spent on AIDS research. His presentation was so powerful, and his name so reassuring, that checks started rolling in: $50,000 from actress Amy Irving and donations from ventriloquist Paul Winchell and actress Estelle Getty.

Heimlich might have been arrogant, but he was never foolish. He kept his malaria treatments well beyond the borders of the United States — and beyond the jurisdiction of the Food and Drug Administration — in countries where experimental treatments were less stringently regulated.

A malaria induction-therapy center was set up in Mexico in the late 1980s, where experiments were carried out using the strategy against Lyme disease. Heimlich was enthusiastic about the results, claiming that several patients virtually crippled by the arthritis-like condition have been symptom-free for years. "In certain cases, we've had remarkable results, OK?" he told the *Los Angeles Times* in 1994. "My God, [what] if I told you about a woman who was crawling for several years on the floor because of Lyme disease and she owns 15 horses now and is riding them!"

If he had produced this woman and her medical records, or any of his other success stories, scientists might have taken Heimlich more seriously. But one patient he used as an example of his success, Sallie Timpone, has repeatedly called Heimlich to ask that he stop doing so. Most days Mrs. Timpone can barely get out of bed.

The Mexican malaria treatment moved on to AIDS in the spring of 1993, when Dr. Sergio Perez Barrio — who says he was hand picked for the work by Heimlich — began receiving his first volunteers from Los Angeles. But before the first protozoan could enter the bloodstream of the first patient, Heimlich abruptly moved his treatment facility to China, saying that "the costs increased markedly when it became apparent that Americans would be involved." He then barred American patients from participating in the Chinese study.

None of this seems to have discouraged Heimlich's Hollywood supporters. "No question he's one of the great geniuses of our time," said Joanne Carson. "I expect he will receive a Nobel Prize."

The delusion is partly a reflection of a Hollywood mindset, the same mindset that drove Steve McQueen to Tijuana for infusions of dried and liquefied apricot pits as a cure for cancer. Esther Williams once said, "There's something about making movies that makes you believe in miracles."

It's not just Hollywood, of course. Americans are firmly wedded to the concept of miracles, whether they occur on Thirty-fourth Street or in the appearance of the Virgin Mary's image in rural Georgia. They appeal to a uniquely American naiveté. They help maintain the illusion that nature is a relatively benign force.

Choosing miracles over medicine is nothing new. Americans have been eschewing traditional medical advice for centuries, opting for vitamins instead of antibiotics and chicken soup rather than antihistamines. And the lure of the magic cure hasn't diminished since the days when snake oil cured rheumatism. In fact, as distrust for authority has become a national obsession, Americans are dismissing their physicians with almost as much enthusiasm as they are replacing their political leaders. It is hardly surprising that the same people who take a leave of absence from Catholicism or Judaism to dabble in Buddhism would be attracted to acupuncture or Chinese herbs. Americans are on an anti-establishment binge, and medicine — with doctors who have become corporations — is the ultimate establishment.

The belief in miracles — and its money-making potential — extends well beyond so-called miraculous cures. If the American market is good for medical miracles, it is even better for miracles themselves.

The first guru of AIDS miracles was Louise Hay, an ordained minister in the Church of Religious Science, who began preaching to AIDS patients in January 1985 that "love is the most powerful stimulant to the immune system." In Hay's public workshops and "healing circles," in books, audiotapes and videotapes, Hay sent the message that AIDS is a physical manifestation of self-loathing and lack of love, that if patients could learn to love themselves — if they could purge themselves of resentment and fear and self-hate — they would be healed.

It worked — at least for Louise Hay, who claimed to have healed herself of vaginal cancer by overcoming her resentment at childhood sexual abuse. She began with six patients in a small group. Early in 1988, six hundred were showing up for her weekly sessions, dubbed Hayrides, in West Hollywood Park's auditorium. By the end of the year, eight hundred people were packing into the meetings and healing circles became a virtual national franchise. HIV-positive men and women who were terrified by their illness tried to regain power over their lives by clinging to healing towels, supposedly endowed with the magical and mystical properties of love. They lined up for their turns at healing tables, where they received the postmodern version of the laying-on of hands. Like New Age revival meetings, the Hayrides and the healing circles around the country were filled with young men testifying to their miraculous revitalization.

No one talked about what happened to the Hayites who fell ill. One Miami television producer lived with HIV and almost no immune system for years. He credited his continuing good health to the love and self-love he had learned at the weekly healing circle. When he was diagnosed with pneumocystis pneumonia, he wound up not in a hospital AIDS wing but in a padded room. He blamed himself for becoming sick. Other young men have told of falling ill and being shunned by other followers of Louise Hay, who asked, "What did you do to yourself? How could you have loved yourself so little?"

Meanwhile, Louise Hay became her own industry, based around her Santa Monica, California, publishing company, Hay House. Her book *You Can Heal Your Life* spent thirteen weeks on the *New York Times* paperback bestseller list in 1988 and sold more than 300,000 copies. It remained at the top place on the *Publishers Weekly* paperback list for months, just two spots above an earlier book, *Heal Your Body,* which has sold half a million copies and been translated into a dozen languages.

Where Louise Hay sold hope, Marianne Williamson, Hollywood's favorite spiritual pop icon, peddled hype. The former waitress and cabaret singer from Texas created a mélange of glitz, good work and a spirituality rooted in Christianity and in supermarket women's magazines. Williamson became America's new guru, a symbol of alienation from traditional religion and of a deep desire for inner peace.

"The Marianne Faithful," as they were called, included Anthony Perkins, Lesley Ann Warren, Tommy Tune, Cher and Roy Scheider. David Geffen listened to her on tape and solicited her advice, Barbra Streisand invited her to lunch and Liz Taylor asked her to officiate at her eighth wedding, on Michael Jackson's estate.

Williamson began with the latest bible of the miracle-hungry, the blue, gilt-embossed 1,200-page *A Course in Miracles* — a spiritual how-to bestseller allegedly dictated to an emotionally distressed psychologist by Jesus himself. Only $40 a pop to change the world by changing the mind. Williamson used the book to parlay herself into a miracle worker, then into a celebrity author, speaker and counselor to the stars. When her first book, *A Return to Love: Reflections on the Principles of "A Course in Miracles,"* was published in 1992, Oprah Winfrey grabbed up a thousand copies and gushed that she had experienced 157 miracles after reading it. Hundreds lined up to pay $7 for an evening of "spiritual psychotherapy" with the slim and stylish woman at the Harmony Gold auditorium on Los Angeles's Sunset Boulevard or at the Unitarian Community Church in Santa Monica.

Williamson's fame began in the gay and AIDS community, where she quickly established herself as a designer-clad Mother Teresa of the New Age crowd. The weekly HIV support group at her Los Angeles Center for Living was guaranteed to attract a steady following. "People who attend support groups who have been diagnosed with a life-challenging illness live on average twice as long after diagnosis as people who don't," she said, with no scientific basis whatsoever. "The AIDS virus is not more powerful than God," she assured the desperate in her throaty voice. "The spirit is impervious to illness." And anyway, dying is simply "transition to another plane."

Williamson quickly became an icon among gay men in Los Angeles. Couples in crisis flocked to her lectures. She was hailed as a healer of everything from homophobia to hemorrhoids. Her heroic status advanced still further in 1989 when she founded Project Angel Food. By September 1992 the group was serving four hundred hot meals a day to AIDS patients and offering them counseling, all courtesy of the celebrity enthusiasm Williamson generated. Anthony Perkins and his wife, Berry, became volunteers. David Geffen, Barry Diller and Liz Taylor's husband, Larry Fortensky, joined the advisory board. Bette Midler, Meryl Streep and artist David Hockney attended her fundraisers.

But there was trouble brewing even in La-La Land's center of love and peace, just as trouble had brewed with other cult leaders from Jim Bakker to David Koresh. Williamson was a notorious control freak who didn't hesitate to blow up, even in front of her sickest clients. When criticized, she acknowledged that she came across as "a bitch for God." Many believed that she crossed the line into thinking herself divine.

The first organizational explosion occurred in New York, where appeals to the principles of New Age management carried little weight. Cynthia O'Neal, an actress and the wife of actor and restaurant owner Patrick O'Neal, had been an early Williamson follower. When the guru opened a Center for Living in Manhattan, O'Neal offered her support, bringing her friends Mike Nichols, Stephen Sondheim and Jean Halberstam onto the center's board. Soon, however, Williamson grew unhappy with the New York style of reaching out to AIDS patients. It wasn't sufficiently miracle-centered, so she fired her board. O'Neal started her own organization to provide services to people with AIDS, Friends in Deed.

Then, in the fall of 1991, the collapse in California began. After months of tension between Williamson and her board there — especially with producer Howard Rosenman and photographer-producer Michael Childers, who had been two of her most important conduits to the stars — Williamson summarily dismissed most of the members and reorganized it into a smaller group.

Despite these changes, her Center for Living was still not a happy place. The executive director, Steve Schulte, a veteran gay activist and former mayor of West Hollywood, didn't buy into Williamson's spiritual program. Schulte just wanted to run the center professionally and feed people with AIDS. Williamson did not approve. He actually wanted business plans; "I pray and ask God for wisdom of the heart," Williamson said. Schulte was clearly having trouble fitting into an organization in which Williamson's followers tried to "heal" malfunctioning computers.

On January 7, 1992, Schulte, who was overwhelmingly popular with the staff, became the third executive director to be fired in the group's five-year history. The staff revolted and moved toward unionization. Williamson was livid. "I'm very opposed to the unionization of volunteer organizations," she said, and promptly resigned.

A professional management consultant was brought in to run the organization. He canceled the center's counseling program, leaving two hundred AIDS patients without psychological services, and promptly cut the staff from twenty-two to fourteen. Among those ousted were the pastry chef and the director of the meals program. Williamson's minions were delighted. "This is just a karmic payback for pushing Marianne out of the picture," said R. Morgan Many Feathers, a volunteer who had been recruited through Williamson's seminars.

The consultant insisted he had to streamline the organization because it was suffering financial troubles. Schulte was shocked; the Center for Living had more than $600,000 in the bank when he'd departed.

Anyway, he asked, what had happened to the $750,000 the group netted from Williamson's Devine Design auction, an event that attracted all the requisite Hollywood power brokers? "Where did money go?" Schulte asked pointedly.

Schulte never got an answer.

Most of the money made from AIDS comes not from peddling miracles or miracle cures but from business as usual in a country that rewards entrepreneurial spirit in any form. A new disease is a new opportunity that no good business person can ignore.

Some moneymaking schemes involve direct fraud, the classic take-their-money-and-run swindles that have regularly bankrupted elderly Americans. But others seem too logical to be illegitimate. How many Americans could have entirely resisted investing in latex gloves in the age of AIDS? Everyone knew that gloves were being used by the millions — a new pair for every blood draw, every physical examination, every dental cleaning. So it wasn't hard for four con men to convince investors in Missouri, Texas and Oklahoma to empty their bank accounts to help build latex glove factories. It wasn't until June 19, 1989, that prosecutors in Missouri uncovered what they believed to be the nation's first big AIDS-related investment scam and filed charges of securities fraud against the men. The investors discovered that there were no latex plants and that they were out $500,000 each.

Most of the profits from AIDS, however, have gone to legitimate businessmen taking advantage of someone else's misfortune. In 1987 the president of the company that makes LifeStyles condoms, John Silverman, said it so bluntly that he was actually chastized as an insensitive lout by his own advertising agency. "AIDS is a condom manufacturer's dream" was his honest assessment.

For a while it looked as if he was right. Latex barriers had been pronounced protective against the transmission of HIV, and government and nonprofit agencies began spending millions to distribute condoms in clinics and AIDS information centers around the world. As Americans became increasingly aware of the mounting epidemic, and increasingly worried that they, too, might be at risk, condoms — a commodity that languished on drugstore shelves after more convenient and sex-friendly forms of birth control were introduced — found a new market niche and new marketing tool.

For years, television stations and magazines refused condom advertisements out of concern for the sensibility and prudery of the American viewer and reader. Suddenly marketing executives had a new, almost noble rationale for toppling the opposition. By June 1988, 120 magazines had agreed to accept advertising for Trojans, up from fewer than a dozen just three years before. Television networks that aired steamy sex scenes in movies remained timid about allowing the commercial promotion of latex, but local TV stations and the new Fox network sold time to companies willing to gear their messages to disease prevention.

Ansell Corporation hired Dr. Ruth Westheimer, the reigning elf queen of the sex show circuit, to endorse LifeStyles condoms on her cable television and radio programs. Schmid Laboratories launched the Excita Fiesta line — condoms in bright colors — and turned up the heat in the condom wars by sending an airplane over New York beaches with a banner reading, "Plan ahead with Ramses."

Carter-Wallace Corporation got hip and replaced the ancient-warrior image on its Trojans with a picture of a loving couple strolling happily into the sunset — a clear response to women's concerns about AIDS. For the macho market the company sponsored a Trojan race car. During spring break in Daytona Beach, they held a parade of the "Trojan Army."

The best advertising, of course, is free: public service announcements by Surgeon General C. Everett Koop and safe-sex education in schools and churches. The best plug of all came when Magic Johnson announced that he was HIV positive in November 1991. The next day Carter-Wallace stock began trading with an $8-a-share rise. His infection was a gold mine for Umoja Sasa Products, the Baltimore marketer of an "Afrocentric" condom packaged in a red, black and green matchbook with an outline of Africa on the back with the translation of "umoja sas," Swahili for "unity now."

Sales soared. Trojans' rose 10 to 15 percent in 1985. The sales of all condoms, in all colors, soared 27 percent for the twelve months ending April 1988, then went up 40 percent, even 50 percent by the end of the 1980s. The market, and the profits, seemed limitless as condomania seized the nation.

It didn't last, though. Within a year of Magic Johnson's announcement, sales were increasing by only 5 percent and were actually falling in some cities. Public health officials blamed heterosexual denial of AIDS and the decline of safe-sex practices among gay men. Marketers blamed the continuing ban on advertising by the three major TV networks.

Nevertheless, there were dozens of other ways to make a buck off the plague. Pharmacies began specializing in AIDS, marketing themselves to the specific needs of the gay community. The American Preferred Prescription mail-order outfit not only offers mail delivery in plain brown wrappers but guarantees an "HIV-sensitive staff." They carry homeopathic remedies and offer their own line of vitamins. Their walk-in branch, the APP Community Pharmacy, in Manhattan's Chelsea, even boasts a computer terminal for patients interested in reading from medical data banks before taking their medicine.

San Diego's Priority Pharmacy has long been the cornerstone of the city's AIDS community. It filled the first local prescription for AZT. It helps sponsor AIDS benefits, and a senior executive was selected as grand marshal of AIDS Walk San Diego. The customers know pharmacist David C. Zeiger. If they don't meet him at the counter, they see him racing around town in his 1988 Ferrari Testarossa, his 1990 Jaguar or his 1990 Chevy Corvette. His vanity tags read PILPUSR.

Community Prescription Service advertises in gay publications with a photograph of its cofounder, Stephen Gendin, "AIDS Activist HIV+ for 9 years." It not only fills prescriptions but provides information on alternative therapies, new treatment and drug trials.

Many of the pharmacies are part of the fast-growing mail-order drug business, whose total sales soared from $100 million in 1981 to $4 billion in 1993. Service is fast; they usually bill insurance companies directly; and, most important for many with AIDS, service is confidential.

Profits are also extremely good. In 1993 a typical neighborhood drugstore charged $141 for one hundred AZT tablets. Yet Priority Pharmacy billed insurance companies $265 for the same prescription, Stadtlanders charged $227 and APP $171. The drug wholesales for $120. For Bactrim DS, the standard medication to help prevent PCP, Priority billed at $298, Stadtlanders charged $183, and APP $126.

Even companies that have no special product to offer used AIDS to drum up free publicity in the guise of charity. In 1991 Clairol began its annual National Color Can Make a Difference Day, inviting socially conscious beauty mavens to look good, and do good, by making their hair appointments on that day, when 25 percent of the money for their haircuts and colorings would be given to the American Foundation for AIDS Research. In October 1994 residents of Baltimore were asked to "Eat, Drink, Fight AIDS" by patronizing a specified group of restaurants that had agreed to donate 10 percent of their receipts to local service groups.

Insisting they were just providing a public service, the sportswear company Benetton used AIDS as a marketing tool when it featured a grim photograph of an AIDS patient at the moment of his death, surrounded by his family. The company logo appeared in the corner of the two-page ad that ran in *Vanity Fair* and *Vogue*. Early in 1995, Nike followed Benetton's lead in using AIDS to sell merchandise, but it opted for an upbeat message. The face displayed in commercials for running shoes belonged to an HIV-positive marathon runner.

Entrepreneurs have formed joint ventures with bona fide AIDS fundraising and service organizations — and split the profits. Eclipse Enterprises of California, the same company that brought the nation trading cards with photographs of gangsters and mass murderers, teamed up with Broadway Cares–Equity Fights AIDS, the New York actors' fundraising apparatus. The nonprofit group received 15 percent of the profits from the sale of cards bearing the likenesses of Magic Johnson, Arthur Ashe and Rock Hudson, along with George Bush, Ronald Reagan and Elizabeth Taylor.

Businesses from Tiffany's to art galleries have joined the Red Ribbon Brigade, promising at least a token donation to some AIDS group. Department stores sell the tasteful enameled version of the ribbon, produced by the American Foundation for AIDS Research, with or without rhinestones. The National AIDS Awareness Catalog sells a $27 Christmas tree ornament of Frosty the Snowman bedecked with a red ribbon. When the token signs of AIDS concern became de rigueur for public Hollywood events, the Red Ribbon Foundation was created to offer a rhinestone-studded Evening Awareness pin for $15. The Alternative Gallery in Kent, Connecticut, embedded a red ribbon in a solid block of Lucite — offered at $25, with a promised $5 donation to the People with AIDS Coalition.

The commercialization of caring, as the ribbon mutated from a simple memorial statement to a bejeweled fashion accessory, became so nauseating that a group called Anonymous Queers plastered a retort around New York City in June 1992. "Fuck the Red Ribbon," it read. "Tattoo a bloody handprint on your forehead instead . . . Red ribbons remind me not of the dead, but the rest of us, who live in a world where a mere nod to such unthinkable suffering is considered an appropriate response. A RED ARMBAND WOULD BE MORE LIKE IT. OR A RED GRENADE, SLUNG OFF THE SIDE OF YOUR BELT."

No one ever found a way to market either product, however.

Companies riding the AIDS gravy train haven't been aerse to greasing the wheels. The guiltiest, or most likely to be nailed, are home health care companies and their collaborating physicians. They make a killing on the desire of hospitals to discharge terminally ill AIDS patients and the desire of AIDS patients to receive their treatments at home or in a comfortable outpatient setting.

"Bedside robbery" was the New York City Department of Consumer Affairs' characterization of the practices of these companies and the physicians they subsidize. Patients getting intravenous medication at home routinely receive three or four times the number of intravenous kits — needles, sterile wipes and tubing — they need, jacking up their bills by as much as $50 to $60 a week. They are charged two and three times the going price for prescription drugs. Meanwhile, their cooperating physicians — either through contractual arrangements in which they are paid referral fees or by selling their medical practices directly to the companies — regularly top the national income average even in a profession where that average is an astonishing $170,600.

Infusion therapy is the fastest-growing component of the home health care industry, which is already one of the nation's fastest-growing industries. By 1994 fifty thousand AIDS patients were receiving services from home infusion companies, which were reporting revenues of an estimated $4 billion yearly. The companies defend their profits, pointing out that they save private insurers and the government millions of dollars by providing services at home that would cost much more in the hospital. The insurers are happier, they say, and so are the patients. So what's the complaint?

The major one is kickbacks. One Miami AIDS specialist asked five local home infusion companies for their rates. Prices for a single hypothetical patient ranged from $800 to $2,500 a month. The most expensive included an $800-per-patient monthly kickback to the physician as part of the charges — calling it a fee for the doctor's oversight of infusion services.

The business procedures of many of these companies are so slimy that federal investigators have begun to target the industry. One of the first firms to be investigated was T2 Medical, an Atlanta business started by two medical supply salesmen who dreamed up the concept of turning physicians into partners in home infusion companies. More than two thousand doctors in thirty-one states signed on to what seemed as much a secret society as a business.

For $100 in cash, physicians with good credit and a willingness to refer all their patients to T2 for home health care were given the code to a private telephone bulletin board, access to closed monthly meetings and "referral fees" — a polite term for kickbacks. Their names were a closely guarded secret. Three thousand patient referrals a day generated, for the company and for the doctors, $183 million in fiscal year 1991, a 110 percent increase over 1990.

For the company's founders, who began by hawking their system out of the trunks of their cars, it was a Horatio Alger story. For the participating physicians, it was an ethical and legal quagmire. Medical societies and elected officials denounced them as greedy and self-serving. They were accused of dropping patients who refused to receive services from the companies in which they had a financial interest. The physicians fought back, expecting people to believe that their stake in corporate profits would never color their medical decisions.

"The people involved with T2 are all board-certified, topnotch, trusted by people in the community," said Dr. K. Mike Michaelides, one of T2's first recruits in Georgia. "I cannot believe that a doctor is going to give a patient an extra week of antibiotics just to make a little money."

Plenty of others believed it. The Federal Trade Commission began investigating, and the inspector general of the Department of Health and Human Services wanted to know if T2 had violated a federal anti-kickback law that prohibits doctors from profiting from Medicare referrals.

In fact, it did break the law. On a telephone line accessible only by special code, Dr. Joseph Allegra, T2's chief executive, explained precisely how much profit the company was making. IntraCare, a subsidiary of T2, had just billed Medicare for $278,000 in a single fiscal year, Allegra said. "My best guess," he told the doctors, "is that it cost us from $50,000 to $100,000 to provide that care," suggesting a markup of 178 to 456 percent. Then Allegra acknowledged that Medicare regarded only $30,000 of the charges as justified.

That was hardly surprising. In 1991 the New York State Department of Consumer Affairs reported that drugs and supplies provided by home infusion companies were marked up from 157 to 1,066 percent over retail pharmacy prices. Even those figures are low, since companies like T2 do not pay retail prices for their drugs.

T2 was not alone. In the spring of 1994, Michael Alan Booth, a Georgia man with AIDS, filed suit against Caremark International, the nation's largest home health care company. He accused the company and his physicians of overcharging him by thousands of dollars. Booth argued that Caremark's charges were so high that he was in danger of depleting his insurance, which was capped at $1 million. He had compared Caremark's prices with those of other companies and discovered that the same drugs were available elsewhere at almost half the price. Caremark's charges were inflated by enormous "case management fees" paid directly to referring physicians for coordination and assessment.

Within two months of Booth's filing, the FBI began investigating Caremark for precisely the practices Booth had outlined. What Caremark called a case management fee was widely interpreted as a simple kickback for referrals. Whatever they were called, the fees were astonishingly high. One of Miami's busiest AIDS specialists acknowledged receiving half of her income from Caremark. When one patient tried to switch to a different home infusion company, she refused, saying, "No, they don't pay me."

As companies such as T2 and Caremark come under fire, they're finding new ways to protect their AIDS profits. In October 1994 Caremark announced its acquisition of a medical consulting company that helps physicians organize and underwrite their practices and market themselves to HMOs, employers and insurance companies. As part of that deal, Caremark also acquired a group practice of 270 doctors whose business it would administer for a fee. It was Caremark's third purchase of large doctors' groups in less than a year. Company executives said that they intended to continue purchasing physicians' practices. Physicians who sold them walked away with as much as $500,000 — plus the continuing revenue from their patients.

If AIDS offered old companies new ways to make profits, it also gave birth to entirely new businesses and industries. Most are tiny fish in what has grown into a new ocean. Capitalizing on the hysteria about the danger of HIV-positive dentists, Rod Harris opened a business in Jacksonville, Florida, to test health care workers for HIV and, for a fee of between $100 and $189, provide them with a plaque proclaiming them "free of AIDS." He was in head-to-head competition with a mother-daughter team in Ashland, Kentucky, who ran the AIDS Negative Health Care Professionals, which provided similar certification for $99.

In the summer of 1994, two Florida men — a physician and a pharmacist — founded the High Five Club, a club for the certifiably HIV-negative, complete with a glossy, red photo ID stamped with the date of the member's last negative test. Membership: $35.

Then came the mail-order company you could contact by dialing
1-800-685-URNS for a full-color catalog of urns for the ashes of loved
ones. "By offering the privacy of at-home catalog shopping, LifeStyle
Urns serves those who are ill with AIDS," said the LifeStyle press
release, which included a refrigerator magnet for those not quite ready
to take the big plunge.

This was topped only by Rhonda di Sautel, Alex Ghia and Karen
Leonard, who opened a San Francisco art gallery–cum–funeral show-
room offering coffins shaped like King Tut's sarcophagus ($7,600),
pink and white caskets with silky, wedding cake interiors ($750) and a
wide range of urns, from glass abstract sculptures to "Joe Cool," a
two-foot-tall statue complete with sunglasses and a drawer for ashes.

And Sean Strub — a gay activist who has been making money off
his community for years by marketing mailing lists to companies seeking high-end buyers — founded *POZ* magazine, a glossy faux–*Vanity
Fair* which is dedicated to making HIV a lifestyle. While his editorial
content broadcasts a message of hope, his largest advertisers are members of the most lucrative enterprise that AIDS has created, a new
industry of investors trafficking in "death futures." Brokers of viaticals
— the name comes from the Latin word for the Eucharist given to the
dying — offer people with AIDS who have life insurance policies the
warm comfort of cold cash in their declining years.

Some companies buy policies directly, pay the premiums and wait
for the clients to die in order to recoup their investments and profits.
Others match the dying to individual investors, who follow the same
procedure. For the patient, the system makes sense. Who wants to sit
there, poor and depressed, looking at a piece of paper that will eventually make somebody else comfortable? Why not have the money while
you can still enjoy it? For investors, who pay clients 50 to 80 percent of
the face value of their policies, the rewards can be enormous. But there
are risks. A client can defy the odds and become a long-term survivor.
Or, God forbid, a cure might be found. Then the investor would be
stuck paying premiums for years, with no profits.

Viatical companies take pains to protect their investments. The
medical records of applicants are screened by several physicians who
specialize in predicting the course of the disease. The longer the life
expectancy, the lower the percentage of a policy's face value an applicant is offered. The science isn't exact, but most experienced companies make few mistakes. Of the one thousand AIDS patients whose
policies Living Benefits bought between 1988 and 1994, only 20 per-

cent lived past the company's two-year cutoff, and only 1 percent survived more than a year longer than anticipated.

The $300-million-a-year business is not for the faint of heart, though. Clemente Castro of Los Angeles frustrated his investors for four years. Despite an immune system comparable to that of a cadaver, he refused to die. Finally his phone started ringing with calls from his investors, who had paid $97,500 for Castro's $150,000 insurance policy. "They try to be as roundabout as possible, but they are checking to see if I've croaked," he said.

Of course prospective investors know that Castro's is an unusual case. "Please review this package in its entirety and call me if you are ready to make some BIG BUCKS!" Joe Sowell, the president of National Insurance Marketing of Panama City, Florida, wrote in his prospectus. Don't worry about the risks, he insists, an investment in AIDS death is absolutely safe. "As it stands today, there is virtually no hope for current AIDS patients. The condition is 100 percent fatal."

FIVE

AIDS Inc.

Insurance money and hope were not the only life preservers that AIDS patients, and the activists who purported to represent them, grasped. They also reached out to the federal government for the programs and relief it could grant. But not all of them received an equal measure of comfort.

Doug Nelson, of the AIDS Resource Center of Wisconsin, still remembers the first time he looked at the list of services available to people with AIDS in San Francisco. Medical care, home health care, housing assistance, emergency financial aid, psychotherapy, Chinese medicine, home-delivered meals, groceries, insurance, buddies, client advocacy, day care, dental care, prescription drugs and transportation. Here he'd been juggling his budget, trying to free up a few dollars to hire a counselor to work with residents in Milwaukee's AIDS housing program, and San Francisco was paying for acupuncture.

Nelson skimmed through the endless evaluations of federally funded AIDS service programs around the nation. New York had a program for the deaf, training materials for Native Americans with HIV, sensitivity sessions for prison guards. State officials there were bemoaning the lack of funding for senior citizens with AIDS. In Wisconsin, Nelson couldn't offer hot meals to the homebound.

Miami was paying for vitamins. He couldn't pay for AZT.

Something was wrong, Nelson thought. After all, people with AIDS aren't less needy just because they live in Milwaukee.

When the first federal dollars began flowing into the city, thanks to the Ryan White Comprehensive AIDS Resources Emergency Act — the so-called Care Act, named for the Indiana teenager who died in 1990 — Nelson had been too grateful to notice the inequities in funding. Milwaukee didn't have enough sick people to qualify for the major bucks — channeled through the Care Act's Title I, which gave disaster relief to places like San Francisco, New York and Miami. But Wisconsin, like all states, received Title II funding, which provided essential services to people infected with HIV. Nelson received some of that money at the AIDS Resource Center of Wisconsin to pay case managers, who helped patients get medical care, housing and home health care.

He never questioned the distribution of funds under the Care Act. Written by key individuals from high-incidence cities who knew how to work inside the Beltway, the act gave the lion's share of the federal money to their own hometowns, the centers of the catastrophe. It had made sense in 1990, when the legislation was passed. Those cities were crumbling under the weight of dying bodies and AIDS was still a relatively rare disease in the rest of the nation. But just a few years later the epidemic had shifted. No longer a bicoastal phenomenon, AIDS was moving into cities and states that weren't prepared for it, into places like Wisconsin. They needed help, and help meant more money.

Nelson had worked in health care for a long time. He'd run the Wisconsin Hospital Rate Control Program and lobbied for the state medical association. He took out his pen and began to make a chart. When he was done, he could tell anyone interested — and not many people were — how much money every big city in the country was receiving in Care Act funds for each living AIDS patient.

He was appalled. San Francisco was getting more than $6,000 per person living with AIDS; Milwaukee was getting about $1,000. Pittsburgh and Cincinnati were lucky to see $1,100 per case; New York was receiving $4,500.

The five-year Care Act was coming up for renewal. Nelson decided that it was time to rethink the funding formulas, to establish some sort of equity. He called around the Midwest and found that the people running AIDS service organizations were so overwhelmed by the number of clients asking for help that they'd never thought about formulas, about titles and funding. When Nelson faxed them his chart, they were horrified.

Everyone agreed that San Francisco needed more money. But six times more money per person with AIDS than Milwaukee? It didn't make sense. Neither did the formula for the allotment of Title I funds. Title II money, which went to state governments, was distributed according to the number of people living with AIDS in each state. Title I funds, which went to the original epicenters of the plague, were distributed according to the total number of AIDS cases since the beginning of the epidemic, although 60 percent of that number were dead. That meant everyone could stop dying, even stop getting infected, in New York or San Francisco and those cities would still get the bulk of the Care Act funds.

Nelson heard that the Title I people had been meeting with advocates for the other "titles" of the Care Act — smaller programs for early intervention and children. Together they had formed the Four Title Coalition to plan for the Care Act's reauthorization. The act didn't expire until September 1995, but they hoped to push it through early, presumably to get a head start on lobbying for its appropriation.

Nelson hadn't been invited to the table. It was filled with representatives from the Title I coalition — Cities Advocating Emergency AIDS Relief (CAEAR) — and their full-time lobbyist, who had close ties to the staff of Senator Ted Kennedy, the chairman of the Senate committee handling the Care Act. The CAEAR coalition had spent months negotiating and strategizing to produce a consensus reauthorization document. Nelson heard through the grapevine that they were ready to present it to the AIDS community. On May 4, 1994, he flew to Washington for the meeting, eager to inform the group about the inequities he'd discovered and the formula changes he thought necessary.

He walked shyly into a conference room in the National Conference of Mayors Building. The heavies controlling the meeting sat at a long wooden table. He and others from the public were confined to chairs in the back. "My name is Doug Nelson, and I'm the executive director of the AIDS Resource Center of Wisconsin," he said when the time came for questions from the floor. "I want to talk about fairness, about equity and the Care Act formulas." He proceeded to explain the disparities in funding and the unmet needs of people with AIDS in states like Wisconsin.

He was ruled out of order. The formula was not on the table, he was told. Nelson might have grown up on a dairy farm in Wisconsin, but he wasn't a rube and he didn't intimidate easily. He pressed on, then was cut off again. Nelson didn't know most of the people at the table, but he knew about them. They had practically invented AIDS service in America. The facilitator was Jean McGuire, the former executive director of the AIDS Action Council, the original sponsor of the Care Act. She was one of his heroines; he couldn't believe she wouldn't listen. It had never occurred to him that the meeting really wasn't designed for community input, that it was a pro forma presentation.

The hostility had been palpable. "I'd always felt proud of the solidarity in the AIDS community," Nelson said later. "That was one of the few times since I started to work in AIDS when I felt politics swirling all around me. Their body language said it all: 'We heard you but you don't count.'"

As he walked through the Washington streets after the meeting, Nelson flashed back to the faces around the table. He knew he would never convince the Care Act establishment to support equity. He flew back to Milwaukee with the seeds of a plan in mind.

First he needed credibility, and for that he needed to represent more than his twelve hundred clients and ninety staff members in Milwaukee. Unlike the big boys, he might not be able to afford an expensive lobbyist, but he could at least build his own coalition. For weeks, he called around the country — Indianapolis and Pittsburgh, Topeka, Cleveland, Albuquerque, even Honolulu — building his Campaign for Fairness. It was easy, since everyone in those places felt ripped off after seeing his chart. More than 135 community-based AIDS organizations in 47 states joined him. He was ready for step two: the U.S. Congress.

In the second week of June, Nelson and his public policy director, Mike Gifford, headed for General Mitchell International Airport. Gifford was fresh out of Augustana College, in Sioux Falls, South Dakota. He was twenty-three years old and hadn't been in Washington since his parents took him to see the Capitol and Arlington National Cemetery when he was in the fifth grade. On the flight from Milwaukee, they ate a steak dinner and chocolate chip cookies, then poured each other wine and toasted the United States Senate. "Equity is a principle the Senate will surely support," Nelson declared. When they caught a cab from Washington National to the Washington Hilton, they were scared to death. "What are we doing here?" the two midwestern novices asked each other. "Are we really going to walk into the Hart Senate Office Building and ask a Democrat-controlled Senate to buck Teddy Kennedy?" That was the plan.

In the first months and years of the epidemic, people with AIDS died in the hallways of hospitals, where nurses wouldn't touch them. They were kicked out of their apartments. Insurance companies canceled their policies. Their bosses fired them. They had no idea how to get

Social Security disability payments or Medicaid. They had nowhere to turn for help, for advice, for information on how to cope with a deadly new disease.

In San Francisco, New York, Los Angeles, Miami and a dozen other cities, the gay community rushed into the breach with improvised groups to aid the ailing and the panicked. Volunteers cooked dinner for their AIDS "buddies." Attorneys and accountants worked for free. Bars and restaurants offered their facilities for fundraisers to pay the rent on the modest offices of the new organizations and the modest salaries of part-time employees. Americans were asked to Eat, Drink, Walk, Run, Bike, Dance, and Shop to fight AIDS. And they did.

But when local, state and federal agencies began pouring money into AIDS, the generosity and volunteerism turned into a feeding frenzy over government money. States fought with states over who was the hardest hit by the disaster. Cities argued with states over control of the funds. Municipal officials battled community organizations over how to divide up the spoils. Blacks and gays traded charges of homophobia and racism. Amid the court battles and screaming matches, everyone complained that the federal government wasn't handing out enough.

By the end of 1994, the National AIDS Clearinghouse had compiled a list of 18,402 AIDS service organizations in the nation. "AIDS Inc." has become one of the largest not-for-profit service industries in the country. HIV-specific clinics and community centers, food delivery programs, hot lines, libraries, legal service offices, shelters, apartment complexes, counseling group, drug rehabilitation centers and multiservice agencies can be found in towns and cities large and small, in every neighborhood of every big city, sometimes within blocks of one another. Each service center has its own executive director and staff, its own phone lines, fax machines, copiers, computers and board of directors. Each organization has attracted visionaries and scam artists, idealists and thieves. Each is convinced it accomplishes a unique — and uniquely important — mission. Each fights bitterly to make sure that it, as opposed to some lesser group, secures the public and philanthropic funds it needs.

The biggest trough at which they squabble for their grub is filled by the Care Act, designed to provide a safety net of primary medical care and related services to people with AIDS who are ill-served or underserved by the medical system. The act was the first federal program to underwrite the treatment of a single disease. The Care Act is unique in other ways as well. When the idea of beefing up federal support for the care of AIDS patients was first raised, many suggested channeling the funds through the Medicaid program, giving treatment and care money to patients to use as they needed. Officials of local and state health departments opposed the plan, because they wanted the funds for their own programs. The AIDS community found the concept ironic: local health departments had hardly been on the front lines in helping AIDS patients.

No one trusted the government to deal with the growing number of young men who suddenly found themselves too fatigued to work, go shopping or ride the bus to the doctor. No one believed anyone in power would pay attention to a bunch of queers. The community had been taking care of its own for years, so the captains of the AIDS service industry proposed a different model. Give us the funds, they suggested, to continue our work. Waving the red flag of homophobia, they insisted that the "affected communities" could best handle the needs of their own ailing.

At first no one believed Congress would buy it, but a small group of lobbyists and AIDS policy analysts in New York, San Francisco and Washington were convinced they could win. They created an extraordinary coalition of 150 organizations, representing nurses and psychologists and physicians, mayors, hospital workers, dentists, governors and activists. They designed a bill that would give every member of Congress money for his district, his state. They convinced both Ted Kennedy and Orrin Hatch to lead the charge.

The day before the bill was marked up in the Senate, Ryan White himself was hospitalized for the last time. Hatch was troubled at the thought of the boy's impending death. "Wouldn't it be a nice gesture to attach his name to the bill?" he asked.

Ryan died on a Friday in April 1990. Within the week, his mother was in Washington lobbying for the act introduced in her son's name. She stood outside the Senate chamber, buttonholing one senator after another: "My son would be so proud . . ." she insisted. She cornered Senator Joseph Biden, who had lost his wife and daughter in an automobile accident. They cried together about the tragedy of a parent seeing his or her child die.

Before her arrival at the Capitol, twenty-three senators had agreed to cosponsor the bill. By the time she left, forty-one more had joined them.

The Care Act created a baroque structure to funnel money from the

federal treasury through the Health Resources and Services Administration to states and cities, which were required to convene planning
councils that included representatives from an astounding eleven disparate groups. The councils were charged with establishing policies
and priorities for the division of funds. City governments were supposed to follow those priorities in handing out all contracts.

In practical terms, the system meant that when the money flowed
in, the available service providers could sit down and divide up the
spoils. At first, most of the councils were dominated by affluent white
gay men. By the time the Care Act was passed, groups like the Whitman-Walker Clinic in Washington, the Gay Men's Health Crisis in
New York and AIDS Project Los Angeles had been in the fight for
almost a decade, working on shoestring budgets held together by donations and some local funds. They claimed the federal grants for
themselves as a reward for their against-all-odds endurance, for their
prescience and for their leadership in what had been a very unpopular
cause.

Inevitably, the way in which the federal funds were dispersed created tension. In cities where necessity or ego had given rise to multiple
agencies, each insisted on the superiority of its own programs and
proposals. Municipal governments, charged with overseeing but not
deciding on the division of funds, were frustrated by their lack of
power. In Houston a local judge forced the city to seize control. In New
Orleans the mayor appointed the members of the planning council,
then disbanded the group when it tried to exert its independence.

That was nothing compared to what happened in Newark, where
open warfare broke out between the planning council and the city.
The HIV Health Services Planning Council spent months agonizing
over bylaws and procedures — whether minutes should be kept and
whether meetings should be public. It was September 1992 before the
council got around to dividing up $2.6 million in Title I funds for
grants that were to have begun in January. Not all the delays had been
the council's fault. So many agencies missed the first deadline for sub-
mitting applications — or turned in their applications to the wrong
city office — that the process had to be reopened. Many agencies
missed the second deadline as well; one blamed delays on the elevators
in city hall.

After the awards were made, Newark's director of health and human services, who had attended most of the planning council meetings, abruptly decided that she didn't like the whole procedure — too

many service providers were seated at the table, too many conflicts of interest. She seized control and then dickered with the various agencies for seven months. The city council didn't get around to approving the 1992 contracts she recommended until March 3, 1993. By that time, the federal Health Resources and Services Administration was so disgusted with Newark's record that it denied the city's request for supplemental funding, noting that Newark seemed incapable of spending the money it already had. Every other city that applied received the supplemental funds.

The mayor responded by firing nine members of the all-volunteer planning council. On April 13, while he was swearing in the new members, his attorney was in federal court fighting a lawsuit brought by the ousted volunteers. The council was in limbo for months while the judge listened to pleas and counterpleas and consulted the Health Resources and Services Administration on its regulations.

All this was going on in a city that had the fifth highest incidence of AIDS in the nation.

Throughout the country, the divisiveness grew even more bitter as the face of the epidemic changed. The major service providers tried to change with it. They hired more minority staff and opened satellite offices and clinics in communities of color. Then the turf battles began in earnest. If gay men could have their own groups, why couldn't black men, Hispanic lesbians and Asian transsexuals? Should Hmong-speaking transvestites be forced into agencies run by white heterosexuals? If the spirit of the Care Act was community-based organizations, shouldn't each community get its own?

The AIDS service-scape became a war zone.

On June 21, 1992, African American and gay activists squared off in front of the District of Columbia's Department of Human Services, in one of the crumbling neighborhoods of Washington.

"Black organizations in the city are not getting anything but crumbs," blasted Jim Harvey. "Whitman-Walker continues to get funding, and they are building an empire on Fourteenth Street." Harvey was in a good position to know. He was the former deputy administrator at Whitman-Walker Clinic, the mostly white gay group that had always received the bulk of the District's AIDS funding.

The clinic's supporters were steaming. How dare you accuse us of racism, members of the Gay and Lesbian Activist Alliance sputtered. Our racism isn't the issue, your homophobia is.

An HIV-positive black woman shot back, "This is not about homophobia . . . it's about dollars and cents, and my life. I have the right to live my last days in an environment I choose. We have a right to want the services in our community."

The dollars and cents the woman referred to were the $15 million the District of Columbia received from the federal government for AIDS services. Whitman-Walker Clinic, founded in 1973 to provide medical services to the growing number of gay men suffering from venereal diseases, had received nearly $3 million from the city in 1992 and 1993, along with another million dollars per year to cover its employee health insurance plan. The grants had never been subject to bidding. Whitman-Walker had simply been handed the money, year after year.

The clinic seemed to take the funding for granted. After all, in the early days of the epidemic, its staff had labored with no public funds. They had built up a broad range of support services with volunteers and the charity of the gay community. They had invented AIDS service before anyone else was paying much attention to the disease. But as the epidemic moved into new communities, Whitman-Walker's hegemony was being challenged. Washington's Department of Human Services had announced an open competition for a $100,000 grant for an AIDS awareness campaign targeting the city's black, Hispanic and Asian neighborhoods. Employees of Whitman-Walker insisted that no other agency in town had the experience to administer the grant.

They were probably right. The clinic's dominance had prevented anyone else from gaining any experience — and that was the point. While Whitman-Walker supporters — who'd helped the clinic buy $10 million worth of real estate — thought of it as a model agency with the money and know-how to help the sick and keep the healthy safe, representatives of small, minority AIDS agencies, many of them led by former clinic employees, saw Whitman-Walker in a different light. To them, it was a hypocritical honky institution, one of dozens around the country that had demanded funding for their programs by arguing that communities are best served by community-based institutions. As the color of the nation's AIDS patients changed, however, Whitman-Walker's leaders refused to extend the principle of funding community-based organizations to communities of color.

By 1993, more than 60 percent of Washington's AIDS cases were among blacks, but only 20 percent of the Care Act money was being funneled through black community-based organizations. Although the city's annual AIDS Walk, which raised more than a million dollars a year, was advertised as a benefit for two dozen local groups, Whitman-Walker controlled the split: it was 80–20, with the 20 percent divided among all the other organizations.

The conflict remained a quiet pissing match until Caitlin Ryan, the white lesbian who ran the city's Agency of HIV/AIDS, overstepped her bounds in the awarding of the $100,000 minority AIDS-awareness contract. She wasn't just worried that Whitman-Walker Clinic, her former employer, was in danger of losing the money, which was a token sum in their $15 million annual budget. The competing bidder was the Abundant Life Clinic, a small agency run by the minister of health for the Nation of Islam, a notoriously homophobic group.

Ryan wasn't about to let them get $100,000 of public funds without speaking her mind to the four-member panel making the award. Ryan says she went to a meeting of the panel and expressed reservations about Abundant Life's ability to educate women and gay and bisexual men in the minority community. Others insist that she expressed her concerns less elegantly: "Muslims hate gays."

The precise nature of her remarks was beside the point, which was that according to District regulations, she was not supposed to be expressing any opinions at all, especially not at a grant panel meeting, from which she was legally barred.

When Dr. Abdul Alim Muhammed, executive director of the Abundant Life Clinic, heard about the meeting, he fired off a letter to the mayor of Washington, Sharon Pratt Kelly: "Rather than allow the fairness of the process to prevail, Ms. Caitlin Ryan interfered in the most notorious fashion, literally coercing members of the review panel to alter the award results. Suffice it to say that ALC staff is not only composed of Muslims but Christians, Hindus and others, and a large percentage of our HIV clients are members of the gay community."

Keith Tolver, the vice president for policy research at Urban Inc., which helped Abundant Life prepare its grant application, charged that Ryan consistently steered grants and contracts away from the black and minority communities. "We have to stop recognizing HIV and AIDS in a sexual context. We are looking at this as a social problem and a health threat."

Washington's Mayor Marion Barry, who was then a member of the city council, convened an "action forum" for minority organizations offering HIV and AIDS programs. "There is disproportion in the funding," he declared. "We are trying to break through the political log-jam."

Mayor Kelly placed Caitlin Ryan on suspension pending the results of an investigation into the charges against her. She was fired a month later.

The *Washington Post* treated the conflict as a clash between a strident, liberal white lesbian and the mores of Baptist Washington, or yet another example of the racial tension that is the subtext of virtually all the political infighting in the city.

The war escalated when two *Washington Post* columnists faced off. Courtland Milloy accused Ryan of a racist attempt to recast the D.C. Office on AIDS Activities in her own image — that of a "fierce lesbian warrior" against AIDS. Columnist Richard Cohen shot back with an attack on Abundant Life, wondering "if the federal government would award an AIDS grant to the health arm of the Ku Klux Klan, if it had one, or to any other organization that was indisputably racist and anti-semitic." The city's AIDS programs, he wrote, are "so riven by racial and sexual antagonisms — blacks and whites, straights and gays — as to make Bosnia seem like TV's old Nelson family."

But neither Milloy nor Cohen understood that the fight wasn't really about Caitlin Ryan, Abundant Life or even Washington, D.C., and that it was being waged all across the nation.

By the early 1990s, even gay men of color were chafing at the inequities in funding and services that were leaving communities of color underserved. Minority AIDS organizations formed a coalition to demand a reassessment. Four hundred groups and individuals signed on. "We have to hold the folks who run the community-based organizations accountable," said Alexander Robinson, president of the board of the National Task Force on AIDS Prevention and one of the group's organizers. "Too many programs haven't been rethought since they were conceived. We're missing a large segment of the community, and they have to be brought to the table."

But the invitations were hardly forthcoming.

"What has happened is that gay white men in cities like San Francisco and New York were the first people at the table," said Tim Palmer, a gay man who has worked in the AIDS service industry in Albany, New York, and Boston for a decade. "Once they got control over the table, they closed it off, both locally and nationally. Sure they let a few others come and sit down — but not so many that they can make independent decisions.

"Gay men have gotten ownership of the epidemic and they don't want to give it up. We have the power and the money and we give it to our friends. Gay men have become the Ronald Reagans of the nineties."

The conflicts plaguing the Care Act programs rarely surfaced in the hundreds of documents, studies, evaluations and working papers either sponsored or completed by the Health Resources and Services Administration, the federal agency charged with overseeing the use of the funds. "Grantees, planning councils, consortia and service providers have achieved notable success over the last four years in delivering care to individuals and families coping with HIV disease," the agency announced in one bulletin. That was the party line. It even awarded a contract to a private consulting firm to document "success stories" it could parade before Congress.

The reality behind the boosterism was considerably darker. Take San Francisco, which has benefited from the Care Act windfall more than any other city in the country. For fiscal year 1994, San Francisco received $44.2 million in funds, based on a cumulative caseload of AIDS patients that gave the city the nation's highest per capita incidence of the disease. Grants were given to 62 organizations for 145 programs for dental work, substance-abuse treatment, housing, supervised living, food and nutritional services, Chinese medicine, adult day care, emotional assistance, money management counseling, insurance-reimbursement advocacy, prevention and education. "This city has so many services, it's a dream come true," said Charles Caulfield, a social worker who died of AIDS in 1994. "Nobody in San Francisco who has HIV needs to spend one night on the streets or miss a single meal . . . But people aren't aware of half the services being offered, or what the criteria are for getting services."

In truth, many of the services being offered on paper weren't really available — or if they were, they were barely worth having. When the city began evaluating the programs it was funding, fifty of them — costing $4.4 million — were judged to be unacceptable.

CURAS, a Hispanic group, had received a $73,585 grant to help twenty-six clients. They signed up only eleven. The Bayview Hunters Point Foundation/American Indian AIDS Institute, which got $20,000 to provide health education, delivered just 6 percent of the services it had promised. The institute's records were such a mess that no one was sure whether the group was serving 23 clients or 529. After its board fired eight of its ten staff members, several of whom were HIV-positive Native Americans, the city's health department seized control of the agency and put it into receivership. Native American groups were furious and declared the action "a slap in the face to American Indians, who have endured 502 years of genocide and colonization."

In the spring of 1993, the Shanti Project, the nation's largest AIDS housing facility, was the target of an investigation by the health department because it couldn't account for $2.7 million in public funds. Shanti had no inventory of city-funded property and equipment, no ledgers or other documents to show where the money had been spent. The facility claimed to have spent more than $32,000 in salaries and equipment for a "Housing Network," a computerized clearinghouse of available HIV housing, but no such network existed.

Amid charges that someone had absconded with the funds, both the executive director and his deputy, a San Francisco health commissioner, were fired. The prior executive director had been ousted after he was accused of discriminating against women and minorities in hiring and promotion.

The problems weren't only racial and financial. In the spring of 1994, the cause célèbre was religious. San Francisco has an ordinance requiring groups receiving city funds to certify the race, gender and sexual orientation of their boards and staffs as a guarantee that the individuals running programs actually represent the communities they serve. Catholic Charities, which ran an AIDS housing program serving a client population that was 70 percent gay, refused to comply, explaining that the policy violated their board members' right to privacy.

Melinda Paras, the health commissioner who had just been fired from the Shanti Project, threatened to pull the $640,000 grant that Catholic Charities' Peter Claver Community received each year. No one had ever suggested that the housing project was homophobic. In fact, it consistently received top evaluations. Paras took a political stand that nearly deprived dozens of people with AIDS of a place to live.

Beyond the backbiting and financial shenanigans was the problem of duplication of services. More than fifteen agencies provided case management — essentially the coordination of clients' care and services. Twenty offered substance-abuse treatment, another two dozen emphasized psychosocial support, and seven concentrated on housing. Nineteen groups catered to women, fifteen to Latinos, nine to African Americans and fourteen to Asians and Pacific Islanders. "We have created a job-empowerment program," said Pierre Ludington, a member of the San Francisco Health Commission who was also an AIDS patient and activist. "This has become an industry. We've given a lot of people work."

The industry analogy was apt. The San Francisco AIDS Foundation, the city's largest service provider, had 103 employees, two buildings and an $11 million annual budget. When Tomás Fabregas resigned in May 1994, only three people with AIDS remained on the board, and they were all white. Only six of the agency's staff members were openly HIV positive. The staff had just unionized.

The directors of groups like the AIDS Foundation had joined the bureaucrats running the United Way and the American Red Cross with their six-figure salaries. AIDS Inc.'s Washington presence was maintained by its trade association, the AIDS Action Council. Its members paid annual dues pegged at 1 percent of their budgets. Full membership was reserved for organizations contributing at least $50,000 a year, which bought them a seat on the board of directors. The heavyweights, who paid $150,000 or more annually, were granted two seats.

Not everyone was in it for the money; there were subtler rewards. Mike Shriver, the executive director of the Mobilization Against AIDS, for example, earned a modest salary, but got to fly around the country on expense accounts, organizing and lobbying. He stayed in touch with his office courtesy of a sky pager. The position transformed him from a bad boy of AIDS activism into a corporate and political insider. Back in 1989, as a member of Stop AIDS Now or Else, he helped block the Golden Gate Bridge; nine months later he was arrested in a tense confrontation between ACT UP and the San Francisco police; in 1993 he landed in jail again at a sit-in at the mayor's office. By 1995, however, he was sitting on the committee that doled out the city's $39.2 million in federal AIDS funding; he was serving on the board of the American Foundation for AIDS Research (the youngest member ever, he pointed out); and he was a member of the San Francisco Health Commission. He loved to tell the story of his first meeting with Elizabeth Taylor, who grabbed his wrist and said, "Call me Elizabeth."

San Francisco was hardly unique.

In the summer of 1991, funding for direct patient services in Dallas ran out. AIDS Arms Network of Dallas, an umbrella organization for twenty groups that provided direct care to AIDS patients, had been given $175,000 by the state to pass along to the providers. Rather than turn over the money, AIDS Arms had used it to pay its staff's salaries and its overhead. In Philadelphia, the head of the AIDS Task Force was ousted from his position in April 1994 amid a fiscal mismanagement investigation. A year later he was charged with the theft of $200,000 from his former agency.

The Gay Men's Health Crisis in New York — the nation's oldest and largest AIDS service organization — was rocked by one scandal after another. One of GMHC's 850 employees filed suit alleging, amazingly, that he wasn't promoted because he was HIV positive. In the summer of 1993, employees, many of whom had begun as volunteers, petitioned the National Labor Relations Board for a vote on unionization. That September, the group came under fire throughout the community for proposing the construction of a $20 million office building.

A whistle blower in Miami complained to Dade County authorities that La Liga Contra SIDA, the city's only Hispanic AIDS group, was fudging its records. All organizations that provided case management were required to document monthly face-to-face visits with their clients. La Liga allegedly had asked clients to sign dozens of blank forms during their initial visits. The group was also charged with forging treatment plans and billing for support groups that never took place. The agency, after all, was in an upper-middle-class Anglo suburb with few AIDS patients.

In January 1994 officers of the Cascade AIDS Project in Portland, Oregon, discovered that thousands of back bills hadn't been paid and that the $1.4-million-a-year agency had a $140,000 deficit. They hired a prominent gay attorney to investigate, but two weeks later he was forced to resign from the bar for defrauding one of his clients. When the state's justice department took over the investigation, it concluded that the AIDS Project's former chief financial officer had siphoned off money into his own bank account.

All across the country, the problems arising from the federal government's experiment in community control were legion; the state of disorganization was mind-boggling. Care Act funds were specifically earmarked to support only those services that could not be reimbursed under any other program, but few agencies billed clients' insurance companies or Medicaid for eligible services. One Miami patient receiving therapy at the Health Crisis Network asked why his insurance carrier wasn't being billed. "We're not set up to do that," he was told.

Federal funds were earmarked for patients in need — those who would otherwise have had no access to health care. But prospective clients were rarely asked to prove their inability to pay. In preparing his evaluation of local AIDS programs, a Miami researcher asked all the Title I cities, then numbering thirty-two, how they defined eligibility. Eighteen of the twenty-eight that responded said a client had only to declare himself needy. No proof was necessary.

Records of charges for psychosocial counseling in Miami were in such disarray that no one was sure whether clients were receiving peer counseling, support through a Twelve Step program or individual therapy with a psychiatrist. They were all billed at the same rate. No one had a firm idea what case management meant, so some case managers were meeting regularly with their clients and drawing up treatment plans, while others were available only in case of emergency. Their agencies received identical funds for their work.

All over the country, the plethora of services was so broad, so fragmented and so decentralized that a person with AIDS could spend days going from agency to agency, signing up for disparate or duplicate services. Follow the sojourn of a single person with AIDS in Miami, a city with fewer services than New York or San Francisco. When he was diagnosed with AIDS in 1988, Joel Rapoport's first stop was the Social Security Administration office, where he signed up for disability and Medicaid. Then he waited in line at a different office, across town, to apply for food stamps and then took two buses to Jackson Memorial Hospital, to register for the AIDS clinic and pharmacy. That was just the beginning.

Even with disability checks, Joel's income still didn't cover his expenses. He heard about a rental assistance program offered to people with AIDS. Securing it required a trip to the county Office of Emergency Assistance and a series of "site visits" by a caseworker to the apartment where he lived. When the refrigerator in the apartment broke, Joel was told about a special Medicaid waiver program to help AIDS patients with home repairs, shopping and cleaning. Only one AIDS service agency could enroll him, so he got back on the bus and became a patient on the rolls of Health Crisis Network.

At each agency he visited, a different social worker was assigned to manage his case.

Just when Joel thought he was done — that he had waited at every imaginable office — his food stamp caseworker called: it was time to reregister. Then the county changed the designated AIDS pharmacy, demanding yet another visit to another agency. Finally the state of

Florida agreed to pay for certain anti-HIV drugs, which meant that the drugs were not disbursed by the pharmacy but by a state-affiliated clinic. That, too, was on the other side of the city.

Joel didn't take advantage of all the available services. If he had needed meals delivered, he would have had to visit yet another office. Dental care required a special case manager; dietary supplements like Ensure and Sustacal were handed out at a clinic where nothing else was available; and handicapped stickers for cars were handled by motor vehicle agencies.

At a time when their energy was diminished, people with AIDS faced daunting schedules, all in the name of staying well.

Some patients double dipped, triple dipped and quadruple dipped. Since there was rarely any central recordkeeping, a person who knew how to manipulate the system could exploit it and reap a windfall few homeless, mentally retarded or chronically ill people ever enjoyed.

Virtually all attempts to centralize and coordinate AIDS services, and thus to save money, were resisted. Since much of the chaos was bred by the tiny agencies — many of them minority-run — that often couldn't afford the type of professional staff necessary to administer large federal contracts, health departments and white activists proposed the consolidation of services. They suggested a system of subcontracting, through which large umbrella groups would receive money that they could then channel into small agencies, or "multiculturalism," expanding the traditional, gay white male agencies to serve a wider population.

People of color criticized both approaches as racist and imperialist.

Even where race was not the central issue, consolidation was torpedoed by vanity, ego and distrust. In Miami in 1991, a group of gay men proposed that small agencies at least consolidate physically to avoid the escalating overhead of multiple phone lines, fax machines, copiers, computers and rent. But the opposite occurred. The People with AIDS Coalition moved out of the building it shared with the Body Positive Resource Center so it could have larger quarters — and its own crystal chandelier. The coalition was invited to share space with the Health Crisis Network, but its board members refused that invitation. Some members explained that they didn't want to be around "those people," many of whom were black.

Even suggestions that cities create centralized computer data banks to prevent individuals and agencies from double dipping were resisted. The image of a centralized registry sent panic through a community hypervigilant about confidentiality. The proposal was defeated almost everywhere.

The larger issue was why AIDS patients needed so many separate services anyway. That question was never broached. No one wanted to talk about the fact that poor people with cancer or lung problems weren't receiving taxi coupons or free vitamins, that they rarely had case managers to smooth their way through the maze of public and private social services. No one wanted to discuss the fact that an infrastructure of transportation and food delivery for the disabled and ill already existed in most cities — and that the Care Act funded the establishment of a parallel universe. AIDS service providers lobbying for the act in 1989 and 1990 insisted that AIDS was special, that organizations based in the community needed to create their separate reality because the needs of AIDS patients were different, because mainstream agencies didn't understand gay men or the discrimination inherent in AIDS.

They were, of course, feathering their own nests. And Congress went along with them, not only because the mounting epidemic was having a catastrophic impact on the hardest hit cities and because people were suffering, but because the AIDS community proved extremely savvy at lobbying the federal government for funds. Grasping a fundamental principle about America — politics is more important than fairness — they used Washington connections, the media, civil disobedience and even Ryan White's mother to create the most effective disease lobby in the nation's history.

The bureaucrats running AIDS Inc. complained loudly and regularly that AIDS patients were ignored and shortchanged by an indifferent government. The opposite was true. They received a level of federal attention, support and services that were the envy of people with cancer, multiple sclerosis and heart disease.

"The unlevelness of the playing field is a result of the gay community's initial articulateness and money," said Jean McGuire. "That has come to mean that AIDS has a far greater impact than the number of its victims would dictate."

When Doug Nelson and Mike Gifford flew from Milwaukee to Washington in June 1994, they were pitting themselves against the pros. The Title I coalition — Cities Advocating Emergency AIDS Relief (CAEAR) — was run by the heads of the nation's biggest AIDS service agencies. They were men and women who'd spent most of a decade polishing their political skills and building bridges to key staffers on Capitol Hill. They were led by the lobbyist for the Title I cities, who happened to be the man who'd written the legislation in the first place.

That lobbyist, Tom Sheridan, began his career as a social worker at a group home for mentally retarded adults and wound up in Washington working for the National Association of Social Workers. After two years as a paid staffer for the failed presidential campaign of Walter Mondale, he'd signed on as deputy director of the Child Welfare League of America. In 1988 he joined AIDS Inc. as the director of public policy for the AIDS Action Council, and he was at the helm when the Care Act moved through Congress.

Once it was enacted, Sheridan left his job with its modest salary and opened his own lobbying firm, the Sheridan Group. Why? "The big boys have lots of money, and they hire all the big shots with their $300,000-a-year retainers," he said. Sheridan offered himself as an alternative to the fat cats.

There wasn't much difference, actually, at least in terms of the retainer. Sheridan's fee to the Title I cities for lobbying on behalf of the Care Act reauthorization was $360,000 plus expenses — with a 5.5 percent penalty for overdue payments. Since he was paying out less than $70,000 a year in salaries, including his own, he seemed to have placed himself well in the financial range of the "big shots."

Sheridan also founded and runs the American AIDS Political Action Committee, AIDSPAC, the only political action committee dedicated exclusively to supporting candidates friendly to AIDS issues. But there was rarely any candidate support. During its first year in existence, the PAC reported receipts of $659,195.39. Sheridan received about $65,000 to run the group. Its total donations, to four congressional candidates, were only $3,000.

Sheridan's power lay in the connections he had built to key congressional staff members during the early lobbying for the Care Act. He had worked closely with Senator Orrin Hatch's office and with Michael Iskowitz of Senator Ted Kennedy's office, organizing and lobbying during the annual battles for Care Act appropriations.

Sheridan and the rest of the inside-the-Beltway crowd hardly laid out the welcome mat for a couple of guys from Milwaukee riding into town like Jimmy Stewart in *Mr. Smith Goes to Washington*. But Nelson had nowhere to turn but to Congress after Sheridan and the Four Title Coalition dismissed his concerns. His plan was to do an end run around that group by asking senators to sign a "Dear Colleague" letter to Senator Kennedy, asking for a change in the formula for distributing Care Act funds. His own senators, Russ Feingold and Herb Kohl, fully supported the crusade. On that first trip Nelson and Mike Gifford took to Washington, they carried their letter all over Capitol Hill. In a single week they met with seventy senatorial aides, begging for help. They didn't have to try very hard.

Their pitch was simple and straightforward: everyone living with HIV disease in this country deserves a fundamental baseline of support services, regardless of where he lives. It wasn't hard to convince a senator from Nevada that it was unfair to discriminate against people who didn't live in New York or San Francisco. And since thirty-two states had no Title I cities, and thus received markedly less per capita funding for AIDS services, sixty-four senators had a vested interest in equity. Nelson also never neglected to remind members of Congress that Ryan White, the boy for whom the bill was named, had lived in Indiana, a Title II state that was on the short end of the disparity.

Eight senators, two of them members of key committees, quickly added their signatures. That's when Tom Sheridan panicked. As word got out about Doug Nelson's successes on Capitol Hill, Kennedy's staff warned Sheridan that a "Dear Colleague" letter, a clear sign of disunity among AIDS advocates, could derail early reauthorization of the Care Act. Nelson had demonstrated his political power; Sheridan had to pull him into the process.

On July 10 the CAEAR Coalition's executive committee met in Washington to map out their strategy. They had agreed to meet with Nelson, but they weren't banking on success at the bargaining table. They began calling Nelson's supporters around the country, evidently hoping to breed dissent. Sheridan met with Senator Feingold and told him that Nelson's calculations were questionable. The party line was that the formulas weren't the real issue; the real issue was Congress's insistence on giving greater funding to Title I, to the higher incidence cities, than to Title II, to the states.

Meanwhile, Nelson was also lining up his forces. As chair of the Public Policy Committee of the AIDS Action Council, the powerful national AIDS lobbying group, he brought a new perspective to the council, which had always been dominated by people from big cities on the coasts. At one meeting, he stepped down from the chairmanship and asked the committee to endorse the concept of equity in Care Act funding. The vote was close, but Nelson won. Despite the resistance of the San Francisco AIDS Foundation, even the full AIDS Action Council board voted to support negotiations for a more equitable formula.

So Nelson and Gifford walked into their second meeting with Sheridan's group with a stronger hand than they had had when Nelson had wandered in from Wisconsin in May. At the urging of the AIDS Action Council, a professional mediator had been hired to run the negotiations. Several representatives of each of the four Care Act titles were permitted to attend. Sheridan was there with his staff. Nelson and Gifford came with a single representative of the Minnesota AIDS Project; the other members of their coalition didn't have money in their budgets to fly to Washington for meetings.

When they entered the negotiating room on July 21, Nelson got the picture immediately: twenty people were waiting for them, sitting together. "It was clear that they'd signed a pact, All for one, one for all, all against us," Nelson says. "The onus was on me to deliver a plea that would convince them to change the formula." San Francisco, Los Angeles and New York were represented, and as he made his opening presentation, Nelson finally understood: they had no idea what it was like to have AIDS outside the epicenter cities.

"AIDS isn't as complicated in the Midwest," one person told him. "You just don't understand how much more difficult things are in Los Angeles." They seemed unaware that AIDS service agencies in places like Milwaukee or Minneapolis also had to deal with language problems and poverty, racism, homelessness and addiction. If anything, things were worse in middle America because of the lack of infrastructure, especially in rural areas where there were no physicians specializing in AIDS, no easy way to get food, medicine and other essential services to the dying.

Nelson proposed a straight per capita formula for funding. Each city and state would receive a given sum for each current AIDS case — rather than including the number of dead. He was convinced it was the only way to provide an even blanket of services across the country. Nelson was not inflexible. He recommended that a percentage of the funds be set aside for special needs, but he was firm on the principle, insisting, "The money must go where the epidemic is."

He produced data to show what such a formula would mean for most of the nation. Everyone knew that a per capita formula would help the smaller cities, but Nelson showed that it would increase the funding of most Title I cities as well. While San Francisco was receiving almost $6,500 per living AIDS case, Chicago was getting $2,699, Detroit $2,175, and St. Louis $2,652. Under his proposed formula, those inequities would vanish. Most of the Title I cities — thirty-two of the thirty-six — would gain funds because AIDS patients who had died a decade earlier would no longer be counted in the formula.

Unfortunately, Chicago, Detroit and St. Louis weren't at the table when Nelson met with the CAEAR Coalition. They were represented by San Francisco, Los Angeles and New York, which would lose funding under his proposal. "Are you really thinking about what's best for all your members?" he asked when they balked at his proposal. "Are you thinking about people with AIDS in the entire country?"

He didn't need to hear the answer. He quickly offered to support a "hold harmless" clause that would guarantee the cities likely to lose money that they would suffer no decrease in funding. They could be grandfathered in at their current levels.

"How dare you put a dollar value on a person with AIDS," someone said. Nelson knew he was in trouble. He took a deep breath and said, "We don't put a dollar value on a person with AIDS. We put a dollar value on services for that person, and Care Act funding means services."

Things deteriorated from there. Sheridan said that any substantial change in the bill would stall its reauthorization, endangering the lives of the sick. Regina Aragon, chair of the CAEAR Coalition and public policy director of the San Francisco AIDS Foundation, suggested that if cities like hers were grandfathered in at their current levels of funding, Nelson's proposal would cost $40 million more than the current level of Care Act funding. And what about cost-of-living increases for their employees? She argued that cities that had been battered by the epidemic for years needed extra money to compensate them for earlier neglect. Nelson countered that cities just being hit needed extra money to create agencies from the bottom up.

The Four Title Coalition agreed to some minor tinkering with the Title I formula and an adjustment in Title II funding that would free up $14 million, which could be shared by more than thirty states. But they remained adamantly opposed to any per capita formula. They said it was too risky; it made comparisons between funding for AIDS care and care for other diseases too easy.

Nelson tried to negotiate. He abandoned his insistence on a straight per capita formula but clung to the principle of equity. After two days of battering, the negotiations collapsed — and Nelson was blamed for not cutting a deal.

Over the weekend, the CAEAR Coalition met to devise a new strategy. They were prepared to find ways to give more money to cities like Milwaukee, but they weren't prepared to move toward any sort of national equity. No matter how many new proposals Nelson put on the table, he found no agreement. San Francisco, New York and Los Angeles were defending their high-priced turf.

In public, the CAEAR Coalition spoke in high-minded terms about the importance of maintaining services in San Francisco and New York and about the dangers of disunity. In private, Sheridan was more candid: "Those people have lost sight of the fact that this is a crisis," he said. "They're turning this into a trade association war."

When Nelson flew home to Milwaukee, he drafted a letter to the members of the Campaign for Fairness. "Every meaningful proposal to reduce the inequities in Care Act funding was rejected by the Coalition," he wrote, and it's time to talk with your senators for their signatures on our Dear Colleague letter.

The Sheridan Group and the CAEAR Coalition moved into high gear. They met with Senator Feingold again and demanded that he disavow his own constituents. They launched a phone campaign to the members of the Campaign for Fairness, saying that Nelson didn't know what he was doing, that he was killing the early reauthorization of the Care Act — which by then seemed unlikely in any event. Sample letters criticizing the Campaign for Fairness were drafted by Sheridan's office and mailed out on July 25. Recipients were told to "stop this potential threat to the expeditious reauthorization of the Ryan White Care Act," and provided the names, addresses and fax numbers of the Campaign for Fairness members to whom they might complain.

The worst attacks were personal. Doug Nelson was accused of being ignorant of public policy and refusing to negotiate. When that tactic had no effect, a CAEAR Coalition member called an official of a major Milwaukee corporation who served on Nelson's board at the AIDS Resource Center of Wisconsin. His company had been one of the group's most generous supporters. The caller threatened a boycott against the company's products if the executive didn't stop Doug Nelson.

Observers around the country who watched Nelson's reputation being torn to shreds were not surprised at the tactics. "The CAEAR Coalition is a closed fiefdom, a trade association organized to protect the interests of its members," says Tim Palmer, who was the executive director of the Boston AIDS Consortium. "Like the members of the

Pharmaceutical Manufacturers' Association, some are more worthy of protection than others. If you don't agree with them, they shut you up by telling everyone that if you keep talking, Jesse Helms will get a hold of the record and use it to cut services."

Just as the fight was getting out of hand, the AIDS Action Council interceded, once again. Gradually, in a series of conference phone calls, Nelson sensed some movement. His opponents would not accept a per capita formula, but they did agree to divide up Title I funds according to the number of AIDS cases reported during the past decade rather than the past fifteen years. It was not much, but it seemed like progress. The CAEAR Coalition then moved off dead center on Title II funding, agreeing to adjust the formula for states that had no Title I cities. It still wasn't much, but Nelson was getting tired.

All around the country AIDS activists were charging, as Palmer had predicted, that a protracted fight would draw the attention of Jesse Helms, with disastrous consequences for the Care Act's reauthorization. The end of the congressional session was drawing near, and Nelson wasn't willing to be in any way responsible if the reauthorization bill did not come up for a vote.

He caved in.

On August 18 he announced to the other members of the Campaign for Fairness that the negotiations were over and a partial victory had been won. For Wisconsin, in fact, the victory was substantial. The changes would increase the state's federal AIDS funding by at least 57 percent, although it still left Milwaukee with less money per AIDS case than the major cities received.

Nelson and Mike Gifford went home for a rest. Gifford got married, but before he could settle in, he and Nelson were back on a plane to Washington. They had agreed to help lobby for Care Act reauthorization, and they made good on that promise, hitting as many offices on the Hill as they could.

Despite their hard work, Congress was unwilling to consider the bill while health care reform was still being debated. By the time it was declared dead, the session had nearly ended. Congress was too tired to pay any attention to AIDS.

In December 1994 the Four Title Coalition and the Campaign for Fairness met to plot strategy for the new legislative session. Just weeks earlier, the Republicans had been swept into majority control of Congress, yet Tom Sheridan asked that everyone reaffirm their commitment to the formulas worked out in August and to the bill introduced at that time by Senator Ted Kennedy and Congressman Henry Waxman, the former chairmen of the appropriate House and Senate committees.

"That's not smart," Nelson said. "Kennedy and Waxman are out. They no longer chair any committees. There's a new Congress, with a new leadership. We can't proceed as if nothing changed in the November election."

No one listened.

He and Gifford met with the legislative aides of the new Senate committee chair, Senator Nancy Kassebaum. They had already read a report prepared by the inspector general of the Department of Health and Human Services which criticized the Care Act funding formulas and recommended ways to make them more equitable. Nelson and Gifford negotiated with the aides alone. Tom Sheridan had so infuriated Kassebaum's staff assistants that he had been barred from her office. Then, on January 9, 1995, the CAEAR Coalition met yet again, and Nelson proposed a revision of the previous year's agreement. The balance of power had shifted on the Hill; it tilted in his favor. This time the hostility was greater than ever. No more discussion, the representative from New York declared. Nelson and Gifford were accused of being disloyal, unprincipled and untrustworthy, of undermining the fast reauthorization of the act. After two hours of badgering, the group tried to impose a loyalty oath on the mavericks from Wisconsin. If they refused to pledge their allegiance to the Kennedy-Waxman bill, they would not be welcome to return to the table after lunch.

Doug Nelson and Mike Gifford refused. They were asked to leave, and headed to the Hill to discuss the hearings that Nancy Kassebaum had planned for February.

By 1995, the Four Title Coalition had become largely irrelevant. For five years the group had played on its close ties to Kennedy and Waxman. Now that new players were on the field, the game changed.

The most important of these players is the nation's most unlikely AIDS activist, Shepherd Smith, the founder and director of Americans for a Sound AIDS Policy. Smith is everything an AIDS activist shouldn't be: white, Republican, straight and born-again Christian. Unlike most of AIDS Inc.'s organizations, which occupy downtown office buildings, Smith's domain is a tiny space above an insurance company in Herndon, Virginia. His annual salary is $24,000.

Smith has been on the scene since 1987, when he and his wife,

Anita, decided that you didn't have to be gay or infected with HIV to care about AIDS. His priorities are clear: people need to be tested for HIV; if they are positive, their partners need to be notified by public health authorities; the uninfected need to show more compassion to the infected; the sick need access to health care; and abstinence-based education should be a central part of AIDS prevention.

Perhaps no one is more aware of the lockstep thinking of AIDS activists than Shepherd Smith, since so many of his principles run contrary to theirs. He leads the only national AIDS activist organization in which condoms are not king and which advocates routine testing and partner notification as essential weapons in the war against AIDS. "What we've done by putting all our emphasis on protecting the confidentiality of people with AIDS is driven the epidemic underground," Smith says. "Clearly we have to protect the rights of the infected. But you don't do that by giving AIDS a special status and making it a secret. That only isolates people and creates more fear. Activists are always saying that we shouldn't base public health policies on fear. I agree. But they are.

"We need to normalize the disease process, to treat it like any other disease. I don't blame the activists. They're doing what they think is right. I blame the public health people for not standing up to them and saying, 'Look, we'll protect their confidentiality, but we need to do partner notification.' Maybe our view is different because we work with a lot of wives. All they've done is been faithful to their husbands and they wind up with AIDS. The husbands knew they were infected. Their doctors knew. The public health authorities knew. Why didn't the women have the right to know, so they could protect themselves?"

Those positions haven't made Smith very popular in AIDS circles. He is rarely included in any of the endless rounds of meetings of national AIDS organizations. The AIDS czars have pretended he's not there. Even the press has ignored him — unless they need someone they believe to be a right-wing fanatic to pit against AIDS activists.

Smith is probably the only person active on the issue whose motives have been repeatedly questioned. The possibility that his motives might be identical to those of the directors of the Gay Men's Health Crisis and the AIDS Action Council rarely occurs to people. Activists like to allude to his allegedly shady past, which included a stint in a Martinique jail — although they resent anyone talking about theirs. They are bitter over the impact he has had on various attempts to end the ban on the immigration of HIV-positive foreigners into the country. When President Bush's secretary of health and human services proposed lifting that ban, Smith alerted his supporters and more than forty thousand letters poured in opposing the proposed change. The administration backed off.

Although Smith is a frequent guest on conservative talk shows like *Focus on the Family*, he has almost as many detractors on the right as on the left because he departs from most of the conservative movement on one key issue: he refuses to condemn homosexuals. He clearly enjoys bucking the conservative stereotype. "The only issue we're working on is HIV and AIDS," Smith says with a twinkle in his eye. "I say to groups, 'If you're trying to fight a war against homosexuals, forget it. That's not what we're doing.' This doesn't make me very popular in certain circles."

His insistence on the importance of testing is equally unpopular among conservatives. Christian women resent his support for routine HIV screening of all pregnant women; they are offended even by the implication that they might be at risk. Anti-abortion activists consider him dangerous; pregnant women who discover their infections might opt for abortion. Smith answers them the way he responds to his opponents on the other side of the political wars: this is an epidemic. Don't mix other agendas with this one.

Anita Smith runs a program of Americans for a Sound AIDS Policy which helps families living with AIDS. She consoles women whose husbands are dying, hands out emergency grants when mortgage payments are overdue and wraps countless packages for the eight thousand HIV-positive children to whom she sends birthday and Christmas presents. Meanwhile, Shepherd Smith exercises quiet political clout. For years his role was almost a secret; it would only have done damage to officials at the Centers for Disease Control and in the Public Health Service to be associated with such an infamous character.

Then Newt Gingrich took over on Capitol Hill, and Smith was transformed from a minor to a major player. Republicans have few inside experts on AIDS, after all. When the Heritage Foundation needs a knowledgeable and trustworthy person to brief their researchers on the issue, they call Shepherd Smith. When Republican congressmen find themselves running committees dealing with AIDS research, or Care Act funding, they call Smith for advice.

In December 1994 he took time out from the continuous planning sessions being held by the Heritage Foundation to attend a meeting of Washington AIDS policy activists. The president of the National Association of People with AIDS had demanded his inclusion. No one else appreciated his presence. He was treated like a spy in their midst. Smith was trying to bring them a message: there's been a sea change in Washington and you have to respond. They agreed to meet again in January.

"There's no sense of urgency," he complained. "They don't seem to grasp what a fundamental change is happening on the Hill. They seem utterly clueless."

As the leaders of AIDS Inc. dithered, Smith was meeting with the staffers whose senators and congressmen were rethinking the Care Act. Tom Sheridan's contact in Senator Kennedy's office was assuring everyone that nothing was going to change; Smith was working out a revision of the division of funds that would put more money into rural America and into minority communities. He was helping the Heritage Foundation devise ways to ensure that money wasn't squandered on people who don't really need help. And he was thoroughly enjoying himself.

"The funny part is that activists think I'm the enemy," Smith says. "In fact, they're lucky that I'm there. They don't know these people. They've ignored them for a decade. At least they have someone on the inside fighting for the Care Act and fighting for AIDS.

"Imagine what could happen if they didn't have me?"

SIX

Color Bind

Blacks with AIDS were betrayed not only by the gay white activist establishment but also by their own leaders — and by their own intractable paranoia. In no instance did it flare more disastrously, and sadly, than in the determination to exalt a dubious medicine that emerged from Africa in February 1990.

It was then that Dr. Davey Koech of the Kenyan Medical Research Institute held a press conference in Nairobi to announce that he had succeeded where the combined scientific genius, and funding, of the Western world had failed: he had developed a drug that cleared up most opportunistic infections common to AIDS patients within two weeks and eliminated most symptoms of HIV infection within four.

He reported that more than two hundred HIV-positive patients who'd been suffering from nausea and diarrhea, weakness, weight loss, respiratory infections, pain, fatigue and swollen lymph nodes had recovered within a month of daily treatment with extremely small amounts of a new oral preparation of alpha-interferon, a protein naturally produced by the body. Eighteen of the patients tested negative for HIV after completing the regimen.

"A MIRACLE DRUG AGAINST AIDS — AT LAST!" trumpeted the *Weekly Review* magazine of Kenya.

The American media did not follow suit. What the magazine's editor, Hilary Ng'weno, called "a development of major historical importance" was ignored by the *New York Times* and the *NBC Nightly News*. That was hardly surprising, since American scientists scoffed at the notion that a negligible amount of interferon — less than would normally be found in a liter of human blood — could cure AIDS. They weren't exactly inexperienced with alpha-interferon, which had been touted as miraculous, and then proved to be worthless, in cancer treatment. In higher doses of 10 million units, as opposed to the 200 units Koech suggested, the chemical was being used to treat genital warts and hepatitis. In higher doses still — up to 50 million units, an extremely concentrated dose — it sometimes helped slow the growth of Kaposi's sarcoma, an AIDS-related cancer. Alpha-interferon had even been tested against HIV, and showed no results.

But scientists' dismissals did little to dampen the enthusiasm of a community desperate for good news. AIDS buyers' clubs, small groups of activists who defied U.S. Customs and the Food and Drug Administration, smuggled drugs from all over the world into the bodies of the dying. Koech's preparation, Kemron, became the drug du jour of patients who had already latched on to, and discarded, egg lipids, Chinese cucumbers, Saint Johnswort, the anti-alcohol drug Antabuse, mixtures of deer antlers, licorice, peonies and tortoise shells.

African American newspapers hailed Koech's finding on their front pages, and black physicians and activists beamed with pride that the cure had come from Africa. The enthusiasm grew stronger five months later when the president of Kenya, Daniel arap Moi, called a press conference in Nairobi. Kemron was the long-awaited magic bullet against AIDS, he announced. "Fifty-eight victims have already been cured."

There was a considerable discrepancy between arap Moi's announcement and the data Koech and his colleague, A. O. Obel, published that month in the *East African Medical Journal*. Reporting on the responses of 199 symptomatic and 5 asymptomatic HIV-positive patients to treatment with their new drug, the physicians claimed that weight loss was reversed and immune functions improved, but that fewer than 20 patients were "cured." Nonetheless, *Kemri News,* the Kenyan institute's newsletter, declared Kemron "a miracle drug against AIDS."

For a while, at least, that was enough in a world in which the star of the single anti-AIDS drug approved by the U.S. medical establishment, AZT, had already begun to fade. At its best, AZT did no more than Koech claimed for Kemron. At its worst, it produced severe nausea and life-threatening anemia.

By early July, five hundred New Yorkers were sucking on communion wafers soaked with Kemron, courtesy of the PWA Health Group, a buyers' club that reveled in the irony of that special delivery system they'd devised for the liquid preparation. More than two thousand other patients — who found access to the drug through buyers' clubs in Texas and Florida, or through the small clinical trials being mounted quickly on both coasts — were following suit.

Later that month Gary Byrd, host of *The Global Black Experience* on New York's WLIB-AM, along with Clemson Brown, a minister from Brooklyn, and Dr. Barbara Justice of Harlem Hospital launched their own investigation of the drug. They flew to Kenya with two patients, a woman from Queens and a man named Cedric Sandiford, whose son had been murdered in a racially motivated attack in Howard Beach, Queens, in December 1986. Byrd had read about Kemron in the *New York Native,* one of the city's gay weeklies, and was convinced that the Kenyans had developed an important drug that the American media were determined to ignore. "Geography was clearly playing a role in why this story was not getting the kind of play it should have," Byrd declared. "To not see any coverage — and coverage does not mean endorsement — moved closer to out-and-out racism."

The charge of racism made the politically savvy Dr. Anthony Fauci, director of the National Institute of Allergy and Infectious Diseases, take notice. "We must keep an open mind," he said, although he added, more quietly, "but it's kind of difficult to believe." Other scientists who didn't hold political appointments were more candid. "If you drank thirty-six million units of alpha-interferon, a tiny fraction might make it to your blood, a tiny fraction," said Dr. Robert Spiegel, the vice president for clinical research at Schering-Plough, which manufactures alpha-interferon. "We obviously would have been into it a long time ago if oral interferon led to any blood levels at all."

Spiegel and Fauci both explained again and again that taking alpha-interferon orally made no sense, that it is destroyed in the digestive tract. An immunologist named Alan Richards disagreed, arguing that the drug could be absorbed directly through the mucous membranes in the mouth. Richards, however, was employed by Amarillo Cell Culture, the small Texas company that held the international patent rights for the oral preparation of alpha-interferon that Koech was claiming as his own discovery. In fact, it was a veterinarian at that company who had developed the drug for oral use in animals and who sought out Koech for help in testing it in humans once he had decided that it might have promise for AIDS patients.

While scientists battled over the drug's potential, drug companies fought over the ownership of the vet's preparation. Koech's institute in

Kenya, Amarillo Cell Culture, Hayashibara Biochemical Laboratories of Japan, which actually made the alpha-interferon being used, and Innovative Therapeutics Ltd., the Kenyan distributor of the compound, were so caught up in disagreement that Kemron had become a scarce commodity in Africa. Then a former Amarillo Cell Culture employee handed the formula over to an Australian chemical company, which produced Immunex — which the Kenyan government proceeded to ban.

Meanwhile, research on the drug and the experiences of patients began to make the corporate jockeying irrelevant. One study of Kemron, conducted in Zimbabwe by the World Health Organization, showed the drug to be worthless. Another trial, conducted in five African countries, suggested some moderate relief from AIDS symptoms, but no dramatic improvements or reversals of infection. And the American patients who'd tried it were returning to their prescription drugs or moving on to the newest miracle. "I can't say that we've heard dramatic results either way on the drug," said Derek Hodel of the People with AIDS Health Group, who'd been monitoring the reactions of the five hundred patients buying the drug, "and given how dramatic the reports out of Kenya have been, we should have seen something by now." Dr. Bernard Bihari, a New York AIDS doctor who frequently oversaw his patients' use of experimental treatments, was infuriated by the hype after one of his patients gave up high-dose injections of interferon for his Kaposi's sarcoma in favor of the lower-dose drug — and died.

But the group that had gone to Africa with Gary Byrd was not discouraged. The American underground was getting nowhere, its members said, because they were using a liquid form of the drug, made in the USA, rather than the "Kenyan" version, which was actually a powder made in Japan.

The *Amsterdam News,* New York's largest African American newspaper, went on the attack against white scientists, activists and journalists who refused to acknowledge the importance of the Kenyan drug. The lack of publicity was "curious in view of the fact that the white press swarms Harlem whenever there is a rumor of a riot, or a shooting or a stabbing or a drug bust or of any white person who has contributed two dollars to support anything black."

The volume of enthusiasm was turned up still higher in September, when Gary Byrd called a press conference at the Apollo Theater in the center of Harlem. "When we left New York, Cedric could barely keep up," Dr. Justice said, referring to one of the two patients she'd taken to Kenya. "Today he is responding to the treatment and it looks like he will be okay." Cedric Sandiford wasn't alone, Byrd and the others insisted. Nearly thirteen hundred AIDS patients had been released from the shadow of death and reclassified as HIV negative. "This is the first victory over AIDS and it's coming out of Africa, yet you haven't heard anything about it," said Byrd. The culprit, in his mind, was greed and racism. The inexpensive drug "posed competition for expensive AIDS medications offered by the white medical establishment," and physicians wouldn't pay any attention because of "racially based distrust of African science."

The World Health Organization maintained its skeptical view. Just as Byrd and Justice were touting Kemron's miraculous properties, WHO officials convened a conference on oral alpha-interferon in Geneva and invited Koech, scientists from seven countries, representatives of Amarillo Cell Culture, the FDA and even the leading American buyers' club importer. The international agency's conclusion was that there was no reason to give the Kenyan results any credence because they had yet to be reproduced. But under the barrage of criticism, WHO began to soften its stance. It is "too early to tell whether low doses of interferon-alpha given orally are of any value in the treatment of persons infected with HIV," the agency's report said.

Then the first two American studies of Kemron were completed and also failed to duplicate the Kenyan results. In one trial, the Search Alliance, a community-based group certainly not affiliated with any pharmaceutical company or the U.S. government, had given low-dose oral alpha-interferon to 167 patients. The results: "no profound effect." In another study, Dr. Wilbert Jordan, a prominent infectious diseases specialist at Martin Luther King, Jr.–Drew Medical Center, in Los Angeles, reported slightly more encouraging results. Thirty-seven of forty patients taking the drug gained weight and reported feeling better. But even those modest results contrasted starkly with the rosy reports from Nairobi.

"So far we've not seen anything that would confirm it's a miracle drug," concluded Dr. Joseph Hassett, who was conducting a Kemron study at Mount Sinai Medical Center in New York. He also noted that even the Kenyan researchers had been unable to duplicate their earlier results.

Project Inform, an AIDS information program in San Francisco known to be skeptical of establishment pronouncements, weighed in.

"We do not recommend this drug because we do not see benefits," said Larry Tate, the manager of the group's hot line. "I don't care if it comes from Mars — no one is going to reject an effective drug. If we saw results, we would not hesitate to recommend the drug."

By then, most savvy AIDS patients had become decidedly unenthusiastic about Kemron. Mount Sinai had been unable to find enough volunteers to fill its two studies of the drug. And the PWA Health Group, which had been selling a version of oral alpha-interferon for over a year, was finding fewer and fewer takers. It did not stop stocking the drug but ultimately provided it for free.

That fall Cedric Sandiford, weakened and often delusional, returned to Kenya for another round of treatments. "When he came back, he was a different person," said his wife, Jean Griffith-Sandiford. "It was like he was psychotic or something." Blind and unable to speak, Sandiford died at the Veterans Administration hospital in Brooklyn in November 1991.

But neither the studies' results nor Sandiford's demise dampened the enthusiasm for Kemron in black neighborhoods of Washington and Philadelphia, New York and Los Angeles, where the word was that whitey didn't want you to know about the cure. It was the best publicity the drug could get.

"It has proven successful . . . for some people who went to Africa to receive the treatment," said Curtis Wadlington, the director of Philadelphia's Blacks Educating Blacks about Sexual Health Issues. Black physicians in New York, Washington and Los Angeles continued to tout the miraculous properties of the drug — and denounce the white conspiracy to suppress it. Clinics run by the Nation of Islam offered Kemron for sale.

AIDS treatment activists, mostly white, were livid at how black physicians played on racism to promote Kemron, charging them with manipulating their own people. "When people say, 'We can get it for you and no one else can,' that's exploitation," argued Kiyoski Kuromiya, the editor and publisher of *Critical Path,* a monthly newsletter on AIDS treatments. Most infuriating to the activists were the prices being charged by the black clinics. The Abundant Life clinic in Washington, whose director is the minister of health of the Nation of Islam, charged patients $250 for a one-month supply of Immunex, which was promoted as an improved version of Kemron. A buyers' club in Dallas offered the same drug for $50 a month.

AIDS activists simply didn't get it, failing to understand the chord of response to racism and the long history of injustice that the rhetoric around Kemron was striking. "The racial overtones are very sad in this," said Larry Tate of Project Inform. "Anybody with a sliver of common sense knows that nobody with HIV cares anything about who developed the drug or the race or ethnicity or any other factor about a cheap drug that works."

This kind of response further inflamed Kemron's supporters, especially the Nation of Islam, which had adopted the drug as a cause célèbre. Dr. Abdul-Alim Muhammad, the health minister for the Nation of Islam and a spokesman for Louis Farrakhan, Gary Byrd and Dr. Barbara Justice denounced all criticism of the drug as racist denigration of African science. Black members of Congress, who had been noticeably inactive on issues related to AIDS, suddenly demanded a thorough explanation of the scientific indifference to Kemron and more complete studies of its efficacy.

Accusations of racist conspiracies hit a nerve at the National Institutes of Health, where reputations and rumors can make or break federal funding requests. The discomfort was intensified by repeated references to a decades-long experiment in which scientists in Tuskegee, Alabama, withheld penicillin from a group of African American syphilis patients long after it was known that penicillin would cure the disease. Public outrage over the experiment had forced the federal government to pass more stringent laws to protect research subjects — and had made scientists acutely sensitive to charges of racism.

NIH turned the Kemron matter over to the AIDS Research Advisory Committee, a group of nongovernment experts headed by Dr. Gerald Medoff of Washington University in St. Louis, and asked them to examine all the existing evidence on oral alpha-interferon. They waded through the results of thirteen studies from around the world, including two American studies, and concluded that the treatment was basically worthless. Health and Human Services Secretary Louis Sullivan, himself an African American physician, urged AIDS patients to forget Kemron and seek proven treatments.

But Kemron's advocates were not deterred. Some suggested that the results of studies might have been skewed because most participants were white, and that black patients might respond differently to the drug — although that did not explain why African researchers were getting the same results as their American counterparts. Dr. Barbara Justice maintained that many of her patients, especially those in the early stages of infection, had benefited from the drug — although it seemed difficult to know how she'd seen improvement in early-stage patients, who have no symptoms.

"Let's look at this," Justice said, demanding a serious, government-sponsored clinical trial of the drug. "It's not a cure, it's not a miracle, but it's also not snake oil. Let's take the time to look at this right. The patients deserve it."

Whether the patients deserved it, or the drug merited reconsideration, became unimportant as political pressure mounted on the National Institutes of Health. The nation's African American newspapers continued to editorialize about the racist conspiracy to keep the drug from dying blacks. The Nation of Islam denounced white scientists again and again for ignoring Koech's advance. "If he'd been of a different complexion he would have been heralded by now as having brought about a major development in AIDS," said Dr. Abdul-Alim Muhammad. "In America you always have to take that factor into account."

Dr. Wilbert Jordan of Los Angeles, one of the first American scientists to study the drug, agreed that racism was preventing any serious study of Kemron. He believed the drug might be as effective as AZT, but he was also skeptical of the motives of the Nation of Islam in marketing the drug and arguing that it might halt AIDS. "I hate to see them do it, because the ones they are hurting are black people, by making those claims," he said.

Dr. Alonzo Ellis, a Nation of Islam physician working in a clinic in Downey, California, was careful not to overrate the drug's effectiveness. "We're not claiming a cure because it has not been five years. We want to wait until after five years before we call it that," he said. Yet his patients said that they had been told the medication would halt the progress of the disease, if not eliminate the virus altogether.

Finally Dr. Mohammed Akhter, the public health commissioner of the District of Columbia, got involved. He'd been hearing about Kemron, but he said it was a chance encounter with a cashier outside a Safeway supermarket that convinced him to get involved. "I looked at this poor woman — she probably worked all her life to send her son to college — and now he comes home with HIV," he said. "I decided I had to find out for this poor mother. I wanted to make sure we provide what our community needs . . . If my people want Immunex, then I've got to do what I have to do."

Akhter went to the Abundant Life clinic and pulled the medical records of eleven patients who had taken Immunex. "Three of the eleven showed improvement in their white cell counts," he said. "Five of the cases showed significant symptomatic improvements. One case was new and so we excluded it. The other two cases showed no effect." After consulting with local researchers about the drug, Akhter asked three other physicians to accompany him on a fuller fact-finding mission across the Anacostia River to the clinic tucked away in the Paradise Manor housing project. "Regardless of anyone's good intentions, we have to be very objective to make sure the drug is safe and effective," he said, adding that he might recommend that Medicaid pay for the drug.

Kemron's supporters were elated. "I am pleased to know Dr. Akhter is more open than the FDA . . . If it saves one life we're much better off," said Jim Harvey, a black AIDS activist in the city.

Finally, leaders of the National Medical Association, the nation's oldest black medical group, demanded a meeting with officials from the National Institute of Allergy and Infectious Diseases. Little of the meeting held in October 1992 was devoted to discussions of the data; instead, government officials were blasted for racism and genocide. By the time the National Medical Association was done, the U.S. government had decided to cede to the pressure and finance a full study of oral alpha-interferon. "Clearly, this drug is of interest to the black community," said Marion Glick, speaking for NIAID. "We still feel there is little scientific basis for having an interest."

In December a study panel began planning a three-site trial. The central drug to be studied was ImmuViron, also known as Immunex. Immunex was touted as an African drug, but it is actually an Australian knockoff of the original preparation developed by the Texas veterinarian, based on alpha-interferon supplied by the Japanese.

In March 1993 the panel recommended a traditional placebo-controlled trial. But unlike the AIDS drug studies up to that point, it would be designed not to test the drug's impact on biological markers such as T-cell counts and other blood levels, but on physical factors like apparent symptoms and the numbers of days lost to work, along with "psychosocial" factors like memory, patients' perceptions of their own health and "life satisfaction" — factors usually considered too subjective to measure.

Meanwhile, as plans for the study were proceeding, WHO investigators reported the results of their latest studies of Kemron, conducted in Uganda. Five hundred and sixty infected patients received Kemron or a placebo every day for more than six months during the period from June 1991 to February 1993. The results: "No subjects lost their HIV seropositive status, and the study did not show any benefit to subjects who took the oral alpha-interferon compared to placebo." Dr. E. T. Katabira of Makerere University Hospital in Kampala also reported that he found no difference in survival rates or disease progression, no difference in CD4 counts or body weight, between the two groups.

Undeterred, five weeks later NIAID announced that it would continue clinical testing of the drug through its Community Programs for Clinical Research on AIDS. "The scientific evidence proves [low-dose oral alpha-interferon] products give no benefit in fighting HIV or in improving the immune system of persons with HIV infection," Dr. Lawrence Deyton, director of the NIAID division scheduled to conduct the study, had written in a letter to the division's steering committee. But he added that the interest in the drug by the African American community justified the expenditure of several million dollars.

That decision, surprising but inevitable, defined the AIDS color bind. NIH had no choice but to spend its limited research funds investigating a drug that scientists already knew was useless because it was caught up in a battle that had little to do with Kemron. AIDS researchers weren't just battling HIV but centuries of racial distrust, of resentment for insults, real and perceived; of oppression and paternalism; of neglect and unwanted attention. When AIDS made its way through black neighborhoods on both coasts — through East St. Louis, Chicago's Cabrini Green and the heart of the nation's capital — those chickens came home to roost, and they did so on the graves of thousands.

The faces of AIDS that Americans met on billboards and television, in newspapers, public health pamphlets and charitable requests, were white, gay and male throughout the 1980s. But AIDS was already cutting a swath through the nation's black neighborhoods. Even more than San Francisco's Castro and New York's East Village, the South Bronx, Watts and Newark had become zip codes of disaster where AIDS added to the downward spiral of poverty, malnutrition, poor housing and lack of medical care that had already lowered the life expectancy of black Americans.

By 1987:

- almost one-quarter of the nation's people with AIDS were black, although blacks made up only 12 percent of the American population;

- more than half of the nation's children with AIDS were black;
- two of every one hundred women who gave birth in a New York public hospital were HIV infected; about 84 percent of them were women of color;
- the survival period for AIDS, from diagnosis to death, was one to three years for whites, eighteen to thirty-six weeks for blacks.

And it only got worse. By 1989:

- for every HIV-infected white infant in New York, there were eight black ones;
- fewer than 1 percent of the patients admitted to American hospitals were infected with HIV, but in inner-city hospitals in places like Newark, 30 percent of the black male patients between the ages of twenty-five and forty-four had the virus in their blood.

By 1990:

- almost three-quarters of the AIDS cases reported in women were black and Hispanic, although women of color made up just 19 percent of the female population.

By 1991, the year the nation reached 100,000 dead:

- in New York and New Jersey, AIDS was the leading cause of death among black women between the ages of fifteen and forty-four;
- new black male recruits to the Job Corps, the training program for poor, underemployed youth, were three times more likely than white males to be infected, and black females were ten times more likely to be infected than white females.

By 1992:

- African Americans were falling ill at a rate fourteen times higher than that of white women;
- Republicans and Democrats both featured women with HIV infection at their conventions. Neither was black.

By 1993:

- More than half of the nation's reported AIDS cases were among minorities. The AIDS rate for black men was five times higher than for white men; for black women it was fifteen times higher than for white women.

But the message just wasn't getting out. When black men and women heard the word AIDS, they turned off. Everyone knew AIDS was a disease of white boys. In June 1987 *New York Newsday* polled the city to gauge residents' understanding of AIDS. Only 16 percent of the African Americans queried knew that intravenous drug use was risky behavior.

"There are sections where the epidemiologists can go block by block in central Harlem and say, 'This block will no longer exist in ten years because of AIDS,'" a black social worker in New York said in 1991. "And the community-board leaders in Harlem are saying, 'AIDS is not a problem for us. AIDS is a white man's disease.'"

So while gay men formed outreach groups to deal with prevention and education, African American leaders acted like ostriches. When the Centers for Disease Control convened a meeting in Atlanta in February 1987 to discuss AIDS in ethnic minority communities, Dr. Beny Prim, a black physician who had for years run drug treatment programs in New York, entreated other minority professionals to join him in the battle against AIDS. Yet it wasn't until late 1988 — when it was clear that dying addicts were spreading HIV to women and children — that the Black Leadership Commission on AIDS was formed in New York.

Black leaders clung to their denial with such vigor that when New York Health Commissioner Stephen Joseph appeared on *Tony Brown's Journal,* a talk show on PBS, the host accused him of racism for insisting that black women in New York City were at risk of AIDS. It's not black women as a group, but black women who have sex with intravenous drug users, Brown insisted. Joseph despaired at this message. How many women know the drug histories of their current or former sex partners?

"We've got to stop talking about AIDS as it affects . . . Bridgeport, Connecticut. We've got to talk about AIDS as it affects people in the South Bronx," said U.S. Surgeon General C. Everett Koop. "We've got to find more leadership in the black and Hispanic communities."

That leadership was a long time coming. When courageous white public health leaders like Koop tried to be the clarions of yet another piece of terrible news, they were branded as racists. The more timid were all too happy to give up under the onslaught — real or imagined — and avoid the line of fire. And it was all too easy, since there was little or no community pressure forcing them to pay attention to the dying of Harlem.

Black leaders, after all, were already battling a dozen other forces that were killing black people; AIDS hardly seemed the highest priority. White activists and health care workers might decry AIDS as the modern-day plague that would decimate the nation, but they weren't living in neighborhoods already decimated by drug overdoses and homicides, where the rate of increase in cigarette smoking was sure to cause a surge in lung cancer.

Some of the reluctance to acknowledge and deal with the truth of the new epidemic reflected the black community's ambivalence toward the infected. In the early years, when the individuals succumbing to the new cancers and old pneumonias were the men and women who most embarrassed community leaders, there was in fact considerable relief that the addicts who shot up their streets and entrapped their children might disappear. The graffiti of Harlem sent the message few would dare speak in public: "When will all the junkies die of AIDS and leave us in peace?"

Conservative African American church leaders seemed unwilling to suspend their moralizing about the evils of homosexuality in favor of organizing a coherent and compassionate community response to the epidemic. "This whole community is going to be dead by the time you get them all away from 'it's an abomination,'" warned Kenneth Reeves, the mayor of Cambridge, Massachusetts.

Even those less sanguine about the newest threat to black youth were reluctant to own an epidemic that shined a spotlight on the most embarrassing problems in their neighborhoods, the type of problems that had long given racists ammunition against African Americans. There was too much background noise associated with drug abuse and prostitution, teen pregnancy and homosexuality — too much shame and too much despair. Denial was easier, a comforting refuge from reality. And for the first years of the epidemic, the leadership clung to it tenaciously.

If at times the denial, the blindness, seemed willful, it reflected too the community's resistance to associating itself with a disease for which black people were being blamed. As scientists and epidemiologists trekked around the world trying to unravel the origins of AIDS, white Americans saw this work as a simple matter of curiosity, if not scientific relevance. Africans and African Americans, on the other hand, saw it as an obsession with shifting responsibility for the epidemic onto Africa. Scientific speculation on the origins of HIV was turned into conspiracy theory. The most common explanation, that the virus came from Africa, was viewed as a white attempt to foist off responsibility for the world's newest disaster on people of color.

"Why do they always have to pin everything on Africans?" — this sentiment was echoed from Lagos to Los Angeles. In 1987 the *Ghanian Times* declared research into the origins of AIDS to be nothing more than "a shameful, vulgar and foolish attempt by white supremacists to push this latest white man's burden onto the door of the black man." The governor of the Nigerian state of Borno insisted that the entire discussion was a perfect example of the "colonial mentality which capitalizes on our weakness and underdevelopment to attribute everything that is bad and negative to the so-called dark continent."

When researchers homed in on the unproven theory that HIV had developed from a virus found in African green monkeys, Africans and black Americans were deeply offended. "Are they trying to say that Africans do it with monkeys?" people asked.

Why all the emphasis on Africa? Was it that scientists "found it so difficult to imagine that white people could infect Africans with AIDS and not the reverse"?

The black community was already divided between the "take responsibility" message of Jesse Jackson and the reassuring "it's their evil plot" rantings of Louis Farrakhan. Blacks were all too willing to pretend that AIDS was the white man's latest burden to avoid facing yet another insurmountable catastrophe. A community heavily influenced by doctrinally fundamentalist and socially conservative churches found it easier to deny than to face up to homosexuality, to yet another toll of drug abuse, to frank discussion of the prevalence of prostitution and teenage sexual activity — the sine qua non of confronting AIDS.

In the end, the community had no choice but to face the truth. The mounting number of funerals of twenty-five- and thirty-year-olds and the growing number of AIDS orphans and babies suffering strange pneumonias became too great. But the same leaders who refused to acknowledge the problem in the first place moved on not to realism but to a rejection of virtually all the proposed solutions.

The trend became clear in New York City when public health officials floated the idea of instituting a needle exchange program. It was a straightforward solution to the spread of HIV through the sharing of syringes, a solution that was being tried, with considerable success, in Europe. Something had to be done, after all, because junkies in shooting galleries were passing the virus around by passing around needles, and those junkies, in turn, were infecting their wives and girlfriends, who were infecting their infants. Shooting galleries had become, to black Americans, what bathhouses had become to gay Americans.

Providing intravenous drug users with clean needles was no problem in the thirty-nine states where possession of syringes required no prescription and was not illegal. But in New York City and most other areas where intravenous drug use, and thus AIDS, was most prevalent, possession of needles and syringes was restricted.

The idea of passing out clean needles, or exchanging clean needles for used ones, hit a storm of political protest, especially in the black community. Community leaders who had fought to keep their streets clean and their children drug-free saw such measures as condoning, if not encouraging, drug use. When public health officials proposed small-scale experiments to test whether needle exchanges would send such a message, or would work to cut the rate of new infections, they exploded. "They tell me this is what we must try," said the Reverend Reginald Williams of the Addicts Rehabilitation Center in East Harlem. "Why must we again be the guinea pigs in this genocidal mentality?"

At a community meeting in East New York, Police Commissioner Ben Ward launched into a diatribe against such a program as fundamentally racist. He turned to Health Commissioner Stephen Joseph and yelled, "If you want to do needle exchange, why don't you go up to Scarsdale and do it there" — referring to a wealthy white suburb hardly known for its AIDS caseload.

Needle exchange had enormous support among public health officials, AIDS activists, and leaders of drug treatment programs, who were threatening to defy the law and exchange needles on the street. Black ministers and black elected officials not only opposed them but accused advocates of such plans of evil intent. The *Amsterdam News* declared war on Stephen Joseph and Mayor Ed Koch. "In the name of AIDS therapy, and on the backs of the Black and Latino communities, these two 'hopelessly white' men have unilaterally decided what is best for these communities, and will (they tell everybody) begin to distribute these needles legally in order that heroin addicts can inject with cleanliness an illegal substance." After listing the community leaders against even an experimental program, the newspaper concluded: "Why, then, this dogmatic approach to something that immediately affects communities with which both Koch and Joseph are unfamiliar? This is so hard to answer. Yet, the simplest reason . . . is that somebody had a brother in the needle business.

"What is probably more likely is that Koch wants once more to let Blacks and Latinos know who's boss in this town, and that he can do whatever the hell he wants and get away with it. What Koch is saying is: Your medical community sucks wind. Your community leaders are cowards, and you Blacks and Latinos are dumb as hell."

Yet neither the *Amsterdam News,* the black ministers nor the black politicos offered any meaningful alternative solution to needle exchange. They remained wedded to the Just Say No strategy, which had made no dent in the drug problem in their neighborhoods and had done nothing to stem the tide of new infections.

The same fight was fought, city by city, when public health authorities suggested making condoms available in public high schools. "This is a moral disgrace," said the Reverend Willie Wilson, the pastor of Union Temple in Washington, D.C., who was referring to condoms, not AIDS. "This policy teaches the wrong values in a society already crippled and dying from a lack of morals and values."

When District of Columbia officials suggested providing condoms to prisoners, the Reverend D. Lee Owens, pastor of the Greater Mount Zion Missionary Church, argued that doing so would be tantamount to telling inmates, "'Take our condoms and engage in homosexual activity in a safe manner, but your activity is illegal and if we catch you, you will be prosecuted' . . . Perhaps the fear of AIDS is just what is needed to scare these men straight."

Part of the resistance was a deep-seated suspicion of any solution that any white person proposed for any black problem. Harlon Dalton, a law professor at Yale, expressed it most clearly: "When we want help, white America is nowhere to be found. When, however, YOU decide that we need help, you are there in a flash, solution in hand. You then seek to impose that solution on us . . . Then you try to turn our concerns back on us. 'Don't you know,' you ask us in an arch tone of voice, 'that while you are standing on ceremony, thousands of the very people you say you care about are dying from AIDS?' Struggling to ignore the insulting implication that we are either profoundly retarded or monumentally callous, we respond, 'Don't you know that they are already dying from drug overdoses, Uzis and AK-47s, joblessness, despair and social indifference?'"

There was an even deeper conflict. Despite years of supporting Democratic candidates, of being embraced by liberals intent on flaunting their progressive stripes, African Americans, and especially community leaders, remained deeply socially conservative, a legacy of their religious traditions and their desire to insulate themselves from the breakdown of values in the inner city. AIDS hit just as the community was already fed up with drugs and teen pregnancy and with the pat answers white liberals had devised as solutions to *their* problems.

The people who reached out to the black community to provoke concern about AIDS were the very ones much of the community blamed for the unraveling of the fabric of their lives. Liberal whites might hold southern conservatives and their northern allies responsible for the plight of Black America, but Black America was increasingly including white liberals in that mix. African American professionals were already reconsidering "do your own thing" sex education messages designed by white professionals who told them to "face facts." The facts they were told to face made their children sound like animals unable to exercise any self-control. While white professionals were emphasizing the importance of contraceptive education, abstinence was making a big comeback among their black counterparts.

Virtually unnoticed by the white community — even by white pundits who purportedly noticed everything — black Americans were supporting prayer in the schools and discipline in education. Amid the chaos that was decimating their own community — and destroying their next generation — they were becoming Muslims or Republicans or at least "conservative" independents. They were rejecting the same permissiveness that Newt Gingrich so enjoyed flailing — but as antithetical, and dangerous, to African American values and traditions.

AIDS activists with bleached hair, nipple rings and out-in-your-face attitudes waltzed into that community and widened the breach. Few realized how offensive they were when they tried to be hip. Few knew how many people walked away disgusted when they "took the name of the Lord in vain," since the PC police rarely guard the concerns of the religious. Fewer still understood that in the eyes of many blacks they were just another bunch of white people telling the community it didn't understand what to worry about and what to do about its problems. Convinced of their own impeccable liberal credentials and sentiments, the activists never considered that they might be seen as yet another group of outsiders acting as if black people were too stupid to notice the number of funerals in their own neighborhoods. When the black community circled the wagons against them, those same activists all too frequently wrote off African Americans as hopelessly homo-phobic.

For decades white Americans had ignored or undervalued the wrongs done to African Americans and the problems endemic in their community, just as black Americans had spent decades wallowing in the type of blame that offered no solutions. The script had been writ-ten long before anyone conceived of the possibility that a new epi-demic could take root in the late twentieth century. The dynamic set up by three hundred years of history made it almost inevitable that black America would respond to the new reality, and to the insistence that it "do something," by turning the situation around and finding someone else to blame. It wasn't just slavery, Jim Crow and racism that dictated the script. It was the increasingly common practice of Americans of all races to take the low road of blame rather than the high road of responsibility.

For those most concerned about AIDS, the first target of blame was the media, accused, justifiably, of ignoring dying black people, of not alerting people of color to the dangers of AIDS. But few seemed to catch even a whiff of the irony of blaming whites for not being suf-ficiently paternalistic. Fewer still were willing to acknowledge that mainstream journalists were reluctant to cover the black community because those who did tended to be called racists.

On the streets, the rap for AIDS was parceled out not only to the media but also to the government, for mounting a plot to rid the nation of undesirables, or a biological warfare experiment using blacks as guinea pigs. The reaction was understandable coming from a commu-nity that remembered the Tuskegee experiments. Or the forced sterili-zation of welfare women, especially if they were black or brown. His-tory gave Black America more than enough ammunition to play the blame game.

The reaction was fueled, not dampened, by African American lead-ers who knew better, who packaged and sold paranoid conspiracy theories to a vulnerable population facing death. At a 1987 conference in London on AIDS and Racism, Dr. Frances Welsing, a black Ameri-can psychiatrist, declared that HIV was invented by whites to destroy blacks, to whom whites were genetically inferior and whom whites subconsciously resented for their color.

Welsing was, in fact, elaborating on the speculations of three East German scientists in 1986 that HIV might have been genetically engi-neered, part of a biomedical warfare experiment run amok. The accusation first surfaced during a meeting of the Non-Aligned Movement in Harare, Zimbabwe, in September of that year. "AIDS: USA home-made evil; not imported from Africa," read the headline of *Social Change and Development* magazine. The following month the Nigerian press reported on the "coincidence" of the opening of the first U.S. military installation devoted to genetic manipulation of viruses in 1977 and the emergence of AIDS two years later.

The United Front Against Racism and Capitalism-Imperialism brought the charges to the Third International Conference on AIDS in Washington in June 1987, with a pamphlet, supposedly based on "exhaustive research," concluding that AIDS was a product of "germ warfare by the U.S. Government against gays and blacks."

The conspiracy theorizing was encouraged most effectively by leaders of the Nation of Islam, who suggested that Jewish doctors had mixed HIV into the vaccines given to black children. At a minority conference on AIDS, Dr. Mohammad of the Abundant Life Clinic suggested that AIDS might be the result of experiments carried out at Fort Detrick, Maryland, as part of its biological warfare division and urged the Congressional Black Caucus to convene hearings on the matter. "Genocide is the policy of the government of the United States," he asserted. "AIDS is just one weapon among many. 'How shall I kill thee, let me count the ways.'"

That sentiment pervaded the black community by the early 1990s. Anita Taylor, the director of public policy education for the National Minority AIDS Caucus, heard it every time she went to predominantly black schools to talk about condoms, needles and risk reduction. "The questions I received back were questions about the origin of AIDS, about whether AIDS was planted in the black community, whether this was an issue of genocide in the black community," she said. "AIDS is seen by many, or the handling of AIDS is seen by many, as one more example of the possibility of attempted genocide."

The word genocide, which was spoken of in only a few, highly emotional quarters in Gay America, was batted around like a Ping-Pong ball at nearly every minority conference on AIDS, especially after leaders of the Nation of Islam discovered the disease. The African American community, already overwhelmed by grave problems, seemed almost relieved to yield to the hype.

Ironically, there was plenty of room for blame without flailing about at absurd targets or concocting conspiracies. By the late 1980s, the life expectancy of white Americans was rising while the life expectancy of black Americans was plummeting. A white child born in 1988 could expect to live more than seventy-five years; a black child was unlikely to make it to seventy. Black children were twice as likely to die in infancy as were white children. They were dying of pneumonia and appendicitis, bronchitis, flu and a half dozen other diseases that were easily treated.

The African American community was devastated by violence, drugs, teen pregnancy, decrepit housing, and the breakdown of the family. Many young blacks were choosing the instant rewards of drug dealing over the tedium — and vague promise of future rewards — of school. Racism persisted as a steely set of attitudes, actions and inactions that defied the quick-fix mentality of civil rights legislation.

AIDS activists of color tried to focus the community's attention on these targets rather than the simplistic rantings of the Farrakhans, but they rarely succeeded. Too many black AIDS activists were gay men whose roots were more in Gay America than Black America. They visited the ghetto but rarely lived there.

The disparity between their efforts and the reality of AIDS in the black community could be summed up by the second annual congressional dinner held by the National Minority AIDS Council on April 28, 1994. Called "Our Place at the Table," it was designed to empower a black, brown and yellow coalition of AIDS activists who spent their days struggling with denial, homelessness, lack of treatment and ignorance; to give them access to senior decision-makers in the government; to make them feel appreciated and included in a movement that increasingly operated within the halls of the Capitol.

More than two hundred men and women dressed in silks and satins with Kinte cloth accessories glided down silent, wide hallways past Ted Kennedy's office and Nancy Kassebaum's domain through a marble rotunda into the American Indian Treaty caucus room in the Russell Senate Office Building. The columns were elegantly sculpted marble. The ceiling was gilt. The tables showcased fine china, silver and crystal. The waiters, all people of color, wore perfectly pressed uniforms. Prosciutto con melone sat on sideboards, awaiting their trays.

Paul Kawata, the executive director of the group, was sporting a brilliant blue Versace jacket — the kind that cost $1,200 in Georgetown. He was anxiously awaiting the arrival of the guest of honor, Surgeon General Jocelyn Elders. NMAC's spokesman, Gregory Adams, scurried around in a tuxedo with a cummerbund made from African cloth, a long earring and a headset.

No member of the black press deigned to show up. Nor did any black member of Congress. The only congressman present was Steve Gunderson of Wisconsin, a white Republican who had not yet declared his homosexuality.

Then-Surgeon General Elders and then-AIDS Czar Kristine Gebbie were sandwiched in between Miss America and ABC news anchor Carole Simpson, who used her few minutes onstage to deliver canned jokes about TV news. Miss America offered an off-key rendition of "You are the wind beneath my wings." Kristine Gebbie thanked everyone profusely for including HER at THEIR table and pontificated on the importance of table enlargement before reading a letter from her boss congratulating the group. When Elders rose to speak about the impact of urban violence on the HIV/AIDS epidemic, the crowd applauded enthusiastically the profound insight that both forces were destructive. They cheered when she emphasized networking with church groups. No one seemed to notice that she never uttered the words racism or homophobia.

The setting was too polite and the event too upbeat to discuss such distasteful realities.

While the leadership of the AIDS minority establishment drank wine on Senate property, their clients lined up outside the nation's homeless shelters, languished in the filthy wards and halls of public hospitals and wondered when Social Security would finally get around to declaring them disabled.

But black activists got their place at the table.

Although they seem hopelessly out of step with mainstream Black America, African American AIDS activists have had some success with the white liberals who dominate the AIDS establishment and who are hypersensitive to charges of racism or the realities of their own racist attitudes. Black activists have forced changes in the way the AIDS prevention message is directed to the black community. They have made the Centers for Disease Control and local public health officials broadcast more "culturally sensitive" advertisements that include, as a minimum, black faces. They have succeeded in prying loose some money from the white AIDS service establishment to bring clinics and outreach programs onto meaner streets.

But that still has not stopped the killing. The AIDS establishment — the physicians, prevention counselors, educators and activists who'd come forward to combat the epidemic — lacks the resources to undo centuries of racism and discrimination while trying to keep tens of thousands alive. That is just too much baggage dumped on an already overwhelming epidemic.

In the end, then, in its desire not to be dictated to, yet again, black Americans have remained trapped in history. Their community has wound up collaborating in the growth of the AIDS epidemic, by indulging first in denial, then in resistance to all but facile solutions and finally, most fatally, in blame and counterblame. None of the rhetoric about injustice, past and present, has saved a single life; it has simply diverted attention from the latest injustice, which was preventable. Hundreds of children are born with a death warrant coursing through their veins because there is no agreement on how to mount a community-sensitive, abstinence-based education program quickly. Thousands of young men and women are needlessly infected by needle sharing because Just Say No just doesn't work.

Fourteen years into the epidemic, Black America continues to live and die in a series of deadly Catch-22s, needing to blame whites for the demise of the community's young, thus condemning those same young people to death from a disease that is immune to blame. Gay men have had stellar moments of courage that forced the nation to pay attention to an epidemic it desperately wanted to ignore — and wound up with that attention and a new level of respect for their community.

Black America wound up with Kemron.

SEVEN

Vaginal Politics

Katrina Haslip was an unlikely candidate for a dispute in semantics, but distinctions were a matter of life and death for her.

An African American New Yorker, Haslip found out she had HIV while serving a five- to eleven-year prison sentence for robbery. She'd already lived a series of double lives, from devoutly veiled Muslim wife to junkie, pickpocket and hooker. She'd engaged in everyone's definition of risky behavior but hadn't thought much about AIDS until a prison doctor treating her recurrent vaginitis suggested an HIV test. It didn't make sense to her: AIDS meant pneumonia and strange brain infections. What did HIV have to do with vaginitis? Everything, as Haslip was about to discover.

By the time she was paroled two years later, left to fend to herself, Haslip was seriously ill. Shortness of breath, weakness and diarrhea made it tough for her to work, even to get around well. Welfare counselors in New York City sent her to the Social Security office to apply for disability. With only 47 T cells — 1,000 to 1,200 are the norm — chronic fatigue, severe weight loss and persistent vaginitis, she was undeniably diminished. But in the eyes of the Social Security Administration, not enough so. They wanted pneumonia, cytomegalovirus, Kaposi's sarcoma — the CDC's yardsticks of AIDS. Benefits were denied.

Haslip knew a lot about sexism in the courts, in prisons, even in Islam. She suddenly got a short course in sexism in public health. Lesson one: almost two-thirds of the nation's HIV-positive women were dying without ever meeting the CDC's criteria for AIDS. Lesson two: AIDS was increasingly killing women, but government bureaucrats and scientists were slow to acknowledge their deaths.

In the early years of the epidemic, American females seemed almost immune to HIV. Unlike Africa, where the virus showed no gender preference at all, in the United States it showed a distinct preference for men. Fewer than 100 of the nation's first 800 AIDS cases involved women. By 1985, when the national toll for men was 8,092, it was just 569 for women. But gradually, inexorably, as women had sex with men who shot drugs or who had sex with other men, the numbers of women facing the terror of AIDS began rising. By June 1994, more than 50,000 American women had been diagnosed with AIDS. The numbers of HIV-infected were rising exponentially.

Nonetheless, for years epidemiologists adhered to a definition of AIDS that virtually excluded women, so women were diagnosed later than men. Bureaucrats denied women disability payments, and pharmaceutical researchers barred women from trials of new drugs that might prolong their lives.

It's hardly surprising in a country where gender determines so much that it also governs who gets diagnosed with diseases, what medications are prescribed, whether patients receive disability and how quickly they die. Nor is it surprising that those who die fastest are female: the average white gay man with HIV lives 39 months after his diagnosis with full-blown AIDS; the average woman survives 27.4 weeks after her diagnosis. HIV-infected women are one-third more likely to die without an AIDS-defining condition than are HIV-infected men.

Meet Terry McGovern, a petite and soft-spoken thirty-four-year-old attorney who has made it her mission to change the human realities of a disease whose medical realities are impervious to the law. A graduate of Georgetown University Law School, McGovern is supposed to be cashing serious paychecks from a law firm with mahogany desks and monied clients. Instead, she works out of a tiny office, waging a one-woman crusade to protect the nation's forgotten AIDS patients — poor, black or Hispanic women — and fighting a man-made epidemic of sexism that is killing them even faster than the one devised by nature.

McGovern is a certifiable AIDS heroine, the type of person whose position in the pantheon of AIDS activist saints should have been assured long ago. She has sued former Health and Human Services Secretary Louis Sullivan and brought the Social Security Administration to its knees over its definition of AIDS-related disability. She has done battle with the Centers for Disease Control and won a major expansion in the reporting of AIDS cases. She has forced the Food and Drug Administration into a long series of embarrassing retreats from its established drug-testing guidelines.

If women with AIDS are now being diagnosed and treated early enough in the course of their infection that they can enjoy some quality life before they die, they can thank Terry McGovern. If they receive disability benefits that allow them to keep warm and eat at least one good meal a day, if they have access to the experimental drugs that are the lifeline of people with AIDS, they can also thank Terry McGovern.

Many do. But most of the people with AIDS who've benefited from McGovern's tireless crusade have never heard of her. Male AIDS activists are featured on the cover of *Rolling Stone* and interviewed on *Nightline* and CNN, by Geraldo Rivera and Oprah Winfrey. But McGovern isn't one of the boys. In fact, the boys have mixed feelings about almost everything she does, fearing that what's good for women may not be best for men, sensing that the pie is only so big, zealously guarding their mammoth portion of it.

That's never stopped McGovern.

Her first major foray into the national AIDS wars involved what seemed like bureaucratic quibbling over the definition of AIDS. McGovern stepped into this semantic dispute in 1989, when she was working as a legal aid attorney. Her male HIV-positive clients were routinely granted Social Security disability benefits when they began to fall sick; her female clients received denials just as routinely.

McGovern began checking with other legal service offices around the city. The pattern was identical: the women were sick, but Social Security refused to recognize their illnesses as AIDS. The distinction was critical, because an AIDS diagnosis allowed for presumptive disability, with immediate benefits; a different diagnosis meant months of paperwork and delays.

The Social Security Administration relied on the Centers for Disease Control for its legal definition of AIDS, and the CDC relied solely on the natural history of AIDS in men. No one had studied the course of HIV infection in women, so it was hardly surprising that Social Security didn't recognize abnormal pap smears, chronic urinary tract infections, cervical dysplasia and a wide range of other gynecological problems as signs of HIV progression.

McGovern wasn't just thinking about disability. Thousands of women with severe immune problems that manifested themselves gynecologically weren't counted as AIDS patients, reducing the number of cases in women so drastically that no one could ever be sure how many women had already died of AIDS, or how many were sick. The limited definition meant that the risks to women were consistently under-estimated and underpublicized. Most ominously, it meant that gynecologists weren't warned to consider persistent problems as possible signs of HIV infection, consigning women to late diagnoses and early deaths.

Definitions of diseases are generally straightforward matters. If you break out with certain types of skin problems and have varicella-zoster virus in your blood, you have chickenpox. If you have a swollen lymph node and a pathologist finds certains types of cells when he puts it under a microscope, you have lymphoma. But AIDS is not a straight-forward disease. It is the culmination of a disease process that begins with HIV infection and ends in dozens of different cancers and bacterial, fungal and viral infections that take advantage of the immune destruction wrought by the virus.

When, then, does someone have AIDS rather than simply HIV infection? There's no clear medical answer, since the line between HIV infection and AIDS is essentially arbitrary. The Centers for Disease Control drew that arbitrary line by devising a list of diseases that signaled the severe immune suppression believed to mark the decline toward death. That list, however, was compiled from the medical charts of participants in the CDC's "Spectrum of Disease" study, the research project used to track the natural history of HIV infection. By 1990 only 7 percent of the members of that group were female.

In practical terms, it came down to this: An HIV-positive gay man who felt healthy, who had no pain, no loss of energy or weight, but suffered from a yeast infection in his throat had AIDS, according to the CDC — and was thus eligible for presumptive disability, according to Social Security. An HIV-positive woman who had lost weight, was in chronic pain from pelvic inflammatory disease, could barely get around and suffered from the same yeast infection, in her vagina in-stead of her throat, did not have AIDS, according to the CDC — and was thus ineligible for presumptive disability, according to Social Security.

Throughout 1990, McGovern, a small band of female activists and a group of physicians with large numbers of female AIDS patients inundated the CDC with data on women-specific manifestations of AIDS. At a meeting with CDC officials at the New York City health department in April 1990, they presented records on the number of abnormal pap smears turning up in HIV-positive women and plotted the dangerous rise in cervical cancer among those women.

The CDC published an article on the data in its weekly bulletin but wouldn't budge on the definition of AIDS. Officials there acknowledged that their definition wasn't all-inclusive, speculating that it left out up to 40 percent of those actually suffering from the disease, but they insisted that their definition was used only for surveillance, for their charting of the epidemic. Any change might mess up their math, making it impossible to compare one year's statistics to those of a previous year.

The activists countered that a change was essential to alert gynecologists to the clear warning signs of AIDS in women. The CDC responded that there were other mechanisms for delivering that message. The women came back with arguments about the importance of encouraging research into female-specific diseases. The CDC noted that disease research was the purview of the National Institutes of Health. Finally CDC officials admitted that vaginitis, pelvic inflammatory disease and cervical cancer were showing up more frequently, or more severely, in HIV-infected women. But they asked, with perfect scientific composure, for proof of a cause-and-effect relationship.

The women were dumbfounded. No one had proven a causal relationship between HIV infection and *Pneumocystis carinii* pneumonia, or Kaposi's sarcoma and HIV, when the first AIDS definition was published. If correlation was sufficient evidence in men, why was it insufficient for women? The CDC gave no response.

They couldn't. No such proof could be developed, since the CDC wasn't tracking women carefully, and since NIH's drug research studies didn't even include pelvic examinations.

Exasperated by the intransigence, McGovern filed suit against the U.S. government on October 1, 1990, alleging that the operative definition of AIDS discriminated against women. Many male activists dismissed the suit as one of those symbolic struggles waged by semi-professional victims in a country where there were more pressing problems crying out for attention. For Katrina Haslip and for thousands of women dependent on the CDC's definition in order to qualify for presumptive disability, however, it was the difference between sleeping on a park bench and renting an apartment.

The day McGovern filed her suit, scores of those women and their supporters went to Washington. That evening, commuters packing into Washington's Metro Center, the hub of the city's transportation system, noticed an acrid odor in the air. Looking up to the vaulted ceiling, they saw a fifteen-foot-high banner suspended from helium balloons. "Louis Sullivan, HHS Secretary: Your AIDS Disability Benefits Stink," it read in enormous letters. Stink bombs had been set off to punctuate the statement.

The following morning, the women descended on the Department of Health and Human Services and chanted, "Men with AIDS get benefits just because they don't have tits," and "HHS is just a stunt, Sullivan get off my cunt." Katrina Haslip had been out of jail less than a month and was already parading on Independence Avenue, yelling, "Land of the free, home of the brave is putting women in the grave." She carried a cardboard tombstone declaring, "Women with AIDS, Dead but Not Disabled."

"Women don't get AIDS," she told reporters, "they just die from it."

The Social Security Administration did study the issue. In a March 1991 program circular, Louis Sullivan recognized gynecological complications as potential AIDS-related impairments, but his exegesis was mere lip service to McGovern's complaints. When he added new illnesses to the presumptive disability list, advanced cervical cancer was the only female-specific ailment included — proving yet again that a woman had to be almost dead to receive disability benefits.

Just as McGovern was on the verge of concluding that government bureaucrats were impervious to reason, the Social Security Administration announced a new set of criteria for AIDS-related disability. She was almost afraid to look at the new list. When she finally worked up the courage, she began to cry. The preface openly acknowledged that gynecological problems were more aggressive in women with HIV; the revised list of AIDS-related illnesses included pelvic inflammatory disease and vaginal candidiasis.

Victory was bittersweet. Katrina Haslip had died one month earlier, without receiving a legal diagnosis of AIDS.

McGovern wasn't done. Women with HIV needed more than diagnoses. They needed treatment, and that was a more bitter battle in a country where a woman's reproductive system is a carefully guarded national treasure.

McGovern discovered what happens to women looking for access to experimental AIDS treatments when a woman named Irene walked off the street and into her office, in an old school building on the decaying Lower East Side of Manhattan. With a T-cell count one-tenth of normal, painful genital ulcers and cervical cancer, Irene was desperate to find something, anything, that might help her deteriorating immune system. She had gone to the Gay Men's Health Crisis, the nation's first private social service agency for people with AIDS, looking for information on trials of new drugs. Someone there told her about the latest antiviral, called ddI, and where it was being tested.

Irene trekked across the river to New Jersey and tried to enroll. Dozens of men with similar T-cell counts were meeting with the study nurse and signing up. Not Irene. Unlike the men, she couldn't enroll unless she was using "detectable" birth control, which meant an intrauterine device, an IUD.

That's ridiculous, she told the trial staff. "There's not a chance in hell I'll be having sex." Besides, she said, she had cervical cancer and a host of gynecological infections that an IUD would only aggravate.

The trial staff was adamant. No IUD, no ddI.

Irene schlepped back across the river on train after train and waited hours to see a doctor at a public health clinic about getting an IUD. Forget it, he said. He wasn't worried about her cervical cancer. Instead, he said simply, "You shouldn't be having sex." Irene explained that she wasn't getting ready for a lurid affair; she was trying to get into a drug study. The physician didn't believe her.

That's when she appeared at Terry McGovern's door, her green eyes flashing in fury. "I have AIDS," she said. "I'm going to die very soon. I'm in the final stages. I'm not even thinking about sex at this point in my life. Are they crazy? I can't believe I'm being treated this way."

McGovern tried to persuade Irene's clinic to explain to the ddI study staff that her client had cervical cancer and couldn't use an IUD. For weeks she called, cajoling and threatening. By the time she detected the first bit of movement, the ddI trial was full. Just weeks later, Irene died.

Irene was the first of dozens of women with AIDS McGovern watched die without the treatments men routinely received. Next came a young woman with two children, referred to McGovern by a prominent AIDS specialist. The woman was resistant to AZT, so her doctor had tried to enroll her in a study of a new type of anti-HIV drug, a tat inhibitor. At that point, tat inhibitors seemed a promising approach to slowing HIV's insidious march. No one was sure what the drug would or would not do, but the young woman had no other options.

As it turned out, she had no options at all. The researchers conducting the study for Hoffmann–La Roche, the drug's manufacturer, refused to enroll women who weren't surgically sterilized. McGovern's client wasn't planning to get pregnant anytime soon, but even her doctor agreed that surgical sterilization seemed unwise for someone with a weakened immune system. She offered to use detectable birth control, to undergo regular pregnancy tests, even to sign a waiver or a contract not to sue. To no avail.

McGovern called Hoffmann–La Roche. Why do women need to be surgically sterilized? she asked. Was there evidence that the drug might harm a fetus? Did it seem dangerous to a woman's reproductive system? Was there no reason to believe that it would harm a man's sperm, or even his ability to produce sperm?

"We don't really know" was the only reply. "We're just complying with an FDA guideline."

McGovern had never heard of any such guideline, so she went looking. She finally found a set of regulations written in 1977 in reaction to the well-publicized horror over the birth defects caused by the sedative thalidomide. The late seventies were the heyday of the feminist movement, when women were rebelling against paternalism and against being defined as breeders. But no one had complained when the FDA barred women of "child-bearing potential" from most drug studies to protect their reproductive systems and their potential fetuses. Before a woman, any woman — even a celibate or lesbian — would be allowed to ingest the latest pharmaceutical wonder, the drug had to be tested on female animals to gauge its impact on their reproductive system and their offspring. No mention was made of studying the impact of drugs on male sperm production.

The upshot was that most drugs licensed for the market were never tested on women at all.

There was an exception in the regulations for women facing life-threatening diseases. When McGovern mentioned it, Hoffmann–La Roche refused to recognize it as applying to AIDS. She produced studies completed on related drugs that suggested that tat inhibitors would have no long-term negative impact on women's reproductive systems. Dr. Paul Oestreicher of Hoffmann–La Roche responded that a woman's egg was too vulnerable to take the risk. What about a man's sperm? McGovern asked. Oestreicher declared the relative indestructibility of sperm — although there was a paucity of proof for that position — and refused to allow McGovern's client into the early drug study.

McGovern was helpless against Hoffmann–La Roche, so she took aim at the FDA, which had written the regulations in the first place. She wasn't a doctor, but she didn't need four years in medical school to understand that the 1977 regulations were woefully unspecific. They contained no clear guidelines for the required animal reproduction studies, no timetable for when the studies should be done and no mention of how the FDA would use the results. There was nothing about studying the drug's impact on a man's sperm or on the male reproductive system — although everyone knew that birth defects weren't caused exclusively by females. In McGovern's view, two things were clear from the regulations: the agency was harming women by protecting them from experimental medications, and drugs tested exclusively on men were being sold to both sexes — despite ample evidence that men and women react differently to many pharmaceutical agents.

McGovern had never realized how much work women's health care advocates had left to do. In December 1992 she began her part, filing a citizens' petition requesting that the FDA commissioner amend the 1977 guidelines to end discriminatory practices against women. She was intent on forcing the agency to take women seriously as something more than fetus carriers, to open up drug trials to female participants and to force drug companies to study male-female differences in drug reactions. In concrete terms, she was demanding that the FDA give women and men equal access to experimental drugs, either by waiving all restrictions on female participation in trials or by requiring drug companies to complete animal reproduction studies before giving drugs to human beings of either gender.

Female AIDS patients and activists from around the country rallied to McGovern's support. But reaction from male activists was lukewarm at best. By insisting that the FDA stop drug trials that excluded women, McGovern was threatening their access to experimental medications. By demanding that companies complete animal reproductive system studies before giving drugs to human beings, she might force delays in the distribution of drugs.

The FDA had caved in to the pressure of male activists, giving them access to experimental drugs despite minimal proof of safety and no proof of effectiveness. The men had gained considerable influence at the agency; they used none of it to advance the needs of women with AIDS.

Meanwhile, the FDA didn't even take the women seriously enough to put McGovern's petition on the front burner. In fact, they didn't even reply. Then, in July 1993, the FDA proudly unveiled a new series of guidelines purporting to address women's concerns. "Window-dressing" was what McGovern called them.

The new guidelines paid lip service to the importance of analyzing the safety and effectiveness of drugs by gender, but they did not require companies to test drugs on women. The FDA reserved the right to make such a demand, but made no mention of when it would do so, how the decision would be made, or by whom. It was worse than that. The agency advised that there should be no "unwarranted restriction on women's participation in trials," but failed to define where "warranted" ended and "unwarranted" began. For example, the FDA continued to stress the importance of requiring female trial participants to use birth control. Was requiring an IUD, even in women with a disease that predisposed them to cervical cancer, warranted? The FDA didn't say. Was requiring a lesbian who never had sex with a man to use birth control pills unwarranted? The FDA didn't say. And what if a woman understood the risks but just didn't want to practice birth control? Again, the FDA didn't say.

Despite the new woman-friendly language in the guidelines, the FDA conducted business as usual. The problem was as much capitalism as paternalism. In explaining the agency's unwillingness to require pharmaceutical companies to complete animal reproduction studies before human testing, FDA representatives argued that it would impose financial hardship on business. Since most drugs that enter testing turn out to be worthless, FDA Commissioner David Kessler argued, drug companies could wait until there was evidence that a product might make it to the market before proceeding with another round of tests. Until then, women of "childbearing potential" — premenopausal women not on birth control — should be kept off experimental drugs, not only to protect them and their potential fetuses, but to protect drug companies from future lawsuits over drug-induced birth defects.

McGovern did not share Kessler's concern for the fiscal well-being of multi-billion-dollar companies, and she confronted the FDA's concern about future litigation head-on. "You want to protect yourselves from lawsuits?" she asked them. "You better worry about the one I'll file — and it won't take twenty years."

McGovern pressed her demands for a revolution at the FDA. She wanted an end to a paternalistic system that presupposed that women weren't competent to make decisions about their own bodies; an end to regulations that treated women as incubators and showed more concern for the welfare of often nonexistent fetuses than the health of existing women; and an end to the marketing of drugs that have never been tested on women. She summed it up in one simple phrase: "All protocol criteria must be gender neutral."

The FDA stalled for almost eighteen months.

By the spring of 1994, McGovern was no longer doing battle with the agency as an outsider. A few months before, when President Clinton authorized the formation of a special task force to identify barriers to swift development and approval of AIDS drugs, McGovern was asked to join. She suddenly had a forum that included Dr. Phil Lee, the head of the U.S. Public Health Service, and Dr. Harold Varmus, director of the National Institutes of Health. The recommendations of the task force would carry weight at the presidential level, and McGovern was determined to use her new clout to move the FDA into the twentieth century.

When the task force met in July, at one of the scores of faceless hotels that ring the nation's capital, McGovern gave a lengthy report on women and drug testing and laid out the problems she'd encountered repeatedly with the FDA. When she was done Dr. Lee, the task force chairman, asked McGovern about the status of her petition.

"Nothing, basically," she answered. Kessler was seated across the room with members of his staff. "The new guidelines were a response to it."

Nonsense, retorted Ruth Merkatz, an assistant FDA commissioner. "It is very active," she said. "I guess we spend quite a bit of time each week on that petition — even though you have not received the response from us." McGovern and her supporters wondered how the FDA could have been working on the petition for hours each week without consulting them and without issuing any new guidelines.

Merkatz acknowledged the "growing societal recognition that participation of women in drug trials up until that point was paternalistic, that [the FDA] failed to consider a woman's capacity to make a decision for herself as to whether or not she wished to enter into a trial." She admitted that 50 percent of the drug studies yielded no information on gender differences in a drug's impact.

Yet Merkatz also asserted that the FDA had reformed. McGovern went on the offensive, raising the questions posed again and again by her clients: "If I'm not having sex with a man, if I'm willing to utilize birth control, if I'm terminally ill, how can they do this? Does the government know that if I were to become pregnant or if I was pregnant, the fetus would be damaged, or is this just speculation?"

McGovern went on to attack the FDA with the results of a 1992 investigation by the General Accounting Office that confirmed that 25 percent of all drug manufacturers don't try to recruit women for their trials — and that 50 percent had never been asked to do so. She demonstrated how sexism pervaded every corner of the biomedical research establishment, from the National Institutes of Health to the FDA. As of 1990, she reminded the group, just 6 percent of the participants in drug trials sponsored by the federally funded AIDS Clinical Trials Group were female, which meant that virtually no information was available on the impact of AIDS drugs on women.

She reminded them that AZT, the gold standard against which all other anti-HIV drugs were measured, had never been evaluated for its safety and efficacy in women — and that the animal reproduction studies suggested that it might cause vaginal cancer; that there were almost no women in the studies of ddI, and that the research design required no Pap smears or other female-specific diagnostic tests for the few who participated; that there had been no attempt to study whether ddI caused gynecological problems because researchers had decided, on the basis of no evidence, that it did not; that there had been no attempt to discover whether AZT and ddI were more or less effective in women than in men because researchers had decided, on the basis of no evidence, that there was no possible gender differential.

Terry McGovern had done her homework. She detailed not only the paternalism of the FDA and NIH toward women's health, but also those same agencies' willingness to subject women to risk whenever researchers wanted to study ways to cut down on mother-to-child HIV transmission. In late 1989, a researcher at Children's Hospital in Newark had informed the FDA that his team was kicking around the idea of giving pregnant women high doses of AZT, to test whether the drug might reduce the number of infants born infected.

It was an alarming proposal. AZT is notoriously toxic. No one knew what impact the drug might have on fetal development, but animal studies suggested it might cause cervical cancer in mothers. Two-thirds of the infants born to infected women were HIV negative even without AZT, and cesarean section births promised to raise that figure further. Yet the proposal worked its way through the federal bureaucracies charged with designing and approving new research designs with startling speed and support.

"When they want to stop transmission to fetuses, they aren't afraid to bombard women with AZT," McGovern said, "but when it's for a woman's own health, they're afraid of hurting her reproductive system. It's pretty clear. When it's just a matter of a woman's health, they don't seem to give a damn."

The FDA slinked away from the July task force meeting after promising to respond to McGovern's demands before the panel's next session in October. On the eve of that meeting, McGovern was laying out the next day's battle plan — an attack on the FDA's lack of response — when Commissioner David Kessler offered to provide her with a written response to her 1992 petition, if she would promise not to attack it before his representative could make her presentation to the full committee.

The next day, McGovern's supporters — including women from ACT UP who held up signs reading KESSLER MAKES US SICK and WHITE MALE SCIENCE IS BAD SCIENCE — filled the seats reserved for the public. Janet Woodcock spoke for the Food and Drug Administration. The agency could find no justification for including women in early drug tests, she said, and downplayed the importance of the animal reproduction studies called for in the FDA's own regulations. They were "not predictive" of what would happen in female humans. McGovern was floored by the latter position. "Then why have they been predicating everything on those studies for the past fifty years?" she asked.

The only movement from the FDA was its agreement to amend its regulations to require drug companies to analyze drugs by gender. That sounded good to the uninitiated, but McGovern was very much initiated.

"What do you mean when you say 'by gender' analysis?" she asked. Did the FDA plan to require researchers to conduct specific studies on the differential impact of drugs on men and women, or was the agency going to allow researchers to get away with reporting only the number of women in each trial?

Woodcock would not commit herself. The ACT UP contingent began handing out waffles to the audience.

Finally Commissioner Kessler took over and turned the discussion into an inquisition, with McGovern as the accused. She was thrilled. As he led her through a long Q-and-A about the history of the debate and the actions of the FDA, she recited chapter and verse on every regulatory change and nonchange, on every obfuscation and inconsistency that had characterized the debate for almost two years. When the meeting ended, Kessler and his colleagues left the hotel with a deadline: the task force had agreed to vote on McGovern's recommendations at its January 1995 meeting.

FDA officials weren't the only ones caught between the demands of McGovern and her supporters and the traditional mindset of scientists. One physician who tried to bar all women from a research trial testing the value of thalidomide as an anti-HIV drug was not only a woman but a strong feminist. For Dr. Gilla Kaplan, the drug conjured up the image of hundreds of European children born with undeveloped limbs and organs because their mothers had used thalidomide to fight nausea. In her eyes, it was too dangerous to give the drug to women who might be or might become pregnant.

Although sympathetic to arguments about paternalism, Kaplan and many other researchers saw FDA and NIH regulations as well-meaning attempts to protect the weak and vulnerable. They remembered all too well how Puerto Rican women had been used as guinea pigs in the testing of birth control pills, and how retarded children at the Willowbrook School in New York had been used in hepatitis experiments in the 1960s.

Dr. Kaplan wanted to avoid those disasters. She believed in the government's role as a protective force. And that was the difference. Unlike Kaplan, female AIDS activists and patients — among them lesbians, poor women, African Americans and Latinas — couldn't imagine government agencies as benevolent. They didn't know or care about Willowbrook or radiation experiments. Lesbians who have fought for custody of their children, black women raised on their community's suspicion of all authorities, and junkies who've been hassled by government agents of all stripes knew about government protectiveness, and didn't trust it.

What sounded like well-meaning concern to physicians like Kaplan was interpreted by patients and activists to be the type of white paternalism blacks rejected decades earlier. "I don't need no honky woman in a fancy office to protect me from doctors," said Sonia Singleton, a Miami AIDS activist who died in February 1992. Singleton, an educated African American woman who'd spent years on the streets, sometimes trading sex for drugs, was an early warning voice to black women. She delivered her "Read My Lipstick, Women Get AIDS Too" sermon in black churches, at community meetings and political caucuses. "Doctors who don't live in my neighborhood don't know what I need," she said. "I know what I need. The women I work with are equally competent to make their own decisions if people will only give them the information that everyone else seems to get. Just give me that information, stay off my back — and out of my womb."

Neither side of the dispute acknowledged that they were caught in the tension that has characterized American debate on everything from seat belts and motorcycle helmets to regulation of adult sexual behavior. The nation has never found a comfortable balance between keeping the government off the backs of the citizenry and expecting the government to protect the citizenry.

And no one feels much need to be consistent. The same conservatives who plan to use their new power in Congress to loosen federal control over everything from education to child welfare nonetheless want to regulate abortion or maintain laws declaring same-gender sex illegal. In the name of feminism — a movement that has demanded federal action to protect women from discrimination — Terry McGovern and her supporters protest that the government is protecting women too much.

Wanting it both ways, of course, is hardly unique to feminist AIDS activists. But the reversal of positions has been most ironic in regard to the single issue that holds the greatest potential to save women's lives. Partner notification — the new, more politically correct name for the old system of contact tracing — is a tried-and-true approach used for decades in syphilis and gonorrhea cases. It means that when a physician diagnoses a patient with a disease slated for notification, he or she reports the patient to a central health agency. A counselor there then contacts the infected person and offers to notify his or her sex partners that they have been exposed. The infected person's name is never mentioned, although many of those notified can undoubtedly guess who the person might be. No one is forced to name names, but everyone is offered the chance to warn former partners.

The system relieves the infected individual of the embarrassment and trauma of calling old boyfriends or ex-wives and delivering potentially disastrous news. It means individuals at risk can be warned to get tested. If infected, they can receive early diagnosis and treatment. They can be taught how to protect themselves and others to stop the chain of transmission.

It's not a perfect system. When contact tracing was studied in North Carolina, the results showed that only half of the sexual partners of infected men and women had been notified. But when individuals were left to inform their partners directly, only 7 percent received the information. Nonetheless, public health authorities have shied away from advocating partner notification, and feminist AIDS activists have done nothing to try to modify their position. Both groups seem to be bowing to the wishes and views of gay male AIDS activists, who have feared contact tracing since the beginning of the epidemic. Female activists declared women's access to experimental drugs a right, but they balked on granting the same status to lifesaving information.

Gay opposition to contact tracing made sense in the early years of the epidemic. The idea of a centralized list of AIDS patients conjured up not entirely paranoid visions of a plot to round them up and cart them off to concentration camps. Short of that, gay leaders worried that contact tracing would inevitably violate the confidentiality of people with AIDS. A city official, say, would call the office of an infected person, speak indiscreetly to a secretary or receptionist and wind up letting everyone know he had HIV. Or a counselor would call a patient at home, run into his mother and inadvertently tip her off to her son's sexual orientation. Public disclosure might not hurt people with syphilis or tuberculosis, gay activists said, but there is a stigma to AIDS that drives people into hiding. Contact tracing would only reinforce that tendency, discouraging gay men from being tested, thus negating the very AIDS awareness and prevention that public health workers sought to increase.

Contact tracing was probably irrelevant in the gay community, where the deaths of so many so quickly provided a brutal course in AIDS awareness. Gay men, particularly those in urban areas who'd built their social lives around bars, bathhouses and parks, didn't need public health workers knocking on their doors to discover they'd been exposed to HIV; they already knew they had. And given the anonymity of many of their sexual encounters, few infected men could have produced a list of their partners even if they wanted to.

The combination of that logic and gay political clout was sufficient to dissuade most politicians from pressing for contact tracing. Bills mandating the process were defeated in Congress, and public health officials, in New York and other cities, who continued to support notification were branded as unrepentant homophobes. As a result, for almost a decade the rights of the infected have been declared superior to the rights of the unsuspecting. The confidentiality of an individual's HIV status is protected by a wall of legislation that makes disclosure an offense punishable by hefty fines or imprisonment. In almost all states the burden of notifying partners rests solely on the infected individual — although few have been willing to bear it.

The opposition to partner notification is so strong that attempts to notify spouses of dead people have been roundly defeated by civil libertarians and activist zealots less worried about the privacy of the dead than about allowing any chinks in the armor of total confidentiality. The first proposal for spousal notification of the deceased came from New York City medical examiner Charles Hirsch, who'd been performing HIV tests during autopsies since 1989. He'd been using the information to track the course of the epidemic and eventually realized it might help the living as well. Why not turn the names of HIV-positive corpses over to the city health department so they can at least inform wives and kids?

Hirsch's suggestion quickly got lost in one of those political quagmires endemic in New York City. The incoming mayor, David Dinkins, shelved the plan and turned the matter over to a task force appointed by his new health commissioner for full analysis of its myriad legal, ethical and political implications. A year later, in March 1991, the task force's report cautiously endorsed Hirsch's proposal and, in addition, recommended expansion of the city's tiny, little-known, voluntary contact-tracing program. "Informing all women — not only some women who are identified by partners as being at specific risk — must be the priority," the report said. The task force undid its own recommendations, however, by insisting that no resources be diverted from existing programs to finance either effort.

In some states, exceptions are made that permit physicians to inform spouses — or ask the city's partner-notification officer to do so — if they have clear reason to believe that the infected mate will not warn his or her unsuspecting partner. But physicians are not stupid. Violations of the confidentiality laws can carry $5,000 fines, and few doctors have been willing to risk overstepping their bounds even with the spousal-notification exception written into the law. In New York, for example, not a single physician had referred a name to the city's contact-tracing office by 1993.

Total confidentiality has been one of those sacred cows that no one with any ambitions to political success or widespread credibility has dared touch. But by 1990, if not before, the face of AIDS had changed too drastically for old truths not to be questioned. Gay men who'd lived in the fast lane knew they were at risk. Men and women who'd shared needles while shooting drugs had learned they had something new to fear. But the fastest-growing group of infected Americans, heterosexual women, were frequently clueless — and impervious to all messages of caution. When they were finally diagnosed, such women repeatedly asked, "Why didn't anyone tell me my husband had AIDS? Didn't I have the right to know?" Obviously, new approaches were warranted.

"The voices that have dominated the debate so far have been male, coercive, public health voices at one end and ACT UP at the other," observed Catherine Lynch, the director of women's issues for the Gay Men's Health Crisis. "And guess what, they're all boys. No one's looked at women's stake in this issue."

Women's stake was clearly high, and growing. New York City health officials estimated that one-third of the state's twenty-five thousand infected women had acquired the virus through heterosexual sex. Few had been aware of the risks to their lives.

- Catherine Burling hadn't really thought about AIDS when she fell in love at her Vermont college. She was 19. It was summer, the flowers were in bloom, the romance was whirlwind and the engagement was announced in late August. Then the young man disappeared, leaving behind a cryptic note declaring that Cathy was "the only woman" he had ever loved. The bereft teenager didn't understand the implications of the phrase until she received a hefty phone bill for calls to a 900 number that turned out to be a gay sex line, until she answered the phone one afternoon and heard a man demanding money, saying that her fiancé was bisexual, and a junkie to boot. Six months later — two days before her 20th birthday — Cathy Burling, who had never known any junkies, and didn't quite understand the prevalence of bisexuality, received a legacy of the relationship: she was diagnosed HIV positive.
- Marie Tulman never thought about AIDS when she remarried in 1983. Her husband had been an intravenous drug user in the 1970s, but he'd been clean for two years when Marie met him in 1982. Even when the epidemic hit the front pages, Marie still never considered that she might be at risk. She was diagnosed by accident — when she gave blood during a Red Cross drive at work. "I married into the virus," she said.
- One New Yorker learned she was playing the 1990s version of Russian roulette only after her infant died and was diagnosed with

AIDS at the autopsy. When the woman received the results of the coroner's investigation, she was confused and hysterical. It made no sense. She called her husband at work and begged him to come home. "So you have AIDS," he barked at her when he stormed into the house, blaming her for murdering their child. He insisted she'd been infected by her first husband, whom she'd divorced twelve years earlier. He was not, in fact, the culprit. It was actually her second husband, the man who had ranted at her. He had never told his wife that he'd been an IV drug user.

• A middle-aged Hispanic woman from the Bronx was infected through her own naiveté. When her husband lay dying of a disease no one would name, a counselor at Lincoln Hospital suggested that she be tested for HIV. "To test means I would distrust everything we built our lives on," the woman responded. "I've been monogamous for so many years. I know my husband has never shot up. He's not gay. He's never with another woman. Every time he goes out, he just goes out with one male friend."

Of the 25,896 individuals tested in New York in 1991, only 933 said they had come in because a partner had warned them they'd been exposed. By 1993 strong confidentiality laws and even stronger state and federal laws against discrimination provided sufficient protection against abuses of any partner-notification system. A few timid voices began to suggest that the time had come to reconsider contact tracing.

"This is very much a women's issue," said Dr. Kathleen Toomey of the Centers for Disease Control, citing data from her six-year study of partner-notification strategies. "What we've found is that seventy percent of partners were never told by their sex partners who knew." And most of the partners who didn't know they were at risk were women. For Toomey, partner notification is "as much a matter of ethics as one of public health efficacy."

Some gay male activists have been more moved by the argument. Tom Stoddard, former head of Lambda Legal Defense and Education Fund — and a man who once labeled a San Francisco plan to contact the female partners of HIV-infected bisexuals "Orwellian" — has begun to reconsider his opposition. "Over time, I've come to believe contact tracing may be desirable if it's conducted in a way that's sensitive to all the people involved," he said. "We all tend to see things based on personal experience. My experience reflected the fact that I am a gay man and an advocate of other gay people. I have no or little sympathy for a gay man who doesn't try to protect himself today, at least one who lives in New York, because they have been given every chance to know they're at risk. Heterosexual women are simply differently situated."

But the same female AIDS activists who have fought the Social Security Administration and the CDC, the FDA and NIH to provide women access to drugs and services balk at the single proposal that might help women avoid the necessity for either. "People who advocate partner notification aren't taking the problems of confidentiality seriously enough," says Terry McGovern. "My clients are terrified that people might find out that they are positive. They're afraid of spousal abuse, of losing their children, of getting beaten up by the neighbors."

McGovern is one of many AIDS activists who insist that instead of partner notification, women need better education about the risks of HIV. Ironically, it is the supporters of contact tracing who understand why education alone does not speak to the reality of most women's lives. "It assumes a level playing field between men and women, and it isn't," says Kathleen Toomey. "Women don't have control over how sex occurs and when sex occurs."

In the end, the failure of many female AIDS activists — most of whom are lesbians — to support partner notification reflects their tendency to identify themselves by sexual orientation rather than by gender and their own conflicting feelings about the politics of AIDS, about the attention the epidemic has given gay men and about their own continuing invisibility as lesbians.

The history of lesbian AIDS activism can be written as a tale of noble self-sacrifice. When gay men first began to notice the sick among them, lesbian activists were torn. The two communities had lived apart for decades. Women who remembered how few gay men had raised money for battered women's shelters or volunteered at rape crisis centers asked why they should offer their support to gay male causes. Lesbians had their own serious problems, after all, as women and as lesbians. But in the end they moved into the breach, spending hours tending the dying, donating time and money to build AIDS service organizations and information centers. It is no surprise that the three most prominent private AIDS physicians in Miami are lesbians — a pattern that can be seen elsewhere in the country. Lesbian writers and artists have responded to the epidemic, trying to rouse the conscience of the nation. Lesbians fill the volunteer rosters at AIDS service groups in every city.

Their concern was not entirely selfless: lesbians worried that their sexual activities might put them, too, at risk. But epidemiologists refused to take their concerns seriously; they simply weren't seeing cases of woman-to-woman sexual transmission of HIV. Lesbians were suspicious of this, knowing from long history that lesbian invisibility has a high price. Were public health officials asking the right questions? Were they looking for woman-to-woman transmission? Were they even considering the possibility?

Officials at the Centers for Disease Control insisted they were — and had turned up only one case. It made sense. In heterosexual sex, it is extremely rare for a woman to transmit HIV to her male partner — seventeen times less likely than for an infected man to transmit the virus to a woman. There just isn't much virus in vaginal secretions.

But lesbian AIDS activists were loath to believe the arguments. They leafleted the delegates to the Fifth International Conference on AIDS in Montreal, complaining that only one of seven thousand papers presented concerned lesbians. Another example of lesbian invisibility, they screamed. After all, lesbians across the country were turning up with HIV and AIDS, yet activists seemed determined to ignore the fact that when asked about their sexual behavior and drug histories, almost all the infected women admitted that they'd had sex with men or shot up drugs. Yes, lesbians have AIDS, the CDC admitted, but not because they are lesbians.

In July 1994 Italian researchers published the results of a study of eighteen lesbian couples in which a single partner was HIV infected. Despite regular sexual activity — mutual masturbation, oral sex, anal manipulation, sex during menstruation and sharing of sex toys — none of the uninfected partners later tested positive. That settles that, epidemiologists argued.

Lesbian activists were not appeased. The following month they pointed to the cases of two Texas lesbians who tested positive and said they could not possibly have been infected through needle sharing or unsafe sex with men. Epidemiologists retorted that it was just two people, and anyway, who knew whether they were telling the truth. Lesbian activists who had been quick to dismiss concerns over the infection of a Florida dentist's patients as too aberrant to warrant much attention refused to be dissuaded.

No amount of research stopped their ranting about the risks of woman-to-woman transmission. No amount of common sense quieted their insistence on claiming a bigger share of this epidemic, a higher percentage of the sympathy accorded the dying, a greater role as actors — and not stagehands — in the drama. Lesbians who had watched men turn condoms into multicolored fashion statements had to have their own accessories, from easily sterilized sex toys to dental dams. They demanded funding for lesbian-transmission studies and lesbian safe-sex seminars. They forced major AIDS service providers to set up special programs for lesbians with AIDS. They brought their own contingents to rallies and meetings.

It was not politically correct to mention it, but the lesbians diagnosed with AIDS continued to be women who'd had sex with men or shot up drugs — whether they called themselves lesbians or not. Fifteen years into the epidemic, the number of women infected through lesbian sex remains in the single digits. It has become difficult to escape the conclusion that lesbians demanding more studies of woman-to-woman transmission are suffering from a different disease: lesbian AIDS envy.

"The whole thing has gotten more ridiculous with time," said Dr. Don Francis, one of the nation's foremost AIDS experts. "It's so absurd and has gone on so long that it's hard not to get angry. First they insisted that everything should be labeled gay-bisexual and lesbian. Then they started talking about dental dams, which are expensive and really silly. Saran Wrap is better if you're really that worried . . . Spending energy and money on lesbian transmission is a waste of resources. There are three cases in the literature. I've read them. It's absolutely clear."

Lesbian AIDS envy is an understandable human reaction to a crisis that has given gay men tremendous public visibility. Gay pride rallies have become AIDS rallies. Gay publications, even while adopting more politically correct language that includes women, devote columns to health and disease problems with little relevance to most gay women.

When it became clear that unless they volunteered for infection, lesbians would never have to worry about AIDS, their leadership contrived other concerns. Lesbian journalists began writing about breast cancer as their own epidemic and stormed the CDC demanding more funding for "lesbian-specific breast cancer." No one was sure what that meant, since pathologists never found a rainbow flag, pink triangle or any other symbol of Gay America in breast tissue samples. Although women without children are at increased risk for breast cancer, not all lesbians are childless, and not all childless women are lesbians.

This lesbian response might have been merely pathetic or laughable if it weren't so damaging to women's AIDS activism, a movement they dominate. Pushing a lesbian agenda where it had no place, they have managed to undercut their own effectiveness in promoting a wider women's agenda that is urgent. They have made women's issues a joke while women lay dying.

Nowhere was the problem more obvious than at the moment when the women's activists, including Terry McGovern, got their meeting with one of the most powerful people in the nation.

Donna Shalala, the secretary of the Department of Health and Human Services, seemed to be at ease in her new domain as she entered her conference room on Friday, April 23, 1993, with her minions in tow. She wore the uniform of an executive in a less than hip corporation. In her tailored black suit and black-and-white-patterned blouse, she looked crisp, and in charge.

For Shalala it was just another in the endless series of meetings that were the daily round of a senior government official. For the fifteen women who sat around the enormous conference table awaiting her arrival, it was a momentous occasion. For years they'd watched the male AIDS activists walk into the inner sanctums of power and emerge with their demands translated into new realities. After four years of arguing, demonstrating and shouting, they'd finally reached the pinnacle of power — a meeting with the woman who controlled the Centers for Disease Control, the Public Health Service, the Social Security Administration, the National Institutes of Health and the Food and Drug Administration.

"We wouldn't be here if you had addressed the situation adequately," said Mary Lucey, a lesbian with AIDS who seemed oblivious to the fact that the woman across the table had been in office less than three months. "We would like to talk, you can listen." Their blue jeans and leather jackets, metal-studded leather bracelets and radical buttons were an in-your-face statement: we're not going to kowtow to you and your power. They'd brought their own camera team to record the event. Shalala ignored the challenge and reminded the women that her time was tight.

Serious, life-threatening problems confronted women with AIDS: denial, husbands who cheated and boyfriends who lied, ignorant gynecologists, recalcitrant scientists and paternalistic regulatory agencies. Some scientists were suggesting that estrogen might hasten the development of AIDS; no money had been targeted to explore the possibility. Few of those issues were mentioned except in passing. Here's what the activists chose to highlight:

Dorothy, a young blond woman from San Francisco, complained that the CDC had listed her in its case reports as a heterosexual woman, not a lesbian. In fact, the federal agency maintains no list of the sexual orientation of people with AIDS, just a record of the means by which HIV was transmitted to them. Dorothy's real complaint seemed to be that she was invisible — whatever that meant.

Mary Lucey's partner hammered away at lesbian HIV transmission, citing data on self-identified lesbians with AIDS, ignoring the number of those women who acknowledged having sex with men or sharing needles. A Florida woman used her three minutes to complain about the CDC's refusal to track lesbians infected in tattoo parlors. The Seattle representative demanded that Dr. Robert Gallo be fired from the National Cancer Institute for incompetence. Mary Lucey wanted Dr. David Kessler ousted from the FDA and a thorough housecleaning at the CDC.

At the end of the session, as Shalala rose to leave, an African American woman quick to identify herself as a heterosexual — the group seemingly couldn't find a lesbian of color to attend — wanted to talk about housing. But by then no one was paying much attention. The group's parting comment to Shalala was "Don't forget to use the L word."

They never heard from Donna Shalala again.

EIGHT

The Immaculate Transmission

In the summer of 1989, a young Florida woman who was waiting tables during her college break mysteriously fainted on the job. It was her first glimmer of trouble, and the launching point for the most baffling, infuriating and ultimately misunderstood episode of the AIDS epidemic. The whole truth of it would never be told. The whole truth of it would never be known.

By the time Kimberly Bergalis died twenty-eight months later, she had become the most deified, demonized and debated virgin in America. Her defenders attached agendas to her that she was too frail to carry. Her detractors attached epithets to her that she was too guileless to deserve. They called her a slut, a cunt and a pig. Their letters showed up in her parents' mailbox even after her funeral. "Thank God the bitch is finally dead," one read. "She got what was coming to her."

Her treatment was petty, ugly and uncompromising.

It perfectly captured the tone of most discussions about HIV testing in America.

George and Anna Bergalis rushed their daughter to Indian River Memorial Hospital in Vero Beach on December 4, 1989. Kim had been sick for months, afflicted with chronic vaginal infections, a strange white fungus in her mouth and debilitating exhaustion. Just before Thanksgiving, when her puzzled physician examined her yet again, he suggested she might have leukemia.

Now, just a few weeks later, she could barely breathe. A doctor at North Florida Hospital hadn't taken that complaint seriously, thinking her just another hysterical, hyperventilating female. So her parents had rushed to Gainesville, where Kimberly was a student, to bring her home. By the time she arrived at the hospital in Vero Beach, her fever wouldn't budge below 102, and doctors warned that she might not last the night.

When the hospital laboratory performed its tests, they found *Pneumocystis carinii* pneumonia in her lungs, an immune system in virtual collapse — and HIV in her blood. "Your daughter has AIDS," the doctor solemnly informed George and Anna Bergalis.

It was hardly the news that this kind of family expected to receive. George was the finance director for the city of Fort Pierce, and his wife was a public health nurse. With three daughters, they were raising what they thought of as a normal American family, immune to disasters like AIDS.

Kimberly had just finished up at the University of Florida and was staying on there to train as an actuary. Except for her addiction to Barry Manilow, she seemed a pretty typical recent college graduate. She loved Tom Hanks movies, and watched *Continental Divide* — the 1981 John Belushi–Blair Brown attempt to go Tracy and Hepburn one better — whenever it came on HBO. At night in her dorm room, she cut her girlfriends' hair and traded gossip. When she came home on vacations, she and her sister Allison would buy bread and walk to the beach to feed the birds.

"Have you had sex?" the Bergalises asked their daughter. Even though Kim was twenty-one, intercourse was still not a comfortable topic of conversation in their strict Catholic family.

"No," Kim said quietly.

"Used drugs?"

"Never," she responded.

"What the hell is going on here?" they asked each other.

The family tiptoed through the possibilities. Kim had never had a blood transfusion. She'd never stepped on a needle at the beach. No acupuncture. No tattoos. No surgery, except for those two teeth she'd had pulled two years before.

They thought about that dentist. He'd been sick a lot recently. His office had been closed for weeks at a time. His staff had told his patients he had cancer.

The Bergalises had long assumed that Dr. Acer was gay. They hadn't cared. He was a good dentist. But suddenly, as they looked at Kim, pale and wasting, the thought of a gay dentist with cancer began to have a more ominous ring.

• • •

Kimberly Bergalis's case report arrived at the AIDS Program Office in Tallahassee within days. Such reporting is the law in every state. Her physician sent in all the usual information: name, address, race, age, date of diagnosis and illnesses. The only item missing was risk factor — the most vital piece of information for epidemiologists trying to track an epidemic. "NIR," the physician had checked off: No Identifiable Risk.

That was hardly unusual. Hundreds of AIDS case reports came in with NIR checked off. Sometimes patients died before their physicians could quiz them about their sexual histories or drug use. More often, patients just lied. But Kim's report caught the eye of the people in state government whose job it was to track AIDS. She was out of the ordinary for an AIDS patient: young, female, white, middle class and claiming to be a virgin. This last characteristic was perhaps the most peculiar.

Florida had been trying to beef up its AIDS surveillance operation and sent Nikki Economu in to investigate. An aggressive young woman who'd worked as a private detective, Economu didn't seem to buy Kim's story, and neither did her bosses in Tallahassee. It wasn't just that there weren't that many virgins graduating from the University of Florida. It was also that Kim's teeth had been pulled only two years earlier. Two years was a very short time in HIV infection. Most of those infected show little or no immune damage in that period, and less than one in twenty is sick.

Kimberly Bergalis must have had a lover, Florida health department officials concluded. They grilled Kim. "Did you ever have an intimate relationship? Were your clothes on or off? Did you ever have oral sex?" They queried her friends. "Did she sleep around? Did her father abuse her?" They quizzed her old boyfriends and tested them — even the one in Central America — for HIV. They even showed up at her house unannounced to ask Kim if she ever had sex with animals.

Kim explained that she hadn't even been allowed to date in high school and that she had decided years earlier to be a virgin when she married. She gave investigators a list of her friends and acquaintances, her ex-boyfriends, even some guy she'd dated just three times.

"Enough," Kim declared after yet another grilling.

But they didn't give up. Which was odd. By then, more than 4,000 Americans reported to have AIDS were listed as NIR. Few of their cases were treated as full-scale investigations.

Florida officials insist that they were simply trying to solve a medical puzzle. But her former colleagues say that Economu was hot to prove a new mode of HIV transmission. Everyone knew that health care workers could be infected by patients. Couldn't the infection travel in the opposite direction? No one had charted it yet. The person who did would draw career-making attention.

Like a good detective, Economu began by trying to poke holes in Kim's story. She insinuated herself into the family, becoming a friend and confidante. She persuaded Kim to talk about old boyfriends. But the stories were about how they took her to church every week or cooked her dinner. There was kissing, yes, and petting, but no intercourse. Economu became so aggressive that the Bergalis family finally decided that she didn't believe their daughter, and kicked her out of the house.

While epidemiologists puzzled over case #242284, the Bergalis family began their own private nightmare journey through AIDS. Kim was frightened that if word of her illness leaked out, her house would be spray painted and the family cars pelted with eggs. "I was afraid this would disgrace her and the other children," George said. "I thought people would believe that we were all a bunch of sleazy characters. I thought we should just let her die her painful, wasting death at home and not let anyone know what was going on." The Bergalises told everyone that Kimberly had a rare blood disorder.

David Acer was one of thousands of gay men who'd spent his life cowering in the closet.

Born and raised in Ohio, he'd set up practice in Jensen Beach, Florida, in 1980 after a three-year tour in the air force. His office in the First Union Bank building was always filled with patients, referred to him by a local HMO. In less than a decade, he built up a large practice of three or four thousand.

But no one in town seemed to know him very well. Acer didn't sink roots into the small, conservative community. He didn't gossip with his patients. Like gay men in small towns all across America, he traveled two hours for his fun and romance, hoping that no one in Fort Lauderdale's gay bars would recognize him as the dentist from the Treasure Coast.

Acer's secretiveness deepened in 1986, when the reality of AIDS began to filter into his life. A former sexual partner told the dentist that he had tested positive; Acer might want to get tested too. He didn't follow the advice. That was common practice among gay men in the days before medicine seemed to offer any hope to the infected, and when discrimination seemed a lethal force.

Acer eventually did find a doctor, but he traveled eighty miles to Fort Lauderdale for his medical care. Even then, he registered under the assumed name of David Johnson.

In September 1987 his secret became harder to keep. Lesions appeared in Acer's mouth, and he drove forty miles to West Palm Beach to consult with another dentist. The biopsy was conclusive: Kaposi's sarcoma. David Acer's name — the real one — was added to Florida's AIDS registry.

For months, the thirty-seven-year-old dentist drove back and forth between Jensen Beach and Miami for treatment at the Veterans Administration Medical Center. Radiation therapy cleared up most of the lesions, and breathing treatments helped ward off pneumonia. But even as he continued filling cavities and pulling teeth, David Acer was trapped in confusion. "Ethically and morally, I think I should not continue with my work without telling anybody," he said to a social worker. But he knew central Florida too well to be naive about the implications of the revelation. He decided to sell his practice, and keep quiet until then.

In June 1989, however, things began to collapse. His lesions had returned in profusion, not just in his mouth but also down into his lungs. His chronic dry cough turned out to be a symptom of *Pneumocystis carinii* pneumonia, and he was hospitalized. By the time he was released, Acer was too weak to continue working. His parents moved down from Pittsburgh to care for him. He sold his dental practice and announced to his patients that he had cancer.

On March 29, 1990, Dr. Carol Ciesielski, a medical epidemiologist for the Centers for Disease Control, told David Acer about Kimberly Bergalis — the implication was clear. No way, Acer insisted. He went over his medical history with Ciesielski, acknowledging himself as bisexual. He told her that he'd had about a dozen patients he suspected of having AIDS, but insisted that he had practiced standard infection-control procedures in his office — masks and gloves and alcohol disinfectants. After he was diagnosed, he'd added an extra cleanup person and began heat-sterilizing instruments he'd just wiped down before. Ciesielski asked for a blood sample so the CDC could try a new type of test to see if his virus's DNA matched Bergalis's.

David Acer agreed without hesitation. He was sure he hadn't infected his young patient.

· · ·

On July 26, 1990, the Centers for Disease Control printed a terse notice in its *Morbidity and Mortality Weekly Report* announcing an investigation into what officers there believed to be the nation's first case of HIV transmission from a health care worker to a patient. The patient was described as a young woman who had had surgery performed by a dentist who'd been diagnosed with AIDS three months before the operation. The CDC did not reveal the location of the case, the name of the patient or dentist, or how transmission occurred, only that the patient's past had been probed thoroughly and no other risk factors were found.

"The possibility that the patient may have been infected through another mode cannot be entirely excluded," the report said. But the CDC did offer a bit of tantalizing proof: the DNA in the dentist's HIV had been compared to the DNA in the patient's; they were nearly identical.

The next evening, as she lay on the couch in her living room in Fort Pierce watching the *NBC Nightly News,* Kim had her moment of vindication. Working from the CDC's publication, Jane Pauley announced the nation's first case of HIV transmission from a health care worker to a patient. The report never mentioned her name, but Kim knew who the patient was. She called her parents into the room to watch the report. Then she sat back in relief. "Thank God. Now everybody will believe I'm a good girl."

Everybody did not.

"Was the patient's hymen intact?" asked skeptical reporters who called the CDC to follow up on the story. "Yes," they responded flatly. "Any signs that she'd had anal intercourse?" others continued. "That's an inappropriate question" was the odd response. "Any indications of other sexually transmissible diseases?" the reporters pressed. "The patient's medical records are confidential."

It seemed a puzzlingly incomplete report for such a momentous announcement. The American Medical Association, when asked to comment, rejected it. "The AMA does not accept this as having been proven," said Dr. M. Roy Schwarz, the association's senior vice president for medical education and science. "They have given us no absolute answers."

Dentists wanted to know what had happened. Had the dentist worn gloves? Had he cut his hand on an instrument or stuck himself with a needle? The CDC offered no answers.

Physicians wanted to know about the DNA testing. Everyone knew about using such testing to establish a person's identity in a criminal case, but no one had ever heard of DNA testing to match viruses. How reliable is it? physicians asked. No response was possible. The procedure for testing and matching genetic material in HIV samples was too new for any honest response. The CDC had compared Bergalis's and Acer's viral DNA map with one another and with samples from around the country. They were more like each other's than they were like the control group's DNA. But what did that mean?

Unlike the kind of DNA tests routinely used in criminal cases, no studies had ever been conducted to verify the accuracy of such matching. The technique was so experimental that Florida health officials had objected to the CDC's releasing of the information. They were particularly concerned about the use of a control group from outside the area where Bergalis and Acer lived. Maybe the virus they had in common was typical of central Florida, they argued, asking the CDC to redo its tests. CDC officials claimed that was unnecessary. "The evidence of transmission is scientifically inconclusive," wrote John Witte, Florida's assistant health officer for disease control, in a final letter to the CDC. His protests were ignored.

When the CDC publicized its conclusion about the unnamed dentist and his unnamed patient, the Bergalis family, deeply hurt by the tragedy in their lives, began their battle for revenge. Robert Montgomery was the general they chose to lead them. One of the most decorated personal-injury lawyers in the country, his spoils included a West Palm Beach mansion, Picassos and a Rolls-Royce. He avoided losing at all costs.

Kim Bergalis was the client of his dreams: mediagenic, tragic and innocent, facing a dentist with $3 million in malpractice insurance and an HMO that had made her referral. The lawsuit was not her idea. Kimberly didn't want people to know she had AIDS. She wasn't looking for a public platform to promote a cause. She just wanted to go quietly without any of her old friends from college finding out she had AIDS. It was her sister Allison who pushed her to take legal action and go public. "It just seemed so unfair that someone could do this to my sister and cause all this pain to my family," said Allison, now a law student.

Allison and her mother made an appointment with Montgomery on their own. At the last minute, Kimberly agreed to tag along and Montgomery offered her a chance to avenge her honor. Within weeks the suit was filed against Acer and the HMO, with the names of Kimberly and Acer coded in initials. When local reporters found the lawsuit, the area was electrified by the news. Who was the patient? More important, who was the dentist? They didn't have to wait long for the answers.

In late August state health department officials met with David Acer for the last time. He was extremely frail. He was clearly dying. They asked for permission to contact all his former patients and offer them HIV testing. Just as they were discussing how to proceed, Acer slipped further toward death. His lungs collapsed and he was readmitted to the VA hospital in Miami. Four days later, on August 31, 1990, he was transferred to the Hospice of Palm Beach County. From his bed there that first night, he wrote a letter that was mailed to two thousand of his former patients for whom authorities had addresses and published in a paid advertisement in local newspapers a week later.

"I am David J. Acer, and I have AIDS," the letter began. "It is with great sorrow and some surprise that I read that I am accused of transmitting HIV virus to one of my patients. I do not understand how such a thing could have happened, and I do not believe it did happen." He nonetheless urged his patients to get tested, and concluded, "Please try to understand. I am a gentle man, and I would never intentionally expose anyone to this disease."

Three days later, David Acer died.

Four days after that, Kimberly Bergalis held a press conference at the Palm Hotel in West Palm Beach and revealed herself as the innocent victim of the dentist with AIDS. Her parents and her ten-year-old sister, Sondra, were at her side. "What we've gone through is an injustice," she said. "If this can be prevented, if new guidelines can be established to prevent this from happening again, then I think that's what needs to be done. If I can protect other people from what happened to me, then I have to do it." Kim ran through the history of her diagnosis and talked about her life with AIDS.

"Now I take it day by day. I try not to think about it. I don't dwell on it. I watch TV, read, write letters, do laundry, run errands. But I have nausea and vomiting throughout the day. I'm in bed by 8 or 8:30 most nights. I don't have much of a social life."

By then the young woman was already fading. After months of experimental and conventional treatments at the University of Miami

Medical School, her immune system was worse than ever. She'd lost thirty-one pounds. Her mother described the situation bluntly: "If there is a hell on earth, we're here."

Kimberly became a celebrity, the innocent young woman whose life had been tragically cut short by the cruelest accident, of fate or social neglect. *People* told her story. Larry King and Phil Donahue called. She appeared on *CBS This Morning* and NBC's *Today* show, calling for mandatory testing of health care workers. When she told a group of schoolchildren that she'd always wanted to go riding in a hot air balloon, *A Current Affair* flew her out to the Grand Canyon.

None of the attention changed the harsh reality: Kim was dying.

September 1990 was a nightmare month for public health workers in Martin County, Florida. An epidemic of St. Louis encephalitis was sweeping through the area, and nothing seemed to kill the mosquitoes. Prisoners in the local jail had been hospitalized with food poisoning. Giardia had broken out in a child care center. In the middle of the chaos, hundreds of David Acer's former patients lined up at the county health department to be tested for HIV. By the time they were finished, five hundred people had been counseled and tested — and told to return.

Two weeks later, reporters heard rumors that two more of Acer's patients had turned up positive. Richard Driskill went from the health department right to Robert Montgomery when he received the bad news. A thirty-one-year-old supervisor at a juice plant, Driskill had seen Acer three times since 1984. Even before the CDC declared that DNA testing had confirmed the link, he was sure why he was sick.

The other patient, Barbara Webb, held her counsel. The sixty-three-year-old retired schoolteacher, mother of three and grandmother of eight, was still in shock after meeting with the health department worker who had told her of her infection. She and her husband, Bob, who'd retired from Otis Elevator in New Jersey, still couldn't believe the news. She waited anxiously for the result of Bob's HIV test, which was negative. Then she hid at home and watched the suspicion swirl around Kimberly Bergalis.

When the CDC knocked on her door, Webb cooperated. She told them about the affair she'd had years before and about the surgery she'd undergone that might have involved a blood transfusion. But even before the results of her DNA matching came back, she was convinced it was Acer. Between December 1987 and August 1989, she'd seen the dentist twenty-one times. He had virtually rebuilt her mouth. She still remembered the time he'd filed two of her front teeth to razor points to anchor a new bridge — and the blood that flowed when she touched them with her tongue.

I wonder if he did it on purpose, she thought. Maybe he and God picked me for infection because I defy the stereotype about AIDS patients. It was a horrible thought. Crazy, she concluded.

Robert Montgomery drew up his battle plan to win Kim's lawsuit against Acer's estate, his malpractice insurer and the family's dental plan, CIGNA Dental Health of Florida. Personal-injury cases are rarely won in court. The pressure is in the publicity, and Montgomery was a master. His consultant on the suit was an old friend he'd represented in a legal dispute with Good Samaritan Hospital in Palm Beach. Dr. Sanford Kuvin was a maverick physician with the kind of ego Montgomery could appreciate. Kuvin was retired from practice and no longer a board-certified internist. He'd never been certified as a specialist in infectious diseases. But he billed himself as the "global authority" on the dangers of infection in health care settings. He'd been beating the drum on the dangers of hepatitis B for years, but was widely ignored.

Kuvin worked himself into a frenzy over things like the dangers of HIV transmission from a *mohel* — a person who performs ritual circumcisions — to an infant. He even tried to whip up concern in Israel over this unlikely possibility. To Kuvin, it all was a plot: powerful homosexual rights advocates had taken over the public health establishment and were endangering society. Mandatory testing was essential, but the CDC was reneging on its responsibility in the name of patient confidentiality. "You cannot treat public health as a civil rights secret disease," he told both Montgomery and the Bergalis family.

Kuvin's crusade gave structure to the Bergalises' grief; it gave them the comfort of blame. The argument also struck a chord with Montgomery, who also had a personal AIDS crisis on his hands. His son Scott was gay, and had found out he was positive. Montgomery believed that Scott's lover knew he was infected but did not tell him.

The defendants in the David Acer case didn't sit by helplessly while Montgomery bashed them in the press. A private detective, a former

FBI man, combed the campus of the University of Florida, looking for Kimberly's friends and possible lovers. Attorneys took depositions from them, picking apart their stories. Kimberly was forced to undergo a complete gynecological workup, a measuring of her vaginal opening and an examination of the state of her hymen. After all, millions of dollars were at stake.

In Atlanta, the Centers for Disease Control was caught in a maelstrom. For years they had known about the risks of infection in hospitals and physicians' offices. At least forty nurses and doctors had been jabbed with dirty needles and wound up with HIV, but the threat to patients had always been theoretical. Suddenly the threat had a name, along with an angelic face and tender voice.

When the Bergalis case hit the media, doctors and hospitals across the country began advising patients of individual medical practitioners to come in for testing. New York State health authorities began probing the office practices of a Long Island dentist who'd continued working during the four years before he died of AIDS. In Georgia, state medical officials suspended the license of a Savannah dentist, although no infections were linked to his office.

Hysterical patients lined up for HIV testing. None turned out to have been infected by their doctors, but the panic continued as the nation's HIV-infected health care workers went public: a surgical resident in northeastern Ohio, a dermatologist in Wisconsin, a heart surgeon in West Virginia and the only dentist in the small town of Nokomis, Illinois.

Why doesn't the CDC do something, people asked frantically.

It wasn't just patients. Hospitals were desperate for a national policy they could follow to protect themselves legally. "We are in a policy vacuum," said Hamilton Moses III, vice president for medical affairs at Johns Hopkins Hospital. In November Hopkins's top breast cancer surgeon had died of AIDS, and more than six hundred former patients were being screened for HIV. Two had filed suit, charging that the hospital should have known about the surgeon's infection, and informed them. "We're dealing with an infectious disease that has been politicized to such a degree that rational decisions on behalf of the public's health and health care workers are impossible," Moses said in the wake of the financial threat.

The CDC's AIDS experts held long meetings in a windowless room on the second floor of their Atlanta headquarters to hash out the dilemma. They estimated that more than five thousand health providers with AIDS were still working, yet Acer's patients seemed to be the only ones infected. "We have evaluated the risk thoroughly for patients, and it just isn't there," concluded Mark Barnes of the New York State AIDS Institute.

But the CDC had to respond to perception as well as reality, to fear as well as to science. The scientists began writing guidelines to restrict the practice of medicine by HIV-infected health care workers. Even before they could issue them, the agency was inundated with complaints from the American Medical Association, the American Dental Association and a dozen other associations of health providers. Just as the CDC's experts seemed about to resist the outcry — to release recommendations restricting infected physicians, dentists and their assistants from working — they were headed off by the threat of a lawsuit from the American Civil Liberties Union.

Health professionals insisted that the CDC was writing a political prescription for a public health issue which seemed to be an anomaly. Mandatory testing was a meaningless sop to a hysterical public, they argued, since a negative test wasn't proof a person was uninfected. Given the average six-month window between initial infection and a positive test, mandatory testing would only create a false sense of security.

In February 1991 the CDC called yet another meeting. For two days, leaders of professional associations, unions, public health organizations, and patient advocacy groups screamed at the CDC about mandating testing of health care providers. They dubbed the CDC's proposals ineffective, unfair, counterproductive, expensive, cruel and, perhaps, illegal. Dozens of questions arose. Should all physicians be tested, even psychiatrists and administrators, who posed no conceivable risk? How frequently should they be tested? If doctors knew that testing positive meant the end of their careers, would they care for AIDS patients, running the risk of being left penniless? Who would police adherence to the policy? If patients had the right to know the HIV status of their physicians and nurses, shouldn't health care workers have the same rights in regard to their patients? Should they be allowed to refuse to fill the cavities of HIV-positive men, or to deliver the babies of HIV-positive women?

One anesthesiologist angrily asked, "You want to force me to get tested? Fine. I'll get tested. But you're going to get tested too. And if you're HIV positive, I'm not going to touch you. Because there's a chance I can get infected by you, and if I do that's the end of my ability to earn a living and support my wife and children."

How serious was the problem, after all? Nobody was sure, but the only known case was David Acer. The CDC presented its statistical estimate that 128 Americans had been infected with HIV by their dentists or surgeons — the figure was one of those computer-simulation numbers the CDC likes to churn out. "Where are these people?" a chorus of opponents of mandatory testing asked, deriding the agency's math.

Even if that estimate was accurate, it meant that the probability of a repeat of the Acer case was about 1 in 2.6 million. "Many more people will die in car accidents driving to their dentist's offices than will get HIV from their dentists," said Victoria Sharp, the director of AIDS care at St. Clare's Hospital in Manhattan. "We have, in the 1990s, become a country that wants absolute safety. Well, sorry. There's just no concept anymore of bad luck."

Bending to the political winds, both the AMA and the ADA reversed their earlier positions opposing interference in the rights of infected doctors and dentists but remained opposed to mandatory testing. Their compromise position was a formal recommendation that all health care workers be tested regularly and, if found to be positive, stop practicing without informing their patients.

Montgomery's adviser, Sanford Kuvin, was the only person at that meeting to testify in support of mandatory testing. "The first duty of the physician is to do their patient no harm," he said. "How can he know that he will do no harm if he or she is a carrier?" Kuvin was booed by the audience. His remarks were later disavowed by the National Foundation on Infectious Diseases, on whose board of trustees he sat.

In the end, the arguments and statistics were largely meaningless. The shadows of Kimberly Bergalis and Dr. David Acer loomed over the meeting like specters, rendering all rational discussion irrelevant.

In July the CDC published a dry set of guidelines in its *Morbidity and Mortality Weekly* calling on doctors and dentists who performed surgery to be tested for HIV. Those who turned up infected should cease all invasive procedures — abdominal, gynecological or heart surgery, tooth extraction or root canals — unless a board of experts approved their work, and their patients were warned. The guidelines were not mandatory.

· · ·

While the CDC dithered, Kimberly Bergalis and her attorney stepped up the pressure for mandatory testing. By then, that demand and the vindication of her reputation were inextricably entwined. She released a letter she had written to Nikki Economu but never mailed.

> Well, I lived Nikki. I have lived to see my hair fall out, my body lose over 40 pounds, blisters on my sides. I've lived to go through nausea and vomiting, continual night sweats, chronic fevers of 103–104 that don't go away anymore . . . I lived to see white fungus grow all over the inside of my mouth, the back of my throat, my gums, and now my lips . . . AIDS has slowly destroyed me. Unless a cure is found, I will be another one of your statistics soon.
>
> Whom do I blame? Do I blame myself? I sure don't. I never used IV drugs, never slept with anyone, and never had a blood transfusion. I blame Dr. Acer and every single one of you bastards. Anyone who knew Dr. Acer was infected and had full-blown AIDS and stood by not doing a damn thing about it. You are all just as guilty as he was. You've ruined my life and my family's. I forgive Dr. Acer because I believe the disease affected his mind. He wasn't able to think properly and he continued to practice.
>
> Have you ever awakened in the middle of the night soaking wet from a night sweat — only to have it happen again an hour later? . . . Do you know what it's like to look at yourself in a full-length mirror before you shower — and you only see a skeleton? Do you know what I did? I slid to the floor and I cried. Now I shower with a blanket over the mirror.
>
> P.S. If laws are not formed to provide protection then my suffering and death was in vain.
>
> I'm dying guys. Goodbye.

By then, Kim's weight had dropped from 132 to 70 pounds. She could no longer walk. Her speech was slurred by weakness and painful blisters inside her mouth, she hadn't eaten solid food for two months and she spent her days in agony, drifting in and out of consciousness. Four months earlier, just days after the CDC reasserted the accuracy of its DNA testing, Acer's malpractice insurer settled with Kim for $1 million. "It's not going to buy me a cure," she'd responded. Then, in March, the family's dental insurer, CIGNA Dental Health of Florida, anted up an even larger check. Kim had celebrated the victory by buying herself a new red Corvette. Within a few weeks, she was too sick to drive.

In July the governor of Florida dropped by to see her. It was like being in the "presence of a saint," he said gravely.

One month after Kim's settlement, Richard Driskill and Barbara Webb both filed suit against Acer's estate. Driskill's immune system was deteriorating rapidly. Webb had already been hospitalized for pancreatitis, but she seemed to be holding her own. Their cases, and causes, were bolstered still further in July, when the three became five.

John Yecs hadn't planned to go public. He'd seemed satisfied to remain the CDC's Patient G. But he'd landed in jail for shoplifting, and a tabloid offered to post his bail in return for his story. His face was soon plastered over the nation's supermarket checkout counters: another Acer patient infected. Yecs was neither a virginal young woman nor an elderly grandmother. A crackhead and drifter, he'd been a resident of a drug rehabilitation center in 1988 when a tooth started aching and he'd been sent over to Dr. Acer. He'd tested positive for HIV in 1990, when he attempted to sell his blood. Insisting Acer was his only possible source of infection, he demanded DNA testing. By that method, the strain was a 99.997 percent match with Acer's, the CDC concluded.

Lisa Shoemaker's face didn't run in the tabloids. She was too embarrassed at how fat she'd become under the stress of living with HIV. She'd tested positive in 1989, after she broke up with her boyfriend in Florida and moved home to Michigan. As it happened, he'd been infected already, so she hardly puzzled over the source of her infection. But when she read about Kim in *People,* she thought about her twelve visits to David Acer. The CDC ran genetic tests on her virus and reported that they'd found no match with her boyfriend's. The source of her infection, the CDC said, was David Acer.

But Yecs and Shoemaker didn't share in the malpractice bounty. In August 1991 Webb and Driskill settled with Acer's insurance company for $999,999 each. By the time the two latest patients filed suit, only $2 remained in his account.

"It felt almost like a rape," Shoemaker said when she heard the news. Both her attorney and Yecs's had tried to cooperate with Montgomery, hoping the five could share in the settlement, but he was matter-of-fact. "For all practical purposes the well is dry," he said.

After the first round of public panic, fears began to subside. All across the country, patients had been told that their physicians and dentists had died of AIDS. The patients had run to be tested and none had turned up positive as a result of that contact. War had broken out in the Persian Gulf. Saddam Hussein and Iraqi terrorism had become the new American obsession.

But Robert Montgomery and the Bergalises didn't end their crusade. Although the media had gotten bored with the story, Washington had not. If the CDC wouldn't force infected health care workers out of their offices, Congress could try.

Sanford Kuvin introduced the Bergalises to a group of Washington activists who advocated rewriting national AIDS policy to steer it away from protecting the confidentiality of the infected in favor of aggressive action to identify the infected. Shepherd Smith, of Americans for a Sound AIDS Policy, flew down to Florida with Colonel Robert Redfield, head of the U.S. military's AIDS programs. They linked the family up with Mike Franc, a staffer for California Congressman William Dannemeyer, long a supporter of mandatory HIV testing.

"I think they're being very opportunistic," charged Dr. John Witte, Florida's assistant health officer for disease control. "They're using a very sick girl to their advantage. And exploiting somebody to the degree she's been exploited raises a lot of ethical questions."

Kim didn't feel exploited. She cheered in July when the Senate responded to the CDC's voluntary guidelines by passing overwhelmingly, 81 to 18, a bill introduced by Jesse Helms that slapped ten-year jail terms and $10,000 fines on HIV-infected health care workers who performed invasive procedures without revealing their infections to patients.

But the battle wasn't so easily won. The same day, the Senate also passed a bill, introduced by Senators Robert Dole and Ted Kennedy, giving the CDC's voluntary testing guidelines the force of law. The denouement would be fought out in the House of Representatives, and Congressman Dannemeyer pulled out the big guns, naming a bill mandating HIV testing for all health care workers and patients the Kimberly Bergalis Patient and Health Providers' Protection Act.

On September 24, 1991, Kimberly Bergalis waited on the Amtrak platform in Okeechobee, Florida, for the train to Washington, D.C. It would be her first train ride. She could barely stand. Her father, George, cuddled the shrunken woman in his arms. For years she'd dreamed of traveling by train, but she spent most of the twenty-hour trip curled up in a sleeper in a T-shirt and pajama bottoms. She walked off the train at Union Station only with the help of two Amtrak conductors.

She was too weak to appear at the press conference arranged by Dannemeyer. With Dannemeyer and Congressman Dan Burton of Indiana at his side, George Bergalis spoke for her. "She knows this is a political decision not to treat AIDS as a disease but as something other than that," he said. "She knows it's going to be a political decision that's going to be necessary to correct that wrong," said George Bergalis. "However, she also knows that political decision is not going to be made . . . unless the American public lets these people know they want to see something happen." The passage of the Dannemeyer bill, he said, was "her dying wish."

That afternoon, members of the House Subcommittee on Health and Environment filed into a hearing room as forty camera shutters clicked. CNN was broadcasting the event live. Kimberly Bergalis, looking like an image from Dachau, was wheeled into the room. The only color on her face was the light gloss of lipstick and blue eyeliner.

"AIDS is a terrible disease which we must take seriously," she said. "I did not do anything wrong, yet I am being made to suffer like this. My life has been taken away. Please enact legislation so that no other patient or health care provider will have to go through the hell that I have. Thank you." Fifteen seconds was all Kim could manage. She was wheeled away to Dannemeyer's office, where she lay under a blanket on a couch and watched the rest of the hearing on television.

"Kimberly is your shame," George Bergalis roared at the House members, "all of Congress's shame . . . She is the result of your unwillingness or inability to deal with this monster that you've created."

Opponents of the bill were given time to respond.

"Here we are at this circus, being pitted against each other," said David Barr, an HIV-positive activist employed by the Gay Men's Health Crisis in New York. "We are not enemies. We are all innocent victims here. We are dying from the same neglect." Kimberly was no longer listening. She had been whisked off to the White House, where she hoped to meet President George Bush and his wife, Barbara. They were both at home, but neither descended to the infirmary to greet her.

One week later the House and Senate resolved their differences and passed a compromise bill requiring states to implement the CDC's nonmandatory testing policy or equivalent guidelines, acceptable to

the CDC, for health care workers performing "risk-prone" procedures. Failure to comply would mean the forfeiture of federal public
health grants.

It was a bitter loss for the Bergalis family, and it was not the last
one. As the CDC tried to define what procedures were risk-prone and
thus subject to the new regulations, the compromise unraveled. Having failed to stave off congressional guidelines, the medical establishment tried to torpedo them by nitpicking at the definition of which
procedures would be included.

Professional associations refused to cooperate with the CDC in
defining precisely which procedures might create risk of HIV transmission. We have insufficient data, they argued, adding that strict adherence to safety precautions would be sufficient to eliminate what was,
in fact, a risk akin to decapitation by a garage door. Less than three
months after Kim Bergalis's gripping testimony before Congress, the
CDC surrendered. It issued a new policy, asking health care workers to
have themselves tested for HIV. Their professional futures would be
decided by local advisory boards.

Kimberly Bergalis never knew how completely she had lost her
crusade for mandatory testing. By the time she returned home from
Washington, she was close to death. Throughout the fall, she simply
wasted away. She died at home on December 8, four days after the
CDC gave up on any meaningful national policy on HIV-infected
health care workers.

In the five years since David Acer became a national villain, no other
cases of patients infected by health care workers have arisen. The CDC
spent twenty months and more than a million dollars trying to solve
the puzzle, without any success.

For a while, the most popular conjecture was that internal parts of
one of Acer's dental instruments had become coated with the blood or
saliva of an infected patient, and that those fluids were passed along to
the uninfected. That seemed unlikely. The amount of virus that could
be retained in a hand piece would be minuscule, and HIV is a fragile
microbe that doesn't live long outside the body. Furthermore, the DNA
testing suggested that Acer, not an anonymous patient, was the common denominator in all of the infections.

Most people preferred the simple explanation that Acer had cut
himself and bled into the open wounds of the patients. But it seemed
unlikely that the dentist would have injured himself, not once but five

times, and bled into the open wounds of patients on all those occasions — and that he could have done so without the patient or his assistant noticing.

The CDC and the press investigated the theory that Acer had passed the virus to his patients by having sex with them while they were under anesthesia. That didn't wash either. None of the infected patients had had general anesthesia.

When all other explanations failed, the media seized on the possibility that Acer had infected his patients intentionally. Dr. John Hardie of the Canadian Dental Association floated the idea at a CDC meeting in February 1991, suggesting that the dentist had added his own blood to Novocain injections. Health care workers liked the suggestion — it got them off the hook — but it was sheer speculation. Acer's staff, patients and doctors all agreed that he was neither vicious nor malevolent.

That didn't stop 20/20 from sensationalizing that possibility. In October 1993 the show aired an interview with Edward Parsons, who claimed to be a deathbed confidant of the dentist. Parsons repeated every word of a conversation Acer allegedly had with him. "Well, you know, when AIDS finally infects a young person and when it starts hitting grandmothers and people like that, then maybe the government will do something," Parsons claimed Acer had told him. Then Acer supposedly turned to the topic of Webb and Bergalis, and commented, "I guess I've got their attention, don't I?"

Parsons was clearly a liar. Acer never knew Kimberly Bergalis's name. When he died, Barbara Webb had yet to be tested for HIV. The *New York Times* ran the story nonetheless, under the inflamed headline "Was It Murder?"

In 1994 a Harvard researcher refined the theory. Dr. Leonard Horowitz published a lengthy study in which he concluded that David Acer had all the personality traits of a serial killer. He'd never met the dentist, but insisted he had reviewed the relevant medical and legal documents in the case, as well as published and videotaped interviews. He concluded that the infected patients were victims of "sexual homicide" motivated by Acer's anger against the U.S. government for infecting gay men with HIV. According to Horowitz, the CDC was fully aware of the murders but had covered them up at the behest of Hillary Clinton and Janet Reno.

Every alley the CDC followed led to a dead end. Harold Jaffe, deputy director of the AIDS division, finally admitted that the CDC had no idea precisely what had happened, and probably never would. About this much, however, he had no doubt: the source of all of the patients' infections was Dr. Acer. The DNA testing presented irrefutable proof.

Or did it?

From the first reports of the DNA matching, Dr. Lionel Resnick was skeptical. The Miami Beach physician, who had worked as both clinician and virologist in AIDS research studied the CDC reports with care. Their procedure — which compared the differences between Acer's and Bergalis's viruses to the differences between Acer's and a national control group — didn't make sense. Why not use a control group closer to home, he wondered. So did the state of Florida, and when they pushed, the CDC used blood from patients in Fort Lauderdale and West Palm Beach. With the same result.

Not good enough, Resnick argued, insisting there might be a strain common to patients in Stuart, where Acer, Bergalis and the others all lived. The CDC refused to test in that focused area, arguing that the control group might be skewed by other patients of Acer or by the sex partners of some of the infected.

Resnick wasn't buying that argument. Working with Acer's insurance company, he took blood samples from men in the local gay bar and from AIDS patients receiving services from local support groups. The results, he says, are dramatically different from the CDC's. He claims to have found five individuals with no connection to Acer — but with virtually identical strains of HIV.

AIDS specialists elsewhere are puzzled by another aspect of the DNA testing. Constant mutation, a hallmark of HIV, means that each individual has multiple strains of the virus and that strains evolve that are specific to different parts of the body. Yet the reports on the testing in the Bergalis case speak of only one strain. Which is curious, if not impossible.

Overarching these particular concerns was a broader one: DNA matching of HIV samples is too new a technique to be at all credible. The Acer case was the first time it was used to try to determine whether HIV transmission occurred between two specific individuals. Several attempts to duplicate the technique using HIV-positive mothers and their infected infants did not reveal a match, although the linkage is irrefutable. "The CDC overestimated the strength, the certainty, they attached to the DNA evidence," concluded Dr. Ronald DeBry, a biologist at Duke University.

The Centers for Disease Control has long maintained that it does not know what happened in David Acer's office. They insist that they are interested in all pertinent information, but they have ignored both Resnick and DeBry. All suggestions that Kimberly might have been used by a greedy lawyer and a bureaucracy of epidemiologists with a clear political agenda have been dismissed.

The Acer case was officially closed in May 1992.

But not before Kimberly Bergalis could become the most debated virgin since Mary. Her sexual history was dissected on the front page of the *New York Times* and deconstructed on *60 Minutes*. Politicians lionized her as the quintessentially innocent AIDS victim; AIDS activists branded her a lying slut who hid the truth from an overbearing mother.

Kimberly was key among Acer's infected patients because the others had clear risks for contracting the virus outside Acer's office and could be dismissed as greedy extortionists looking for money from Acer's insurance company.

Although Richard Driskill was described as a devoted family man, a husband and father of two, he was also well known for having sex with anyone willing in Indiantown, Florida — a fact even his attorney does not deny. Driskill had sex with women. He had sex with men. He had sex with prostitutes, at least one of whom tested HIV positive.

John Yecs had told the CDC he had no risk for HIV other than his appointments with Acer. "I never dreamed I could catch AIDS," he'd said. But Yecs was a former intravenous drug user, an alcoholic and a frequent patron of prostitutes. One hooker swore in a deposition that Yecs had routinely traded crack for sex with her roommate, who had AIDS.

In 1989 Lisa Shoemaker told Acer's receptionist that she was HIV positive and had been infected by her boyfriend — although she didn't repeat that story to the CDC. Sherry Johnson, the last patient to come forward, admitted that she'd had sex with a number of men while she was still in her teens — which seemed a more logical route of infection than a single appointment with Acer for a routine cleaning.

And Barbara Webb, the white-haired grandmother, admitted to having had an extramarital affair, although the CDC never tested the man. In her first interviews, she also reported that she'd received blood transfusions during surgery in the 1980s.

All the infections could be explained by some drama that didn't star Acer — except Kimberly's.

The possibility that neither her honor nor her hymen was entirely intact was first raised at the February 1991 CDC meeting. Dr. Stanley Weiss, the chief of AIDS epidemiology at the University of Medicine and Dentistry of New Jersey, revealed that a gynecological examination of Kimberly Bergalis in 1990 indicated that she had genital warts — the result of a sexually transmitted virus. The examination had been performed in November 1990 by Dr. Phyllis Toon as part of the investigation conducted by Acer's malpractice insurer. Toon noted that Bergalis's vaginal opening was wide and that her hymen was "irregular at 3 and 9 o'clock," conditions she characterized as "consistent with prior intercourse." She also found lesions; a biopsy showed them to be human papillomavirus #18.

Bergalis's attorney, Robert Montgomery, was livid. "Looney Toon," as he called the gynecologist, had sold out to the insurance company. He sent Kimberly to another gynecologist, who, he argued, found no papillomavirus. That physician was, of course, paid for by Montgomery.

In early 1990 Kim did admit that she'd had two sexual encounters, but insisted that in neither case had she been penetrated. She was more explicit in a videotaped deposition in which she described being in bed with an unidentified man.

"Has anybody ever performed oral sex on you?" she was asked.

"Yes," she answered.

"Was there more than one episode?"

"Mm-hmm, yes," she responded.

"And was — was he ever trying to — to get to penetration?"

"He had — it was close to the area, but he had never penetrated."

The detective for Acer's insurance company has said that Kimberly's friends all seemed sure she was lying and that she had had sex with at least one of her boyfriends. A coworker at the Pic 'n Save said that Kimberly slept at her boyfriend's house at least two or three times a week. A recurring pajama party seemed unlikely.

Even the CDC acknowledged in its final report that she "is concerned that if she tells us her risk, her mother would find out" and that there would be "serious negative impact." A report from her therapist noted that Kim said her mother was "hypercritical and rejects all of her daughters."

In November 1993, a few months after the death of his own son, Robert Montgomery financed and produced a $250,000 lobbying and media blitz called The Right to Know. "Do you know that you can be required to take an HIV test to join the military or get health insurance?" he asked, on camera. "But there's no law that requires reporting the AIDS virus among doctors and patients." The film cuts to an image of Kim, beautiful in a pair of shorts and a sweatshirt. "Shouldn't Kimberly have had the right to know? And shouldn't you?"

The battle over the right to know should have had nothing to do with Kimberly Bergalis's virginity. That would be like deciding whether emission controls are necessary on the basis of one Chevrolet. The battle should not be about HIV-positive health care workers either. Mandatory testing in hospitals and doctors' offices won't save many, if any, lives.

The right to know is really about the need to know — about the need for HIV testing to become a normal part of the landscape of American medicine. It's not about who is or was a virgin, innocent or otherwise, or about who might infect whom. It's about the idiocy of treating a serious medical issue like a state secret when lives are at stake. While most Americans were still leery of their dentists, that's what Nettie Mayersohn was worrying about.

Nettie is one of those classic New York Jewish liberals who'd gone into politics to become the bane of upstate conservatives like New York's governor, George Pataki. A state assemblywoman from Queens, she's so pro-choice and pro-woman that she was named legislator of the year by the state chapter of the National Organization for Women in 1989. She has a near-perfect voting record of support for every bill that fights every conceivable kind of discrimination.

Then she became involved in AIDS, and became a pariah.

In 1993 Nettie Mayersohn discovered that New York was testing all infants born in the state but keeping the results secret, even from the mothers. Huh? If the state is going to go to the trouble and expense of testing all those kids, Nettie asked, why not tell their mothers if they're positive so the babies can at least get some treatment?

We can't, state health authorities explained. Infant testing in New York, as in most other states, is blinded to guard confidentiality. That means that the number of infants testing positive is tallied, but that no one is permitted to keep any record of their names, or give their mothers the results of the tests unless they explicitly request HIV testing for their children. By law, the women are guaranteed the right to refuse testing for themselves, and testing an infant is tantamount to testing its mother.

Mayersohn had supported legislation protecting HIV confidentiality without understanding the practical implications of the ironclad safeguards: between three and four hundred children each year were being sent home without their mothers' knowing they were infected with HIV.

"I didn't believe it," Mayersohn says. "They are just letting babies go — so long, kid, take care of yourself — and telling mothers that everything is fine when both the mothers and the babies are infected."

In 1993 she introduced a bill in the state assembly mandating that all newborns be tested for HIV, just as they are routinely tested for syphilis, hepatitis, sickle-cell anemia and a host of other conditions. Parents of HIV-positive infants would be notified of the results whether they requested HIV testing or not.

Nettie knew she was stepping on a land mine when she took on the issue. The AIDS lobby does not treat threats to HIV confidentiality lightly. But the explosion was beyond anything she could have imagined. As soon as her bill hit the floor, Mayersohn became a fascist, a racist, a homophobe, a woman hater. She was accused of advocating mandatory testing.

When the bill's opponents stopped attacking Mayersohn personally, they began berating her proposal as a violation of the civil liberties of women. Theirs was a knee-jerk reaction against the word "mandatory," with its images of strapping people to tables and forcibly extracting their blood. But sacrificing infants on the altar of a woman's right not to know her HIV status was shortsighted and illogical. Infected women would inevitably find out about their own, and their children's, infections. The only question was whether they would find out when they were close to death or when it was still early enough to take advantage of the life-prolonging treatments for which AIDS activists had fought so hard.

The next weapon against the bill was slung. "I think Nettie Mayersohn's bill will kill minorities' babies and poor women's babies," said Melinda Katz, another assemblywoman from Queens. "People will stay away from clinics, therefore not getting prenatal care, if they are afraid that the baby will be tested mandatorily."

There was no evidence that women would flee the health care system rather than allow their infants to be tested, so the advocates of silence went far afield to find grounds for their dire prediction. "When the state of Illinois instituted a mandatory testing program for those applying for marriage licenses, people fled Illinois in droves to file elsewhere," said Kelli Conlin, executive director of the New York State affiliate of the National Abortion Rights Action League.

The comparison seemed strained to Mayersohn, but she was more taken aback by its source. She had expected opposition from gay and AIDS activists, but the attacks from her old allies at NOW and NARAL caught her off guard. They vigorously declared they were defending women's right to privacy. Others suspected that their real concern was that giving an infant the right to be tested at the expense of the mother's rights would be a victory for the rights of fetuses.

Opponents of informing mothers of their children's HIV status didn't dare suggest that there was no problem. The evidence was too clear. By 1994 more than eighty thousand American women of child-bearing age already had HIV in their bodies, and most were unaware of their infections. More than half of their infants went undiagnosed until they turned up with pneumonia. At that point, their mean survival time was three months.

Mayersohn's opponents suggested that the problem could be solved by more effective counseling of pregnant women. "The issue boils down to a basic trust in women to make the right decision for themselves and their newborns if they are provided the counseling to draw them into the process, and to make clear that they themselves will be tested as well," said Kelli Conlin. Conlin and her supporters pointed to the High-Risk Pregnancy Clinic, where about 95 percent of the women consented to HIV testing after thorough counseling.

Elsewhere, however, the figures were abysmally low. Studies by the CDC suggested that two-thirds of infected mothers nationally refused testing for themselves and their babies, despite vigorous counseling. Throughout New York, even in hospitals that had two counselors per pregnant woman, almost 60 percent of all infants born HIV positive left the hospital without the mothers knowing they were infected.

To many pediatricians, counseling simply wasn't realistic, given the tempo of HIV infection in babies. "If we know the mother is HIV positive and the infant is too, we will not lose the child in the first months," said Dr. Aditya Kaul, director of the Pediatric Infectious Disease Clinic at Bellevue Hospital. "If we don't know, the baby dies."

Ironically, neither Kaul nor other advocates for the rights of babies were criticized for not going far enough. But in fact, protecting babies really means testing them not at birth but inside their mothers' wombs, when transmission of HIV can be prevented. Doctors had a pretty clear idea of how to do that by 1991. They knew that most infections occurred either during birth or from breast-feeding, and that cesarean sections and bottle feeding could cut transmission in half. Studies have suggested that the use of AZT, and even vitamin A, during pregnancy and birth could further inhibit transmission of HIV from mother to infant. Testing pregnant women, then, would be sound medical practice.

"If I had brought that up," Mayersohn says, "they probably would have shot me."

They would have been a wider group than she might have assumed. NARAL, NOW and AIDS activist organizations weren't the only opponents of routine testing of pregnant women for HIV. Anti-abortion activists were even more vehemently opposed. They feared that infected women might decide to terminate their pregnancies.

For more than a year, during 1993 and 1994, New York legislators fought the battle of the babies. In the first year, Mayersohn's bill didn't make it out of committee. In the next, she got an unexpected boost from New York newspaper columnists, and even former U.S. Surgeon General C. Everett Koop, who'd become a hero in the AIDS activist community for his candid discussion of the disease despite the opposition of his boss, Ronald Reagan, lent his support. "You have to get rid of the older laws that prohibit the testing of children," he said. "It's thirteen years since we realized we had AIDS. And a lot of things that were problems then are not problems any longer. The best weapon is knowledge. That's how we should face this."

Initially, the state medical society agreed, but in May 1994 they reversed themselves and fought just as hard on the other side. NOW, both nationally and in New York state, maintained its opposition, although the Ulster County chapter broke ranks, calling for routine testing of all pregnant women. In early June, gubernatorial candidate George Pataki threw his support to Mayersohn. Governor Mario Cuomo continued to study the issue.

Physicians working in the field were divided. "We don't have the person power to provide intensive care and follow-up for all the 130,000 kids born in New York City every year and their mothers," said Dr. Lou Z. Cooper, the director of pediatrics at St. Luke's–Roosevelt Hospital. "I can deploy the resources to provide such care for those that are positive. The problem is, I don't know which ones they are. It's ridiculous that you aren't allowed to screen for something that runs in an incidence of one out of fifty babies in our hospital." Dr. Carolyn Britton, a member of the New York State AIDS Advisory Council dealing with the issue, disagreed. Care couldn't be mandated "through coercion," she said.

Eighty-two activist groups spent more than a quarter of a million dollars to lobby against Mayersohn's bill — energy better conserved for other fights — and to remind legislators that they were facing re-election in November.

On the evening of June 28, Democratic state senators and assembly members debated the proposal for an exhausting four hours as assembly speaker Sheldon Silver tried to forge a compromise. Silver's plan was to mandate counseling but to allow women to forgo the test by signing a consent form.

"It's condescending," said Laura Murray, a lobbyist for the New York Civil Liberties Union. "It sets up a scenario where mothers are treated as if they don't understand the consequences of health decisions they make for their children."

The senate dithered all day Saturday, July 2. Early the next morning the body adjourned without voting on the bill.

"Last week, with a great fanfare and a slap on the back for ourselves, we passed a much-needed domestic violence law," Mayersohn said as the session closed. "I submit to you that our failure to pass a mandatory HIV testing bill makes us accomplices in domestic violence in its cruelest and most obscene form: the abuse and neglect of the most neglected children in our state."

It was a sensible statement that went unheeded for the simple reason that it was impossible to sell. It didn't summon any fancy personal-injury lawyers. It didn't pose any immediate threat to the adults who enact laws and elect lawmakers. It didn't create the right cast of characters, the right balance of villains and victims. The Bergalis case managed all those feats and many others, and thus transformed an unremarkable young woman into a remarkable icon of undetermined and bitterly contested meaning. What got lost in the process was any sense of who she really was, along with any real benefit from her suffering.

She died in vain.

NINE

Lights, Camera . . . Death

Teenagers hanging out on Washington Avenue pointed and stared as twenty-six-year-old Sean Sasser sauntered around Miami's South Beach. Twentysomethings on Rollerblades — the terrors of the sidewalks — stopped to say hello. Strangers in restaurants sent waitresses over to ask for his autograph.

"How's Pedro?" everyone wanted to know.

Sean gritted his teeth and muttered, "Hanging in there."

The truth was that at that moment in October 1994 his partner, Pedro Zamora, was lying in bed in a corner room at Mercy Hospital, paralyzed on his left side. He could no longer speak. He would no longer eat. Sometimes his friends and family could pull him out of his semiconscious state, but only with difficulty. Even then, when he opened his eyes and held on to the nearest hand, no one was entirely sure that Pedro knew where he was or who his visitors were. His physician said that only 10 percent of his brain was functioning.

The kids on Rollerblades and in trendy cafes already knew the full details of Pedro's condition when they accosted Sean. Pedro's imminent demise was the lead story on the local news, complete with the kind of graphic that stations design for continuing coverage of an event. "Pedro's Final Battle," Channel 4, the NBC affiliate, called it. The accompanying photograph of his once devastatingly handsome visage bore no resemblance to the gaunt death mask Pedro's face had become.

Despite Pedro's ordeal, no one in a neighborhood where Sylvester Stallone and Sandra Bernhart are regulars hesitated to pursue Sean. So what if Sean was in town for a wake and a funeral, not a day at the beach and a night posturing at the nation's hippest clubs? They could touch him, feel connected to a myth and go home and brag to their friends. Sean and Pedro weren't people, after all. They were stars. And this was the price they were paying for that stardom, a stardom based on Pedro's imminent death.

Pedro Zamora and Sean Sasser were America's first tragic romance of AIDS. Both men had spent years of their young lives trudging from classroom to classroom, from PTA meeting to political caucus warning young people of the dangers of AIDS. Pedro, a high school track star and honor student with a poise and sense of public duty decades beyond his years, got his start the afternoon he walked into the office of his high school counselor and suggested that Miami's Hialeah High School should begin AIDS education.

"That's a really good idea, Pedro," said the counselor, trying to be supportive of student initiative but unable to conceal entirely the condescension creeping into his voice. "But it's not necessary. We don't have that problem here."

Pedro, always polite and dignified, responded in a calm voice. "Yes we do," he said. "I have it."

Sean's career as an AIDS educator began the day he was due to ship out for training in the U.S. Navy's nuclear program. He stopped by the recruitment office to pick up his file and board the bus for the airport. His papers weren't with those of the other men. The woman behind the desk found them in a different box and, with a pained look on her face, sent him into another room. "You're not eligible for enlistment," a medical officer told him sternly. "We found HIV in your blood."

Sean had been having sex with older men, but with the brash self-confidence of an adolescent who believes himself invulnerable to disaster, the bright young man — he was a student at the University of Chicago — he had never considered the possibility that he might become infected. The Detroit high school from which he had graduated in 1986 never bothered to mention AIDS in its sex education or health classes.

Once they had turned their personal tragedies into an opportunity for education, both Pedro and Sean drew honor and praise from the small communities of the AIDS-aware across the nation. Pedro spoke before the U.S. Congress. Sean was photographed by the celebrity photographer Annie Leibovitz. That portrait became an AIDS poster in San Francisco that read: "Testing HIV positive was a wake-up call for me. Today I have a clearer idea of who I am and what I want from life. I think everything will be okay. I have no plans of disappearing any time soon."

At some point along the way, Pedro and Sean also became commodities, in a process so subtle and seductive they could neither fully register nor resist it, a process that sometimes distorted or completely obscured their initial message.

Maybe that point came when MTV realized that an HIV-positive gay man might sell more Ikea furniture than just another nouveau clubby, and invited Pedro to join the rotating cast of the hip and glam station's *Real World,* a cross between a documentary and a soap opera, created by throwing seven people in their twenties into a house and chronicling their interactions and adventures. Pedro's courtship of Sean was filmed in full color and aired to an audience of 1.5 million viewers whose demographics made advertisers drool. His visits to schools were broadcast, as was his growing illness. When Pedro went to the doctor, MTV was in the examining room. When Pedro was diagnosed with pneumonia, MTV was in the hospital.

He was featured on the cover of *POZ* magazine, molded into a sexy symbol that HIV does not equal ugly. Before he fell ill, a modeling agency had been looking for the ideal product match. *Real World* aired Pedro and Sean's commitment ceremony — the best a Cuban refugee and an African American from Detroit could manage in a country still unable to cope with the concept of two men marrying. After Pedro was hospitalized, agents and producers began planning the made-for-TV movie.

Pedro never had any money. After graduating from high school, he sold suits at Burdine's department store, then lived on a $300-a-week stipend from Body Positive, a Miami AIDS resource center. When he arrived in San Francisco to begin filming *Real World,* his wallet was empty. His salary from MTV came in a lump sum at the end of his five-month contract.

He could hardly begin to spend it in the few months before he found himself dying in a bed at Mercy Hospital in Miami, and his growing celebrity brought benefits he could no longer enjoy. Mercy Hospital moved another patient out of the prime corner room on its AIDS wing to give their most famous patient the most commodious accommodations. President Bill Clinton called. The local archbishop, a fervent anti-homosexual zealot, dropped by. Mary Fisher, who barely knew the young man and whose distant affection for him was decidedly not returned, flew in from Washington. After coming out as HIV positive at the Republican National Convention in 1992, she had fashioned herself a kind of Miss Congeniality of the AIDS pageant. This duty went along with the crown.

So many strangers called and stopped in for a chance to see a bona fide celebrity buckling under a big-time disease that the hospital had to give Pedro an alias. Middle school students who had heard Pedro's speeches pooled their lunch and video-game money to send to his trust fund. Hollywood dressed up in red ribbons and held a gala fundraiser.

Curiously absent were the MTV cameras. The station would hardly air scenes of nurses changing Pedro's diapers hourly to remove the diarrhea that poured out of his body, or scenes of family members gasping and crying as Pedro suffered yet another set of convulsions. They would hardly have complemented his image as the nation's HIV poster boy, so his death seemed as melodramatically unreal as the final swoon of Marilyn Monroe.

Pedro Zamora, a shy kid who left Cuba on a trawler in 1980 and became the Person with AIDS that young America embraced, died on November 11, 1994, five years and one day after he learned he was infected with HIV. It marked the loss of an extraordinary individual, but not an end to his ruthless commodification.

Congresswoman Ileana Ros-Lehtinen took public credit for Pedro's deathbed reunion with his Cuban relatives. His physician, Dr. Corklin Steinhart, held yet another press conference, enjoying the best free advertising a doctor could imagine. Two of his MTV co-stars hired an agent to help them build mini-careers on the lecture circuit off their friendship with Pedro. Reverend Fred Phelps, a Baptist rabble-rouser who had been disavowed by most of his fellow fundamentalists, staged a protest at Pedro's memorial service. And millions of Americans cried, convinced that because they'd had a crush on Pedro, they had compassion for AIDS.

I guess I could say that I discovered Pedro Zamora in that strange way that Columbus discovered America or a Hollywood talent scout takes credit for the existence of a nubile, young starlet.

I learned about Pedro from a tip, the kind of lead that feeds hungry newspaper reporters in competitive markets. "Have I got a story for you," Joel Rapoport announced one Saturday afternoon in the fall of 1990. Joel was the city's most knowledgeable AIDS activist, but he was infamous for his hyperbole. That afternoon he outdid himself. A gorgeous young man — "and I mean GORGEOUS" Joel said — had joined the support group he attended at Body Positive, a resource center for people with HIV. He was a powerful speaker: composed, articulate and funny. He was Cuban, just eighteen years old.

I'd been looking for a teenager with HIV to put a face and a family on the growing problem among south Florida's youth. No one in Miami was talking about the number of young adults turning up with AIDS — thus the number of adolescents being infected. Joel was sure he had found THE ONE.

The next day I waited anxiously on the patio of a café by the ocean, wondering if I'd be able to pick Joel's wunderkind out of the crowd of greased, oiled and meticulously maintained bodies. A young man with perfectly chiseled features walked up the steps and glanced over the crowd. He was wearing a purple Izod shirt. His eyes were penetrating. Every head turned toward him. Perfect, I thought, already imagining the color photograph on the front page of the features section.

It was the beginning of the packaging of Pedro Zamora, and I plead guilty to a hand in it. A photographer from the newspaper adjusted Pedro's clothing and placed him in just the right light to capture both his beauty and his power. I crafted my lines carefully to make Pedro into a captivating Everykid. It wasn't hard. Even in his accented English, he knew what to say to reach out to an audience. He took to a camera like a pro.

I could never have imagined that I was helping to turn Pedro Zamora into a star. I could never have imagined that the person — the sweet boy who missed his mother desperately, who had long, intimate talks with his father, who found love just as death was beginning to find him — would get lost in the hype.

Pedro Zamora was hardly born for fame. No one from his decaying neighborhood on the outskirts of Havana had ever made it to national prominence, even on that island. And rags-to-riches, or rags-to-fame, stories are hardly the true-to-life fare of late-twentieth-century America.

He was just another anonymous immigrant among the 125,000 Cubans who were packed into yachts and trawlers in the spring of 1980 when Fidel Castro opened the port of Mariel and invited the island's "scum" to depart for capitalism's shores. Pedro's father, Hector, who worked in a warehouse, accepted the invitation for himself and his wife, Zoraida, for eight-year-old Pedro, fifteen-year-old Milagros, twelve-year-old Jesus and their grandmother.

Pedro often said that May 30, 1980, the day of his journey, was the worst of his life, even worse than the day a nurse sat him down and told him he was HIV positive. It wasn't just the press of thieves, rapists and crazies who were his fellow passengers on the thirteen-hour trip to Key West on the *Cynthia D.* It was saying goodbye to the five brothers and sisters who stayed behind, to the familiar, to the warmth of enormous family dinners and parties and outings.

It will be all right, Hector had reassured his youngest. By next year Castro will be gone and we'll all be together again.

It never became all right. Castro didn't fall, in one year, in five, or ten. Pedro mastered English and became yet another of the thousands of Miami Cuban kids who translate the realities of America for their parents. They all delighted in the luxury of knowing that the supermarkets always had food on their shelves, but the breakup of the family was a gnawing pain. When Pedro's mother had one of her crying spells, it fell to her baby to dance with her.

Then, in the spring of 1983, the pretty mole that Hector had long admired on Zoraida's face began to change. In June she was diagnosed with cancer. Two years later, without cooking any more of her famous dinners, she was dead.

Four years later, Pedro received a letter asking him to call the Red Cross about the blood he'd donated during a drive at Hialeah High School. He ignored it. He received another letter. He ignored that as well. He finally screwed up his courage and went to the family doctor. He'd heard of AIDS; he vaguely remembered a lecture on the disease from when he was in seventh grade. But it seemed to have nothing to do with the lives of junior high school students in suburban Hialeah. He'd put the handout on AIDS with his other classroom notes and forgotten it.

He was stunned when the doctor told him the news, although he shouldn't have been. Soon after his mother's death, promiscuity became his escape from reality, and embraces from strangers became a sad substitute for hugs from his mother. In Pedro's case, the strangers were the older men he found in the bars and bath houses that he used as refuges from grief.

An awareness of AIDS did not accompany him there. "I could never connect a face with the disease," he said in an interview just months after his diagnosis. "No one ever sat me down and talked about AIDS. Our parents and teachers told us to have safe sex, but no one ever explained to me how. If they had, maybe I wouldn't be in this situation now."

Several weeks later, Pedro delivered the news to his father. "I looked at my son, my beautiful son, and saw a corpse," said Hector Zamora, who had spent his entire time in the United States caring for his dying wife, worrying about his children in Cuba and cutting grass, working construction and struggling in factories. "I thought, why can't it be me. I'm old. I've lived my life. Please, God, let us trade places."

After his mother's death, Pedro had buried his sorrow in a frenzy of school activities. If he kept himself busy, he could sometimes forget his mother's death. By the time he turned thirteen, he was a star athlete and student — president of the science club, Student of the Month in the city of Hialeah, captain of the cross-country team, member of the honor society. The teachers loved him. The girls were crazy for those eyes that seemed both wise and incredibly sexy. He'd become the family's hope. Pedro would never dirty his hands with the manual labor that had kept the Zamoras going. He'd go to college and be a doctor, a lawyer, an executive.

By the time he received that fateful letter from the Red Cross, Pedro had adjusted to the loss of his mother. He was no longer spending his evenings looking for somebody, anybody, to give him affection.

But it was already too late. For Pedro, AIDS meant death, so he prepared himself for the end. Within four months, the seventeen-year-old had worked himself into such anxiety that he wound up in the hospital — not with any AIDS-related ailment but with shingles, from the stress.

By the end of his two-month hospital stay, he discovered an antidote to the stress and the despair — anger, "at the government for not caring, at people for not seeing us as real people with a real disease, at society for not teaching us anything about AIDS," he said.

Pedro never planned to leverage that anger, or his diagnosis, into celebrity status. He didn't make any plans at all. Things just seemed to happen to a boy who was extraordinarily handsome and couldn't abide ignorance. During summer school just before his graduation, Pedro sat in a classroom and heard one of those typical student discussions of gays. The word "faggot" cropped up. Pedro tensed. One boy bragged about gay bashing. Pedro exploded, although in the hushed tones his intensity always demanded.

"I'm gay," he announced. He began talking about his life as a gay man, about being HIV positive. He didn't stop for the remaining four years of his life.

Pedro had no talent for the kind of righteous indignation that fueled most activists. Yelling simply wasn't his style. Talking was. He was acutely aware of his heavily accented English, of being an immigrant kid who'd lost his mother and his family, who'd been sexually abused as a young child and sexually used by forty-year-old men at the most vulnerable time in his life.

But when he opened his mouth to speak to journalists, elementary school students, even members of Congress, he was dazzling. "He never clears his throat, repeats the question or employs any of the standard stalling-for-time tactics," said Hal Rubenstein, the *New York Times* reporter who interviewed him for *POZ* magazine in 1994. "His speech is devoid of hmms, huhs, let-me-thinks and, sometimes, when he's really zooming, even breath."

Pedro was pulled into a vortex that overwhelmed him. At first the pull was merely local. Pedro would take time off from his job selling suits at Burdine's to talk to public school kids about HIV and AIDS. Warning them was both a mission and personal therapy. "The anger, the pain," he said. "I don't want anyone else to have to feel this way." After his story appeared in the *Miami Herald,* the demands on his time overwhelmed the suits and Pedro became a professional AIDS educator, receiving a salary from Body Positive to expose himself to public view. He was in constant demand at schools, synagogues and churches. He spoke to civic groups, to businesses and their employees' children. Gradually, the requests began coming from farther afield, from northern Florida and Georgia, then Washington, D.C., and overseas.

He thought about going to school so he could learn to be a counselor for the dying, about creating some balance in his life so that he'd be more than "Pedro Zamora, wonder teen with AIDS." But the bookings kept coming, the honors rolled in. He was asked to appear before Congress. He was invited to give plenary addresses. The U.S. Public Health Service selected him as a poster boy, to deliver the national AIDS message.

For the most part, Pedro revelled in the celebrity status, as anyone his age would. He'd always wanted to meet President Jimmy Carter, the man who opened America to the young Cuban refugee; AIDS paved the way. He loved flying around the country, staying at fancy hotels and being cheered. But acutely aware that his immune system was deteriorating, he also fought desperately to find a way to fit the fragments together, to have a normal life like a normal young man. He tried to carve out time to watch *Star Trek* in the apartment he shared with his boyfriend Angel or spend time with his family. But there wasn't really any time. There was always another plane to catch, another speech to prepare, another interview to give. Time was running out, and racing around blurred that truth as effectively as promiscuous sex had blunted the reality of his mother's death.

Finally, in 1993 a new director at Body Positive tried to transform Pedro from a full-time speaker into a part-time clerk. He balked. That wasn't what he wanted to do, needed to do. He turned in his resignation. Lost and broke, Pedro tried the commercial lecture circuit. It wasn't his world. Then he heard that MTV's *Real World* was looking for new cast members. He was chosen from among the 30,000 other applicants. An articulate, handsome HIV-positive gay man was almost too much to hope for on a program that thrived on the conflict bred by diversity.

"His message was, 'Look at me. I'm twenty-two years old, I look healthy, I look vibrant . . . but there's a killer lurking inside of me and it can come up and grab me at any moment,'" said Doug Herzog, MTV's executive vice president of programming and production. The drama was beyond MTV's wildest dreams. They even spiced it up some more by refusing to tell the cast members which one of them had HIV. The producers decided that the revelation, when it came, would look great on film.

When Pedro moved from Miami to the house on Russian Hill in San Francisco that MTV used as the real-life stage set for the program, he moved from one fantasyland to another. Life as Wonder Boy with AIDS became life as Wonder Boy with AIDS being filmed almost twenty-four hours a day.

Cameras followed him to his speaking engagements. They captured his clash with his roommate Puck, a scab-picking bike messenger who refused to eat with utensils. They were there on his first date with Sean Sasser. For five months Pedro enjoyed a love-hate relationship with the camera. He was a dyed-in-the-wool ham who turned on a magical electricity when the red light came on. But when he fell ill with pneumonia, taping became a nightmare. His mission was to project a positive image of having HIV — the image of living with the virus, not dying from it. He escaped to Sean's apartment for two weeks. But then it was back to the cameras, to the speaking engagements, to the pressures of being the perfect AIDS poster child.

When the filming wrapped up, Pedro flew to New York for an interview on the CBS morning show. He'd been complaining about headaches and promised Sean that he'd slow down. Like most twenty-two-year-olds, he wasn't much good at pacing himself. He had to visit his family in Miami, to confront their confusion about his marriage to Sean and his decision to move to San Francisco. He had a full booking of speaking engagements and offers from a modeling agency.

The night before his CBS interview, however, he was more than just stressed. His head was throbbing. He was strangely upset that he had to change rooms in the hotel, that his shirt wasn't pressed and that the hotel laundry service was shut down for the night. He called Sean in California. "Cancel the interview," Sean told him. "Just tell them you're sick."

The next morning, Pedro didn't appear at CBS. He didn't call. He just disappeared. When he returned to the hotel, his room key wouldn't open the door. With uncommon aggressiveness he demanded that a cleaning woman let him into his room. She gave in to the request, and reported the incident. The hotel manager thought he was dealing with yet another weirdo and he called the police, who charged Pedro with trespassing. Finally an MTV producer showed up. "Look, he's Pedro Zamora, a guest in the hotel," he explained. Pedro had been trying to get into the wrong room. It seemed like an odd mistake, but mistakes happen, he figured. Then Pedro asked to make a phone call before leaving for the airport. He didn't come out of his room. When the MTV producer went in, he found Pedro sitting staring at the phone, unable to remember the number he wanted to call.

By the time he was admitted to St. Vincent's Hospital, he had no memory of anything that had happened — where he had gone in the morning, his altercation with the maid, his failed attempt to make a phone call. Something was seriously wrong. Doctors examined the confused young man, checked out his blood and ran scans on his brain. They couldn't be sure, but they suspected that Pedro had two simultaneous brain infections.

Sean flew in from California. Toxoplasmosis would almost be good news, he knew, since it was relatively easily cured. But PML would be a disaster, the nightmare of every AIDS patient. A poorly understood viral infection of the brain, PML causes confusion and seizures, blindness, paralysis and death. There is no effective treatment. There is no known cure.

One Monday morning a neurologist shaved the side of Pedro's head and stuck a needle deep into his brain. Pathologists examined the results of the biopsy. The PML diagnosis was confirmed.

Two days later, accompanied by Sean, his cousin Oscar and another

Real World cast member, Pedro flew home to Miami — to the bosom of a family that still saw him as their little boy, to the bosom of a community that still thought of him as their wonder teen.

At first, it was easy to maintain the illusion that Pedro would be okay. He still looked gorgeous. He wasn't wasted or feeble. He could still samba with his friends. He took walks with Sean through his family's neighborhood. But one night his friend Ernie came over at dinner time. Pedro looked intently at the piece of ham on his plate, then picked it up with his hands and began to chew it. "Do you want me to cut it up for you?" Ernie asked. "Oh — eh, no, gracias," Pedro answered, picking up the knife and fork he had forgotten. Another night his friends panicked when Pedro locked himself in the bathroom and wouldn't come out. They agonized over his apparent anger, not realizing that their friend had forgotten how to unlock the door.

As Pedro became increasingly helpless, he became increasingly dependent, and the fight for control was waged. His old friends wanted to surround him; his new friends from MTV flew in from California. His family wanted him back in their nest; Sean wanted to lie next to him, to enfold him in his arms. The family spoke little or no English; Sean spoke no Spanish at all. One day Pedro's hand began to swell from the IV dripping into his vein. His sister Milagros removed his wedding ring. Sean never saw it again.

Pedro's speaking schedule had been planned for months before he fell ill. Judd Wineck, another member of the *Real World* cast, replaced him. He didn't speak about AIDS. He couldn't. He spoke about Pedro. While he lay dying, there was yet another AIDS benefit at a fancy Miami Beach restaurant. Pedro was the star — in absentia. His friend Alex was asked to speak. Members of the *Real World* cast were called up to the stage. No AIDS activist talked about Pedro's work. Sean sat, virtually unnoticed, in the audience.

During those last steamy days of fall in Miami, Sean Sasser lived suspended between the reality of the death watch over Pedro's withering body and the fantasyland of chic cafés and sleek bodies on Miami Beach, where he was staying. As he moved back and forth between the two, he was haunted by a distant image, a flashback to his last speaking engagement in a middle school in San Francisco. He'd told his story, yet again, about studying at the University of Chicago, taking time off for a long trip to France and Italy, about joining the army and testing positive. The kids recognized him from his bus shelter photograph and from his constant appearances on *Real World*.

One of the eighth graders sat in the back of the room and scowled. "I don't understand," the boy finally blurted out. "I thought you were trying to scare us about AIDS. Instead, you tell us about going to Europe and becoming television stars because of HIV. You make it seem so wonderful and glamorous."

Pedro had been dead nine days. The anger and grief were still raw as hundreds of friends and family, strangers who had heard him speak and fans who'd fallen in love with the young man on *Real World* made their way to an old theater on Miami Beach's Lincoln Road Mall. MTV Latino had provided a stage manager and an audio system for the event. MTV footed most of the rest of the bill for the memorial service.

Nine months earlier Pedro had gone to the memorial service held for journalist Randy Shilts in San Francisco. It was his first view of the viciousness of Reverend Fred Phelps, whose mission was to expose the evil ways of people with AIDS. Phelps had a long history of picketing the funerals of AIDS patients with signs reading "Fags=Death" and harassing grieving families with letters calling their sons "filthy dead Sodomites." Pedro had been sickened at the sight of Phelps and the family members who always accompanied him parading in front of Glide Memorial Church with signs condemning the filthy face of fag evil. What kind of country is this? Pedro wondered. He hadn't been raised to that kind of hatred.

But the crowds and the passion, the energy of the protest and the tribute paid to Shilts moved the young man who still thought himself immortal. "That's what I want," he said in an offhand comment. A protest, not a solemn wake.

His best friend in Miami, Alex Escarano, had taken the comment literally and supervised the arrangements, because Sean, feeling snubbed and displaced by some members of Pedro's family, fled to a friend in New Orleans. Escarano would grant Pedro his final wish, or at least what he understood it to be. He began making the calls, spreading the word.

The bigwigs and bandleaders didn't need a special invitation. Patsy Fleming, President Clinton's new AIDS czar, flew in from Washington, along with the leaders of Washington's AIDS bureaucracy and other members of the AIDS social A-list. The *Real World* cast was there, along with its groupies. Fred Phelps came from Kansas.

Phelps stood outside the theater, behind police barricades. The filthy face of fag evil he protested that day belonged to Pedro Zamora.

Community leaders intent on avoiding violence, and on demonstrating Gay America's moral superiority, wandered through the angry crowd. "Turn your back on him," they murmured. "It's more powerful not to say anything."

As Ivan Bernstein, a Miami AIDS activist, surveyed this pageant and all the pilgrims who had journeyed to it, he was struck by an infuriating realization: he was the only one on the mall that day who had spent hour after hour, night after night at Mercy Hospital, watching Pedro die. The rest of them knew Pedro in only the most heady of times, if they knew him at all.

Most of them hadn't known him, as Ivan had, when he began his passionate public speaking in Miami, with no aspirations for a glamorous makeover on national TV. Most of them hadn't seen him when the glamour ebbed and he lay catatonic on the brink of death. This service, Ivan fumed, was not about Pedro the activist or Pedro the casualty of a hideous disease. It was about Pedro the star.

Pedro hadn't been in the ground two weeks, and his history was already being rewritten, Ivan thought, burning.

"Fuck you," he screamed at the protesters in particular, but really at everyone. "Go fuck yourselves."

TEN

Pill Pushers and
Policy Makers

Amid all the nasty noise that came
to define the AIDS epidemic, one of the loudest dins was raised at
a demonstration unlike anything that Washington had seen since a
strange mix of hippies and lefties descended on the Pentagon twenty
years earlier to stop the war in Vietnam by levitating the center of U.S.
military might.

Just after dawn on October 11, 1988, more than one thousand
young men and women — with bleached white hair and nose rings,
wearing clothes splashed with simulated blood — surrounded a stark
twenty-story federal building in Rockville, Maryland, screaming, "No
more deaths." Employees had been warned that they were scheduled
for a siege. The men and women who decided to brave the forces and
enter the building were blocked from the walkways and roadways by a
phalanx of helmeted police officers with riot batons and latex gloves,
standing shoulder to shoulder protecting the main entrance.

"Shame, shame," the demonstrators yelled at employees trying to
enter the headquarters of the Food and Drug Administration — renamed, that day, the Federal Death Administration.

"Hey, hey, FDA, how many people have you killed today?" activists chanted as the American flag was lowered and a burning effigy of
President Reagan raised in its place.

"I'm here today because I don't want my name on a quilt in front of
the White House," said Vito Russo, a prominent film historian and
AIDS patient, referring to the AIDS Memorial Quilt, then on display
on the mall downtown. He and demonstrators from fifteen states had
converged on the agency to demand the release of new drugs to fight
AIDS. They seemed convinced that the FDA had some magic potion
locked inside that regulators were refusing to license.

"There's absolutely no reason why these drugs cannot be released," said Daniel Snow, a Chicago AIDS patient who arrived in a wheelchair. "We'll sign releases saying we understand there are risks. But if we don't get these drugs, we are going to die. It's as simple as that."

As police began to lead handcuffed demonstrators away in commuter buses, thirty protesters lay down in the street. The FDA "doesn't want to treat us with the drugs because they don't recognize us as human beings," shouted Steven Gould, an HIV-positive Los Angeles real estate appraiser.

It was less than one month before the presidential election. Vice President Bush and his vice presidential candidate, Dan Quayle, had been riding the deregulatory bandwagon to campaign stops from Oregon to Florida. The Food and Drug Administration had long been at the top of the conservative hit list. As they watched the television reports of the siege of the agency, they smiled.

They had found the FDA's Willie Horton.

In the AIDS activist roll call of dishonor, social indifference to the imminent demise of millions of citizens of the planet has long been public enemy number one. The Food and Drug Administration has always been a close second.

It's an easy target. The sprawling federal agency that regulates nearly everything Americans eat and drink, paint on faces, feed to their cats and buy at the pharmacy has been under fire for years. Pharmaceutical industry profits aren't growing as fast as corporate executives would like; blame the FDA. Liquefied apricot pits aren't available as a cancer treatment; blame the FDA. Children die because drug companies don't report toxic side effects as required by law; blame the FDA. There's no cure for AIDS — blame the FDA for that too.

AIDS activists view drug development as a long pipeline that begins in the secret laboratories of pharmaceutical companies and ends up in hospitals and drugstores. By 1987, six years after the first AIDS cases were reported, that pipeline wasn't disgorging any drugs, miraculous or mediocre. Activists went looking for the blockage in the system. The FDA was targeted for a heavy dose of Drāno.

Sometimes the agency needed it — desperately. Witness the case of ganciclovir, for years the single medication that helped AIDS patients maintain their sight against the ravages of cytomegalovirus retinitis. In 1984 Syntex Corporation alerted the FDA that it had a compound that might fight CMV and asked for approval to release it to patients under a compassionate-use protocol. Such a release wasn't unusual; in fact, an entire class of anti-cancer drugs had long been distributed in this manner.

As ganciclovir reached hospitals around the country, physicians overwhelmed by their powerlessness to treat a dozen diseases believed they had finally found a miracle. Within a week of receiving ganciclovir infusions, even blind patients regained their sight. In a disease in which the home runs have been few and far between, ganciclovir flew out of the ballpark.

Over the course of the next three years, Syntex handed out $25 million worth of ganciclovir to more than five thousand patients without mounting a single clinical trial to prove its worth. Cynics insist that the company had assumed that if it created enough pressure from the patient community, the FDA would be forced to approve ganciclovir without systematic — and expensive — trials. Others contend that the FDA led Syntex to believe the agency would look the other way when approval was sought.

The truth is that ganciclovir got caught in the middle of a patent dispute between Syntex and Burroughs-Wellcome, which had a virtual lock on AIDS drugs with AZT and Septra, Burroughs-Wellcome's version of Bactrim. Neither company was going to invest the millions of dollars necessary to mount a clinical trial for a drug it might not own. And by the time Syntex won the patent, in March 1987, a carefully controlled study was impossible: patients and their physicians already knew ganciclovir worked so no one was willing to sign up for a trial and risk getting a placebo. Even if anyone had been willing, no one believed such a trial would be ethical.

Syntex asked for FDA approval of ganciclovir based on four studies culled from information on the patients who'd taken the drug under the compassionate-use program. The data were a mess. Physicians had given the drug in different doses to different kinds of patients with blindness of differing severity. Some had kept meticulous records; most kept few at all.

When the FDA advisory committee met on October 26, 1987, to consider the application, its members were appalled. "Investigational anarchy," Stephen Straus called the data. But the committee had one other problem: they knew ganciclovir worked. The opinion of physicians who cared for AIDS patients day after day was unanimous. Still, the committee balked at recommending approval on instinct rather than on the data. Only the ophthalmologists on the advisory panel voted for approval. FDA Commissioner Frank Young sided with the majority, saying simply, "We can't accept testimonials."

Patients continued to receive the drug under the compassionate-use exception, although physicians complained about the added paperwork that entailed. Syntex couldn't market the drug. Other drug companies realized the perils of benevolence.

Ganciclovir remained in that FDA-created netherworld for almost two years while Syntex and the agency argued back and forth about how to document what everyone already knew. Syntex eventually caved in to an FDA demand for a clinical trial and turned the study over to the AIDS Clinical Trials Group. It made no difference. No one would enlist. Syntex tried to muscle patients into the trial by canceling compassionate-use distribution. But the ACTG didn't get the study going for months, leaving patients with no source of ganciclovir. It was a Catch-22 leading to blindness. Syntex began handing out the drug once again.

By January 1989 so few patients had volunteered for the trial that physicians admitted full enrollment would take a decade. In despair, the FDA agreed to take a second look at ganciclovir. They saw some new data from trials in San Francisco and France, but were faced largely with the old information dressed up in more professional clothing. The second time around, it was sufficient. Six weeks later ganciclovir was formally approved — five years after its value in treating CMV had been demonstrated.

However, the FDA often got a bad rap, receiving blame that rightly belonged to researchers. That's what happened with the endless struggle over the approval of aerosolized pentamadine, a drug used to prevent *Pneumocystis carinii* pneumonia. The scourge of AIDS patients, PCP was on everyone's hit list as *the* disease to prevent. Physicians already had two treatments in their arsenal. Unfortunately, the approved one, Bactrim, caused severe allergic reactions, and the other, pentamadine, was out of reach.

Used primarily to prevent African sleeping sickness, pentamadine had little market in the United States. It was available only through the CDC's Parasitic Drug Service, which had long imported the tiny quantities needed from England. By the end of 1983, however, CDC staffers were spending their days rushing to the airport to pick up, and reship, the drug to help the growing number of people with AIDS. They finally prevailed upon a small Illinois company called Lymphomed to produce a steadier supply. The FDA rushed to approve the injectable solution in 1984.

The injections, however, didn't work. The drug lingered in the spleen or the liver and barely made it to the lungs. Clinicians needed an aerosolized version of pentamadine, and a new version meant a new drug approval. NIH researchers declared the testing of aerosolized pentamadine a high priority in 1987, but for two years the ACTG seemed incapable of designing a trial. What type of nebulizers should they use? What size particles should be delivered? What dosage should they try? Should they test the drug against a placebo or would that be unethical, since everyone already knew the drug worked?

While researchers debated scientific niceties, people were dying. At their patients' insistence, a group of physicians in San Francisco and New York mounted their own clinical trial. The strategy was unheard of, but the FDA didn't balk. When Lymphomed presented the physicians' data to the FDA, approval was almost instantaneous. The FDA was no villain in the delay; the rap belongs to an inept group of researchers.

FDA Commissioner Frank Young wasn't oblivious. He understood that his agency needed new policies for AIDS. There were too many sick people without medications who needed quick access to experimental treatments. In March 1987 he unveiled a plan to help these patients, creating a category of drugs that could be sold before approval if they seemed safe and showed at least some minimal signs of effectiveness.

Conservatives were ecstatic over this modicum of deregulation. The *Wall Street Journal* heralded the changes as a "giant step for the sick and dying." Pharmaceutical companies celebrated the new precedent: the sale of drugs of unproven value. AIDS activists on the West Coast, the greatest boosters of allowing the sick to take anything — and permitting drug companies to sell it to them — claimed the victory as theirs. They were wrong, of course. The hand moving the FDA belonged to Vice President George Bush, who couched his concern in the compassion he'd gained through his own experience trying, and failing, to obtain experimental medications for his daughter's leukemia. There was clearly more to it: Bush was the chairman of the President's Task Force on Regulatory Relief, which was the conservative's point group for gutting the FDA.

The FDA likes to think of itself as a benevolent agency. The Pentagon might drop bombs on innocent people, the Department of Health and Human Services might force children to read books their parents despise. But the FDA exists for but one purpose: to protect the public from greedy pharmaceutical companies, quacks, hypesters and charlatans. Once upon a time, Americans could eat, drink and medicate themselves with anything they wanted. They could buy any potion any miracle man could convince them to imbibe. But in the inevitable trend toward a government that protects its citizens from forces domestic as well as foreign — commercial as well as military — citizens lost those problematic and sometimes perilous rights to regulatory agencies. To the ultra-individualists, it was a basic violation of civil liberties. To most Americans, it was common sense.

The FDA was the child of scandal, a creature created by Congress in response to the growing awareness in the twentieth century that capitalism is not always beneficent. Stung by muckraking journalists like Upton Sinclair, whose graphic portrayal of the filth of the meatpacking industry made *The Jungle* an instant success, legislators in 1906 bowed to public hysteria and turned a small laboratory at the Agriculture Department into the Food and Drug Administration. Regulation was popular back then. Physicians had been complaining about the adulteration of drugs and the lack of standards in imported medications at least since the Mexican-American War. Freedom was unrestricted, and that freedom had caused deaths.

The FDA of that era did little to oversee the drug industry, or anything else. It tested some compounds and tried to enforce standardization. But deceptive advertising was commonplace since the courts seemed to accept the "I believe it works" defense. There were no warning labels, no explicit directions about drug interactions or how to take a medicine without burning the inside of your stomach. The FDA had no power to keep unsafe drugs off the market. Before the time of big government, after all, no one expected federal regulatory agencies to be proactive.

Then, just as the New Deal winds began to blow, the sulfonamide scandal riveted the nation. Sulfa was one of the first wonder drugs to fight the constant onslaught of human bacterial infections, from meningitis to urethritis. When one enterprising company prepared an oral solution of the drug to administer to children, however, it used diethylene glycol as the solvent. The company didn't have to check with the FDA before selling the new preparation. If it had, a pharmacologist might have told them that diethylene glycol was poison.

More than one hundred Americans, most of them children, died.

Less than a year later, in 1938, Congress passed the Food, Drug and Cosmetic Act, giving the FDA real power to ensure that drugs sold to consumers were not going to kill them. The procedure was simple: any company planning to sell a new drug had to submit proof of safety to the agency. If the FDA didn't say no within sixty days, the drug went out on the shelves.

In the late 1950s Senator Estes Kefauver got into the act, launching the nation's first serious investigation of the pharmaceutical industry. In that era when science and technology seemed poised to cure all the world's ills, Kefauver found little support for a major overhaul of federal oversight of the pharmaceutical industry, until another well-timed scandal greased the way.

Thalidomide — a name the mention of which still sends tremors through the hearts of women who were pregnant in the late fifties, was a sedative widely prescribed in Germany and England to relieve morning sickness. American approval was stalled at the FDA by a recalcitrant medical officer who was, many claimed, just too picky about the standards for safety evaluation.

Her zealousness saved thousands of children. It turned out that thalidomide caused severe birth defects. More than eight thousand European children were born with no arms or legs, with limbs shaped like flippers, blind or retarded because their mothers had taken the drug during pregnancy.

Suddenly the FDA was heroic, and the issue of government supervision of drug testing skyrocketed on the national agenda. In August 1962 Congress amended the Food, Drug and Cosmetic Act and upped the ante. Companies that wanted to sell drugs in America not only had to prove them safe, but effective as well.

The agency had a long honeymoon with a public more suspicious of industry than of government. The idea of being protected by big government was still reassuring to a populace convinced that business, left unfettered, would sell molasses as miraculous if the price was right. The FDA gradually spread its tentacles throughout the American economy. Today, twenty-five cents of every dollar spent in the country goes to purchase an FDA-regulated product: Cocoa Puffs and Twinkies, orange juice, aspirin, antibiotics, eyeliner, silicone breast and penis implants, Puppy Chow and microwave ovens. What began as a small chemistry lab at the Department of Agriculture has expanded to half a dozen buildings inside and outside the Beltway. In 1960 the FDA commissioner had 1,678 employees helping him protect America from fraud and injury. By 1990 the legion was 7,800. By 1994, 9,000.

Not everyone applauded this growing empire, but most of the complaints came either from industry or from ultraconservative academics and politicians — a relatively marginalized group until the congressional elections of 1994. They charged that the FDA was killing American business and American citizens with overregulation. *Forbes* cited the agency's delay in the approval of beta-blockers, compounds that treat hypertension and other cardiovascular disease. The nine years' testing and approval lag was responsible for the deaths of ten thousand or more Americans a year, the business publication charged. "But the victims are usually voiceless. So they don't count."

Academics, often funded by industry, bemoaned the fact that drugs became available in Europe years earlier than in the United States. That was hardly surprising since it took an average of 9.75 years for a drug to move through the testing and regulatory rigors in this country. But other countries had licensed thalidomide. Why should the federal government be in the business of deciding which medicines are effective? they asked, comparing the FDA to an Orwellian Big Brother controlling helpless consumers. Demanding the inalienable right to experiment and take risks, they proposed turning the FDA into a certifying agency without veto power, an empty shell that would provide consumers with information they could use or ignore.

No one took advocates of the evisceration of the FDA overly seriously because they were so clearly more concerned with the profit margins of pharmaceutical companies than with the health of Americans. Their insistence that bad drugs would just fall by the wayside in an unregulated marketplace showed callous indifference to the people who might succumb to false advertising and bad drugs in the process. Their suggestion that pharmaceuticals could be handled through contract law — regulating the market through lawsuits from consumers displeased with individual drugs — ignored the reality that all too many of those disappointed consumers might be dead.

The bottom line is that drug companies are notorious whiners. They have the highest profit margins of any American industry. They peddle their potions in the United States for 60 percent more than they charge in England. They complain endlessly about the high cost of research and testing — an astronomical $230 million for each drug brought to market — but rarely acknowledge that they spend up to twice that amount on marketing, drumming up business by handing out free samples and gifts to physicians. One company even came up with a Frequent Prescriber Plan, whereby doctors earned airline tickets by prescribing its drug.

In their zeal to support industry, conservatives long failed to balance their commercial concerns with human ones — and they are movingly powerful. For researchers at universities and FDA officials, careful testing and firm regulation are sensible — the basic "greatest good for the greatest number." But the sensible global principle obscures the reality of the individual patient dying from liver cancer or Alzheimer's, or the plight of a family facing the stark words "There's nothing I can do." The FDA has protected them from wasting their money, and the even more precious commodity of hope, on worthless treatments. But there is no way of knowing how many patients it may have also condemned by keeping them from life-saving medicines.

AIDS drew fresh, intense attention to that flaw. The young, well-educated and articulate men who first turned up with unusual immune disorders were deeply suspicious of the government's attitudes and actions toward them. They didn't accept the pronouncements of the FDA any more easily than they accepted the conclusions of the Supreme Court that their sexual activities should be illegal. The possibility of powerlessness in the face of death was anathema. These men wanted — needed, perhaps — to believe that miraculous concoctions already existed that needed only to be pulled off the shelf, tested perfunctorily and sped into their bodies. Groups like California's Project Inform and ACT UP published long and ever-changing lists of potions they were convinced had the power to stop death, if they were only made available. Not yet ready to turn on the research scientists, they turned on the FDA.

As they became guerrillas attacking FDA regulators from all sides, conservative deregulators who showed no other concern for the bodies piling up in AIDS wards in San Francisco and Greenwich Village found their thalidomide scandal. Vice President Dan Quayle and his Competitiveness Council were already gunning for the agency, which he believed was plotting against the health of the pharmaceutical industry. "The iron triangle — the seemingly permanent clique of special interests, Hill staff and faceless bureaucrats — is now energized to stop the Competitiveness Council from demanding a serious review of the impact of regulation on our economic productivity," he said. "The council is simply protecting America's greatness from over-zealous regulators." These paragons of overzealousness, in Quayle's imagination, worked at the FDA. When AIDS activists hit the streets, dividing the liberal consumer protectionists of the nation and Congress, Quayle's convoluted rhetoric began to make sense.

• • •

Martin Delaney was the man who made the connection. The founder of San Francisco's treatment information group Project Inform, he began his career in AIDS as a bad boy of the underground helping to smuggle potentially lifesaving drugs into the country. Over the years Delaney managed to parlay his work and considerable bluster into access to power at the highest levels of government. He quickly ended his foray into anti-establishmentarianism and dedicated himself to fighting AIDS by supporting the AIDS research establishment.

Delaney meets regularly with officials of the Food and Drug Administration and the National Institutes of Health as the self-styled representative of the AIDS treatment activism community. When in Washington, he dines with his friend Robert Gallo of the National Cancer Institute. He meets regularly with executives of major pharmaceutical companies, who give generous donations to Project Inform. The potential conflicts of interest have never been explored.

Delaney can't bear to lose; he seems never to have admitted to being wrong. Reporters who write articles with which he disagrees are inevitably called into their editors' offices to read the long, single-spaced, point-by-point diatribes with which he responds. When their facts are unassailable, their motives are impugned.

When the *Chicago Tribune* reporter John Crewdson wrote an extensive investigative piece on allegations that Dr. Robert Gallo had stolen credit for the discovery of HIV from French researchers, Delaney rose to Gallo's defense. He accused Crewdson of creating a "climate of fear at NIH" akin to the research atmosphere in eastern Europe, "where scientists (formerly) operated under a cloud of suspicion." He demanded that the paper reimburse the government for the cost of the inquiry into Gallo's activities. He even reported Crewdson to his editors for staying at a five-star hotel in Paris — although the reporter was a denizen of the Marriott.

San Francisco activists have learned to stay out of his way. "He believes himself to be a demigod," one said. "He might be, for all I know. But believe me, you take your chances when you go up against him." Another was even more candid: "Martin Delaney is to AIDS activism what Jimmy Hoffa was to the labor movement."

When Delaney heard about FDA Commissioner Frank Young's plan to give AIDS patients access to experimental medications, he jumped to Young's support. Delaney knew of a dozen drugs he believed would help the sick, and was relieved to discover that the FDA seemed ready to open the floodgates.

But it wasn't that easy. Young's reforms stunk so acridly of politics that consumer protectionists were immediately wary. Congressman Ted Weiss's staff members began looking for evidence of a deregulatory plot, and found it in documents from the Office of Management and Budget suggesting that drugs should be approved without being proven effective. Consumer advocates made common cause with East Coast AIDS lobbying groups — from the American Foundation for AIDS Research and the People with AIDS Coalition to the National Lesbian and Gay Task Force — who insisted that allowing the sale of unproven and potentially harmful drugs could wind up killing more AIDS patients than they would save. "Don't forget suramin," said the task force's executive director, Jeff Levi, now the assistant to AIDS czar Patsy Fleming. Suramin, which had shown early promise as an anti-HIV medication, was precisely the type of remedy that would be sped into early release under Young's proposals. After more study, it had not only proven ineffective but dangerous: at least two people died during the trial.

Researchers were also worried by Young's reforms. If patients had open access to experimental drugs, they would never participate in controlled drug studies. How will we ever know if the drugs really work? they asked. Delaney argued that he couldn't care less. He wanted "Drugs into Bodies," as the protest chant demanded, even if formal trials collapsed and pharmaceutical companies made millions off *dreck*. He insisted that it was a question of freedom, and he wasn't about to allow a bunch of scientists and AIDS activists to block liberty.

"You're so caught up in liberal Democratic party politics that you can't see where your own interests lie," he screamed at Jeff Levi on the phone from San Francisco. "Out here in the heartland, people want these drugs. They don't give a shit if it's coming from Reagan or anybody else. You're just a goddamned gay bureaucrat. People with AIDS are dying because of FDA bureaucrats. We don't need them to die because of gay bureaucrats." Delaney fired off letters to the members of the boards of national gay organizations, denouncing Levi for "endangering our lives and giving the government an excuse to back away from the most responsive action they have ever taken on AIDS." He vilified the American Foundation for AIDS Research for its accusation that Young's proposal was just another cover for pharmaceutical company profiteering.

He received an infusion of support when ACT UP, newly formed in New York, rushed into the fray in a blaze of activist glory, seducing the media with sexy graphics and perfectly staged demonstrations. Its members became, in essence, the shock troops of deregulation, giving a human face to the price of FDA rules.

Delaney isn't the street-activist type. He prefers being interviewed in a TV studio to being filmed screaming at a demonstration. So he shows up calm and collected, dressed like a businessman, on *Donahue* and *Nightline*. He seems most comfortable dealing in boardrooms, even with conservative deregulators, the very men who tend to blame AIDS patients for their own illnesses or refuse to fund the AIDS research budget. He joined forces with them on October 12, 1987, when he met with Vice President Bush's chief counsel, C. Boyden Gray, at the Executive Office Building and agreed to feed him FDA-busting ammunition.

He even met with the FDA, which was where he met his nemesis. Dr. Ellen Cooper was the agency's gatekeeper for AIDS drugs. A Phi Beta Kappa graduate of Swarthmore College, Cooper had a medical degree and a master's in public health. She was trained in both pediatrics and infectious diseases, was the mother of triplets and a fourth child with Down's syndrome, and took her responsibility for protecting people from drugs that might be poison extremely seriously. She was less than enthusiastic about rushing unproven drugs into already weakened bodies. Delaney collected rumors and anecdotes about new drugs; Cooper preferred scientific data.

Delaney says he hated her on sight. As he tells the story of his first encounter with FDA officials, Commissioner Frank Young was an open, honest bureaucrat interested in responding to the AIDS community; Cooper was a rigid unfeeling cipher. Over the years, he has called her the Ice Lady in public. According to Delaney, whenever Cooper was present at a meeting, Young would hesitate to move forward with bold reforms. In her absence, he was flexible.

Delaney gradually began to attack Cooper personally, suggesting that she was too inexperienced to have so much authority. "She clearly places the needs of the research process above the needs of compassion for patients," he told the press at the time. "We're also concerned about her age. It's difficult to see how someone so young can really be responsible for making decisions that affect lives in such a profound way." Cooper, who was in her late thirties, refrained from asking where a marketing consultant got the experience to critique her work.

Just weeks before the 1988 presidential election, C. Boyden Gray called to ask Delaney for help in a presidency-making attempt to get the FDA to reduce the burden of proof it required to measure a drug's worth. People like Cooper at the FDA were so adamant, Gray said, that they were threatening to tell the public that the candidate was trying to leave them vulnerable to unproven, even dangerous medications.

Delaney rushed to the vice president's defense. "As much as I hate to admit it, Bush — not our traditional allies in Congress — is the only one in the last two years who has taken any steps to correct the problem at FDA," he wrote Jeff Levi.

Three weeks before the election, bowing to most of Bush's demands, the FDA announced a new plan to speed up approval of drugs for life-threatening diseases. Promising to repeat the miracle of AZT — which was licensed within two years of its first testing on human beings — the agency offered to help companies slide through the approval process.

Delaney and his supporters weren't placated. It still wasn't enough. Most people with AIDS, Delaney insisted, didn't have two years to wait. ACT UP was pushing for expanded access, which would allow patients to take drugs that had been deemed safe while researchers continued studies into their effectiveness. Industry leaders were lukewarm to the proposal. They worried about liability and the costs of gearing up for production without any guarantee of licensure. Expanded access, after all, was a consumer's dream, because patients would get drugs for free while drug companies tried to build both their case for approval and the market. FDA approval was what companies really desired, because only then could they start to make a profit.

Delaney threw himself into their cause with zeal. Accelerated approval — the full licensing of drugs with minimal evidence of both safety and effectiveness — became his demand. Any drug was better than none. He seemed to have full faith that industry would provide if the rewards were sufficiently high.

Accelerated approval wasn't easy to achieve with drugs designed to fight a slow and debilitating disease. Researchers couldn't wait for patients on studies to see if a drug was effective; that would mean waiting for years. The solution Delaney and his allies, in and out of the drug companies, proposed was the use of surrogate markers — specific measures of blood levels they believed correlated to prolonged survival.

Ellen Cooper wasn't buying it. On September 11 and 12, 1989, the Institute of Medicine held a roundtable to discuss the use of surrogate markers in AIDS. Eighteen people had been invited to make scientific presentations and recommend guidelines to the National Institutes of Health. Delaney was one of them. Cooper, who was not invited to be a panelist, sat in. Delaney waited nervously to hear Cooper speak.

Delaney says that over the years he has learned to predict Cooper's mood by her tone of voice. She has two voices, he claims: a deep, masculine one for her moments of scientific rigidity and a warm, feminine one that she reserves for times of conciliation. That day her tone was deep and husky. She was not ready to yield on unproven surrogate markers. Delaney was furious that Cooper, whom he considered a mere midlevel bureaucrat, refused to accede to the recommendations of his friend Dr. Anthony Fauci, the head AIDS researcher at NIH. He had lobbied Fauci hard, and won him over, thinking that his support might be critical.

"Who does Ellen Cooper think she is?" Delaney asked regularly, and loudly.

Cooper knew precisely who she was, as did her superiors at the FDA. She was the person who knew more about AIDS drugs than anyone else. Her job was to read every study, examine every statistic and weigh the evidence with every bit of scientific skill and objectivity she possessed. "Even when I disagreed with the commissioner or key people in Congress, they respected me," she says. "They trusted the honesty of my assessments." And her assessment was that surrogate markers made sense only if they had been validated, which they had not.

With the help of Dr. Samuel Broder, the director of the National Cancer Institute, and Fauci, Delaney forged ahead nonetheless. In August 1990 he wrote Cooper a long letter attacking the FDA's alternate scheme of expanded access and arguing that accelerated approval was the only ethical approach the FDA could take. "Privately within the industry, they are saying that the expanded access program has slowed the development of ddI and diverted resources from the development of other promising BM [Bristol-Myers Squibb] drugs . . . The answer has to be regulatory innovation which focuses on early licensure, not just getting drugs to people by convoluted expanded access mechanisms."

It was his declaration of war.

Delaney sent copies of the letter to scores of AIDS activists, scientists and drug company executives. He called on members of Congress to neutralize the consumer protectionists he feared might block his demands. He ran a sample letter supporting accelerated approval in the Project Inform newsletter and urged readers to deluge the FDA with mail. He worked the scientific community by phone and then in person at the AIDS Clinical Trials Group meeting in Washington, D.C., in November.

Finally he demanded that Cooper call a meeting of the Antiviral Drug Advisory Committee to discuss the use of surrogate markers in the approval of new AIDS drugs. Cooper didn't have much choice. Delaney had boxed her in with the scientific community, which was increasingly pandering to activists' demands. Political momentum was building on his side. She scheduled the session for February.

On December 17 Delaney sponsored simultaneous press conferences in eight cities at which Cooper was vilified for a letter she'd written two drug companies questioning the wisdom of early approval, a letter Delaney admits he had not read. Two days later, she scribbled a note to her boss asking to be transferred to another job, turned off her computer and went home.

"The abusive attack on the FDA was the straw that broke the camel's back," said Mark Harrington, perhaps the most knowledgeable AIDS treatment activist in the country. "She felt if she was going to have to take this type of abuse, she'd had enough."

With Cooper out of the way, and her boss, Frank Young, replaced by David Kessler, whose political acumen is legendary, the pace of change increased at the FDA.

In November 1991 the agency announced a series of reforms designed to slash drug approval time in half. Vice President Dan Quayle, who had helped engineer the move, announced that the changes would "save millions of lives and billions of dollars" by speeding treatments, even potential cures, through the FDA pipeline. In a statement that was as self-revealing as it was callous, the vice president declared, "Drugs having a potential cure for AIDS will have a chance to reach patients sooner, thus saving lives. And wouldn't it be wonderful to have a cure for AIDS in the marketplace before Magic Johnson gets AIDS?"

What wasn't trumpeted so loudly was that in order to keep the process moving, the FDA expected to farm out new drug applications to outside reviewers, which raised the dark specter of conflict of interest. "It sounds like an almost Thatcherite solution to the very real problems at FDA," said Mark Harrington of ACT UP, referring to former British Prime Minister Margaret Thatcher's privatization moves.

"What we're seeing here is, 'Oh, look, the public sector doesn't work after we've spent ten years stripping it of staff and funds, so let's dump it on the private sector.' We're seeing the last exhausted pants of an administration that doesn't have any domestic policy." Unlike Martin Delaney, Harrington had never intended to gut the FDA; he just wanted the agency to work faster and be more effective. He wanted consumer-friendly reform, not industry-friendly deregulation. Patients needed drugs but also needed to trust and know how to use them.

The momentum of deregulation picked up, with other, less savvy activists like Delaney, who were still convinced that a magic potion was lurking somewhere in the FDA pipeline, supporting every Republican proposal. They were the strange bedfellows of Vice President Quayle, who even suggested that the United States grant automatic approval to drugs licensed in other countries — in the name of competitiveness. Perhaps both the activists and the vice president were too young to remember thalidomide. Maybe they'd never heard of dilevalol, a drug given to treat heart disease. Approved in England and Portugal but not in the United States, dilevalol turned heart attack survivors into liver disease patients. The Europeans pulled its approval in 1990.

By 1992 the FDA was churning out drug approvals in record time. That year, ninety-one drugs were approved, the highest number since 1986, and the total testing and approval time had fallen to under three years. "It's crucial to have patients have control over their own destiny," David Kessler said. "The FDA has an obligation to make sure drugs are safe and effective. But that involves risk/benefits, and certainly patients can be pivotal in deciding where those risks and benefits lie."

By the time the nation's third AIDS antiviral, ddC, came up for licensing — the first under the new system of accelerated approval — the quality of the research presented, and the standards by which drugs were being judged, had become a scientific joke. FDA advisory committee hearings usually last only a few hours and attract little attention, but when the Anti-Viral Drug Advisory Committee met on April 21, 1992, to consider the ddC application, spectators packed into a ballroom in a hotel in Bethesda. Scores of drug company representatives showed up to see how the new approval process would work. Commissioner Kessler stayed for the full twenty hours of hearings.

"The industry has been very eager to see something like this to cut costs," said Tom Copmann, a regulatory analyst for the Pharmaceutical Manufacturers Association. "We've been after the agency on this thing for years." Company representatives watched as years of required animal and clinical tests disappeared.

Two preliminary tests of ddC were presented, neither of which had been designed to test its efficacy. No data were presented proving that ddC relieved symptoms or extended life; data did show that upward of one-third of ddC users in company-sponsored clinical trials suffered peripheral neuropathy, a nerve disorder that can cause paralysis of the arms and legs.

Hoffmann–La Roche asked for approval based on the drug's impact on surrogate markers — laboratory tests of T cells, which many believed to reflect the value of anti-HIV drugs. Committee members worried about approving a drug on the basis of indicators that had never been validated. "If the surrogate markers don't match up with clinical benefit, well, what good are they?" asked Paul Meier, a University of Chicago statistician. "If industry is sitting out there thinking, 'All we need to do is show CD_4 effects — any CD_4 effects — and we'll get approval,' well, that's a dreadful message and a dreadful lesson."

To Martin Delaney, the quality of the science was of secondary importance. "The issue is choice," he said. "And what is happening now that is so very important is the FDA recognizing that patients have the right and the intelligence to make their own treatment choices." Delaney advocated approving any drug believed to be safe and letting the highly touted "market" sort out the effective drugs from the duds.

A growing number of activists disagreed. Choice is fine, argued David Barr, an attorney working at the Gay Men's Health Crisis, "but simple approval of a drug doesn't make that a choice." Many AIDS specialists were openly alarmed. "We don't have the data, as physicians, to tell us what to do," said Dr. Neil Schram, an AIDS physician and FDA consultant from Los Angeles. "How do you set a standard of care now for AIDS? How do you decide who can benefit from ddI, AZT, from ddC? When? At what dose? What we have is treatment chaos."

The pharmaceutical industry won the day — and enormous savings in testing — when the advisory committee bent to the prevailing winds and voted to recommend approval.

The last straw was the approval, two years later, of the final antiviral drug in the PWA's arsenal, d4T. The efficacy trial for d4T began with 822 patients, but more than half dropped out within five months, so there wasn't enough data to tell if the drug had helped anyone. Furthermore, the data concerned CD4 counts, the artificial yardstick of dubious value. Less than a year earlier, the European Concorde trial had shown that chemically induced increases in CD4 cells bore no relationship to increased health or longevity.

"You may be able to construct a cause for approval, but there's no way to look at the data and tell doctors how to use this drug," said Derek Link, a New York AIDS activist at the FDA hearing on d4T in May 1994. His friend Spencer Cox was more succinct. "I don't know whether this drug would be helping me or would kill me faster." Mark Harrington was chilled at the new reality. Choice without information is no choice at all, he realized. That's what "deregulation with an activist face," in his words, had brought people with AIDS.

Harrington, Link and Cox are members of the Treatment Action Group, New York's elite AIDS treatment specialists. Scientifically and politically savvy, they had already pulled off a coup at NIH, removing the Office of AIDS Research from the National Institute of Allergy and Infectious Diseases — against Delaney's firm opposition. In the summer and fall of 1994, they took aim at accelerated approval, insisting that the drug companies provide at least some proof of the value of their products before approval, and that the FDA force them to conduct the agreed-upon studies after drugs are released to the public.

Timing was critical because a new class of drugs — the first drugs that would be more than AZT me-too compounds — was being tested. "The nightmare scenario is to repeat the mistakes of the past with the next generation of drugs," said Link. "This is a chance to get both drugs and information."

Many people with AIDS agreed with him. "We used to believe that taking a drug was better than nothing," said Carleton Hogan, a Minneapolis AIDS patient and activist. "That often isn't true. In many cases a placebo is the best treatment available — at least it's not toxic. We can't keep flooding the market with drugs without knowing if they work. It robs this generation and the next."

Joseph Fleiss, a biostatistician at Columbia University's School of Public Health and an FDA consultant, said bluntly, "I think the accelerated approval process is a horror. The person who thought of it and saw to its acceptance should be shot."

Instead, the big guns were aimed at the Treatment Action Group. The opposition by pharmaceutical companies, who were enjoying the added profits generated by accelerated approval, was immediate. They spread rumors that drug companies would pull out of AIDS research if accelerated approval was rescinded. Other activists accused TAG of selling out to science. TAG members were branded Nazis, a particularly cruel blow since one of TAG's members is the son of concentration camp survivors.

"Any attempt to slow drug approval may as well be holding a gun to my head," screamed one young man at an ACT UP meeting held to discuss TAG's proposals. "It may as well be putting a mine under my doormat or a fucking bomb under my pillow."

Martin Delaney organized another of the endless "consensus statements" he used to counter the opposition; a long list of individuals and groups signed it to protest TAG's position. Drug companies already aren't making any money on antivirals, Delaney said. And people with AIDS need hope.

Hope is good, TAG responded. Hope based on science is better.

TAG's leading members tried to reason with the AIDS community, explaining that the problem was more than the absence of data. Accelerated approval was providing pharmaceutical companies no incentive to do research on breakthrough drugs. Why should they spend a fortune on real advances, which might require extensive research, when they knew the FDA would approve me-too compounds with little testing?

On September 12, 1994, the FDA's Anti-Viral Drug Advisory Committee held a hearing on the growing controversy over accelerated approval. The meeting room at the Holiday Inn in Bethesda was tense as researchers, FDA officials and activists filed in and took their seats. Ellen Cooper was long gone from the agency, but she was in the audience that day representing her latest employer, the American Foundation for AIDS Research.

Everyone fidgeted, waiting for the TAG members to appear; Delaney's attacks on the group had the room astir. TAG had been caucusing in the coffee shop and arrived, just on time.

FDA staff members presented three case studies on their experiences with accelerated approval and asked committee members and invited guests to raise questions and offer comments. Time was reserved for statements from the public. It was nearly 6 P.M. before Delaney got his chance at the podium. "Many of us resent the fact that the agency and industry ran on for three hours this afternoon, forcing us to speak to an almost empty hall," he began. He was due to have dinner with Robert Gallo that night and was running late. Although dressed in khakis and a denim work shirt, Delaney gave the type of crisp presentation he'd practiced dozens of times when he was still making a six-figure salary working in business.

He dismissed TAG's concerns as the worries of errant children who didn't quite understand the stakes — which was ironic, since most of TAG's members, unlike Delaney, were HIV positive. Choice was once again his demand. He had missed the morning session, where TAG's Rebecca Pringle-Smith had compared the drug choices open to a person with AIDS to the choice one South American dictator offered the men that he tortured: you can have the nails of your left hand pulled out or the nails of your right.

But Delaney wasn't interested in the opinion of TAG members. When one, who was serving on the FDA committee, tried to point out inconsistencies in Delaney's positions, Delaney cut him off. "This is cheap, personal crap," he said. "I know the game you're playing."

Ellen Cooper watched from the far side of the room and smiled coolly.

The debate between the Treatment Action Group and Martin Delaney became moot on November 7, 1994, when conservative Republicans gained control over both houses of Congress. Incoming House Speaker Newt Gingrich had already branded the FDA the nation's "number one job killer." He and his supporters had been gunning for the FDA for years, and in the months after the election, Gingrich and the conservative think tanks that fed him were already sorting through proposals for revamping the agency. In the name of eliminating bottlenecks — a worthy goal to which even Commissioner Kessler subscribed — they began pursuing their wider goal of dismantling federal regulatory agencies and privatizing many of their duties.

The FDA had, in fact, already streamlined to a remarkable extent. Between 1993 and 1994, it cleared up its backlog of safety applications, reducing the total from 2,000 to 500. The delay in processing export licenses had fallen from an average of 60 months to 50 days. But streamlining wasn't the goal of groups like the Progress and Freedom Foundation (the think tank at the heart of what Washington calls Newt, Inc.), the Competitive Enterprise Institute or the Washington Legal Foundation.

These groups, which receive large contributions from the pharmaceutical industry, are more concerned with political philosophy than with practical problems; changing the drug approval process is part of their attempt to reshape the federal government.

The American Enterprise Institute suggests doing away with the FDA's power to approve drugs and allowing any medication, lethal or not, to be sold. Citizens for a Sound Economy wants to turn the FDA's job of screening and approving new drugs over to the drug industry itself.

The foxes, in other words, would protect the chickens.

The American public is notoriously schizophrenic, and easily manipulated when it comes to government regulation. One week's sob story about a dying patient's fight for access to an unapproved treatment sends deregulatory fever through the roof. The next week's tale of an infant condemned to life without arms because of a prescription drug provokes demands for more regulation. The same voters who support the ban on euthanasia demand the right to put drugs that might kill them into their bodies.

The FDA, where politics and science collide in the tension between public good and corporate profit, has been the changeable child of that fickleness. Time and time again, the agency has bent to the winds of public sentiment and political opportunism. Which is precisely the problem. Unlike the Federal Reserve, which has a quasi-independence that allows it to withstand political buffeting, the FDA has never had the freedom from politics essential to protecting the public health. And FDA commissioners have never demanded it. Quite the contrary. They have been utterly political creatures, dancing to whatever tune the American public, and politicians in office, are playing.

That penchant has given enormous power to activist groups and companies that can afford loud bands. AIDS drugs get fast-tracked while a drug for Alzheimer's is sent back for more testing; AIDS patients scream louder than the elderly, after all. Burroughs Wellcome, which seeded both the research and activist communities with grants and donations, received more help from the government, and speedier FDA approval of its drug AZT, than almost any company in history. Corporate giants like Johnson & Johnson and Merck that rally political influence, public support and media headlines consistently watch their products slide easily through testing. Smaller companies like HEM, the producer of ampligen, and ICN, which makes ribavirin —

drugs many believe to be effective against HIV — are shoved into research and approval oblivion.

While Martin Delaney and the Republicans have bashed the FDA for overregulation, they have ignored this problem of systematic favoritism toward large, wealthy companies, a dangerous trend for American consumers. Inevitably, the small companies — like the biotechnology startup firms that are on the cutting edge of gene therapy and rational drug design — don't have a prayer. Their loss is shared by millions of Americans.

Consider the case of two companies trying to secure FDA approval for their products: Epitope, an Oregon corporation with sales of $3.3 million annually and 130 employees, and Johnson & Johnson, the health care conglomerate with sales of more than $4 billion in prescription drugs alone. It owns more divisions than Epitope has employees.

Epitope is one of scores of startup biotech companies that has yet to be profitable. It lost $14.7 million in 1993, almost double the loss of the previous year. That sounds like disaster, but it's pretty common in the biotech business.

All Epitope had was a product with the potential to turn the company into a cash cow and to alter the way Americans are diagnosed for disease. Blood tests have long been the standard: blood is taken from the veins of the terrified and sent off to labs for analysis. In the late 1980s Epitope began to explore a cheap and easy alternative, especially for HIV, using saliva instead of blood. Everyone knew that there was some virus present in the mouths of the infected; Epitope created an HIV test for it.

OraSure was the kind of product companies dream of: a cheap and easy replacement for an expensive and much-hated test. If your doctor wanted to test you for HIV, or, for that matter, a number of other diseases, he could just give you a swab to hold in your mouth, then put the swab in a vial filled with preservative and ship it off to the lab. No needles, no phlebotomists, no careful control of the temperature of the sample. The saliva test would be easy to use with fidgety kids, the elderly who have fragile veins, or intravenous drug users who have no accessible veins at all. Health care workers could go out to community centers, even onto the streets, and take testing to the public. Even more impressive, OraSure could cut the cost of testing drastically because no nurse or phlebotomist would be necessary.

Epitope began testing OraSure in 1990 on hundreds of people

around the country, matching the results of their oral samples with the results of blood tests, and filed for FDA approval in May 1991. In November of that year, the agency asked for more information — the two thousand matched samples it had requested six months earlier suddenly weren't enough.

The company obediently expanded its testing and dealt with the dozens of questions about its analysis and quality control that were raised by the FDA after surprise inspections. Then, after most of the difficulties were resolved, a stock market analyst got hold of the FDA's confidential inspection reports and predicted the imminent demise of Epitope. The company's stock price plummeted. The inspection report received by the analyst was normally a confidential document not released by the FDA. The FDA claimed it was given to the analyst accidentally, and in an almost unprecedented action, the agency's ombudsman actually apologized to Epitope. It was too late. The company had already lost millions.

An FDA advisory committee finally met in December 1992 to discuss the application for approval of OraSure. Although the accuracy of the test was determined to be within 2–3 percent of blood test results, some members balked at the difference. Others were concerned because the test kit was for initial screening only; blood would have to be drawn afterward to confirm any positive results.

Epitope executives held their tongues. They had asked for approval for both screening and confirmatory testing and had withdrawn the latter application at the behest of FDA staffers.

Epitope's supporters among AIDS activists, most of them African American, argued that a saliva test would encourage minorities to learn their HIV status. They presented surveys of people of color which demonstrated a strong preference for a saliva test, even if it was slightly less accurate. Health care workers extolled the virtues of a procedure that posed no risk of needle sticks and reduced client apprehension.

The committee, however, deadlocked on the issue, and kicked the matter back to the staff and the commissioner.

Two months later company representatives went to Washington to discuss approval with FDA officials, and left in total confusion. FDA officials were suddenly worried that OraSure might make self-testing so easy that individuals would try to turn it into a home test kit. Epitope didn't know how to respond. They didn't plan to market the product to the public. All the company could offer was to label the kit

"Not for Home Use." Then the agency raised concerns about how health care workers would learn to administer the test, which required a patient to place a swab between his gum and cheek for two minutes. Epitope agreed to produce an instructional videotape on how to place a swab in the mouth and count 120 seconds.

By the early summer of 1993, Epitope believed it had answered all the FDA's questions and concerns, but OraSure continued to languish in FDA limbo. "I have been told that the FDA is sensitive to the fact that small biotechnology firms risk their very existence on an expeditious regulatory review process," an Epitope official wrote to the agency. "Our survival may depend on the FDA taking action now." By then, fourteen months had passed since the company filed for approval of OraSure.

Throughout the summer, a small group of African American AIDS activists pressured the FDA for a decision and demanded to meet with top officials. In December, when the activists brought President Clinton's director of media analysis with them to a meeting, FDA officials acknowledged that the bulk of their concerns had been met and that they were moving quickly toward approval.

Then disaster struck again. Dan Dorfman, a stock market analyst reporting for *USA Today* and CNBC television, announced that an FDA staffer had told him there was "less than one percent chance of agency okay" for OraSure. The FDA denied that such a comment could have been made. "If such a statement was made by an FDA employee, it was unauthorized and inaccurate," the agency ombudsman insisted.

Dorfman stood by his reporting. Epitope executives wondered who inside the agency was trying to destroy them.

Just after the Dorfman fiasco, the CDC released the results of its own tests of the product, and they were a knockout. In both the screening test and the confirmatory Western Blot using OraSure on hundreds of people, there were no false negative results and very few false positives. The report seemed to make no impression on the FDA.

FDA officials began bringing up new concerns about counseling, about partner notification and the reporting of test results to state authorities. These are central issues when considering a home test kit, but they were curiously irrelevant to OraSure. The saliva product wasn't a test but a collection device handled exactly like a blood sample.

In May of 1994, Epitope received a letter from the agency congratulating the company on its progress and acknowledging that almost all the remaining issues had been resolved. But nothing more happened. By then twenty-four months had passed since the company's application.

The following month, the FDA was distracted by a different testing issue: a home test kit produced by a division of Johnson & Johnson. Johnson & Johnson makes Epitope look like a kid's lemonade stand. The company markets more than eighty prescription drugs, twenty-five of them with annual sales above $50 million. Its 1994 budget for research and development alone was $1.3 billion. From its corporate headquarters in New Jersey, Johnson & Johnson controls an empire of more than 150 companies around the globe. It is a household name. Birth control pills? Johnson & Johnson. Heartburn medication, Band-Aids, joint replacements, diagnostic tests and sutures? All Johnson & Johnson.

For years the FDA had insisted it would not license a home test kit for HIV. Public health professionals seemed to agree that it was too risky for individuals, who would learn the dire results on the telephone — or at least that's what the FDA told Epitope when officials raised the possibility of applying for OraSure's approval for home use.

It's also what the FDA told Elliot Millenson when he tried to submit a home blood-test kit called Confide for approval in 1987. Millenson owned University Hospital Laboratories Corporation in Bethesda, and was one of a small group of entrepreneurs who sensed a market for home HIV test kits. Then, even more than now, Americans were incredibly resistant to being tested for HIV. No one goes looking for bad news, after all, and medicine seemed to offer nothing to help those facing a fatal illness. But that wasn't the only hesitation for the millions of Americans who were Millenson's potential customers. People were afraid to be tested because if they turned out positive, someone might find out.

A home test seemed the perfect solution. It's a simple device, after all. Millenson's test kit, like most, would come with a lance to prick your finger and a piece of filter paper with an identification number on it. If you wanted to know your HIV status, you'd simply prick your finger, drop some blood on the paper and mail the sample off to the company in a prepaid Federal Express mailing envelope. The company would run both a screening and confirmatory test and report the results when you phoned in. If you were negative, you'd get a recording;

if you were positive, you'd be switched directly to a counselor, who could refer you to help in your community.

No names, no office or clinic visits. Total anonymity and privacy.

Millenson's company submitted its application in December 1987, along with the results of tests conducted by the Johns Hopkins School of Public Health and the Medical University of South Carolina. Several similar requests were already languishing at the FDA as staffers tried to decide how to approach home testing. In March 1988, after consulting with the Public Health Service, the FDA ruled that it would not even review any applications for HIV home test kits unless they were to be used by medical professionals in clinics and hospitals and physicians' offices — an obvious contradiction in terms.

Millenson appealed. The FDA declined to reconsider and reiterated its position in the *Federal Register* in February 1989. The only movement occurred after a public meeting held to discuss the question: the FDA agreed to accept approval applications that would allow companies to run clinical studies on home test kits.

The FDA was not just being obstinate. Home testing was still viewed as a risky business, with none of the safeguards built into the network of testing and counseling centers that had been built up to provide confidential — even anonymous — testing to the public. At-home testing for HIV isn't like buying a blood pressure cuff or a pregnancy or glucose test, after all. The consequences of HIV diagnosis are grave.

Activists and experts alike feared that receiving the news of infection on the telephone, without benefit of a trained counselor who could explain the results and gauge a person's reaction, might lead to panic, depression, even suicide. They worried about confidentiality. Couldn't someone prick another person's finger, send in the blood sample and discover whether or not that person was infected? Everyone could imagine abuses in institutions, in day care centers, in workplaces, even in personal relationships.

Millenson became fed up. In March 1990 he filed suit against the FDA and its parent agency, the Department of Health and Human Services, asking the U.S. District Court to force the FDA to review his application. The FDA did just that, at an advisory committee meeting in July, where his application for approval was rejected.

Finally, Millenson sold his company in early 1993 to Johnson & Johnson, which turned it into a new division, Direct Access Diagnostics. Little Elliot Millenson and his small laboratory might not have gotten anywhere with the FDA, but Johnson & Johnson was a different story. In less than a year — and without any cogent explanation — the FDA began to reconsider its eight-year opposition to home testing and scheduled a public meeting to discuss it.

With Johnson & Johnson now leading the charge, the number of sophisticated advocates with refined — and sometimes ludicrous — arguments rose exponentially. During a mind-numbing thirteen-hour session at the Holiday Inn in Gaithersburg, Maryland, on June 22, 1994, dozens of health professionals and activists, many long-time opponents of home testing, rose to support the drug giant. They harped on the importance of encouraging Americans to be tested. Early knowledge, they argued, encourages early intervention, which can prolong life. That same knowledge, furthermore, could prevent HIV-positive people from passing on the virus. J & J's supporters predicted that in minority communities, where the stigma of infection was still palpable, the rate of testing would skyrocket. That Puerto Rican single mothers without the time to go to clinics could test themselves at home. Migrant workers wouldn't have to worry about moving on before their test results were ready at health centers. Men and women in rural areas would have access to totally confidential testing.

"We believe that the benefits of home-access HIV testing far outweigh the modest and mitigatable risks," said Bruce Decker, the president of the Health Policy and Research Foundation. "It is time to get HIV testing out of the closet and onto the grocery shelf." Decker was speaking for a group of thirty "veterans in the war against AIDS," representing "an accumulation of three hundred years of wisdom and experience" in the epidemic.

Sean Strub, the publisher of *POZ* magazine and a New York activist, presented the results of his survey of community interest in a home test kit, which suggested that almost three-quarters of the population wanted a home test for HIV. The results might well have been biased by the fact that his marketing company, Strubco, and its mailing list were heavily weighted toward Gay America. In fact, 70 percent of the people returning his survey cards had already been tested.

Mary Fisher, the HIV-positive scion of one of the stalwarts of the Republican party, spoke movingly about her kids. "I suppose it's too late for me," she told the panel. "But my children are now six and four, and they represent a generation that is not yet lost. Not yet."

The highlight of the hearings was the testimony of former Surgeon General C. Everett Koop. "Despite our best intentions, AIDS has become the all-American epidemic and the weapons we wield against AIDS are both too few and too feeble," he said. "Testing is all we have. Therefore, testing is what we must do."

It was quite a show, staged for the committee's edification by Johnson & Johnson. In accordance with FDA testimony requirements, Bruce Decker later acknowledged that the company had paid his travel expenses, but he didn't reveal the full extent of his involvement: he was the chairman of J & J's community advisory board, a group he put together singlehandedly. ("I appointed them," he said. "This is an oligarchy.") Sean Strub admitted that he was a paid consultant to J & J, which had retained his services to conduct the survey to demonstrate community support for its product. Although unwilling to disclose precisely how much money he'd received, Strub acknowledged that 5 percent of the total income of his companies came from Johnson & Johnson.

Koop himself acknowledged being on the company's payroll as a consultant. Fisher, founder of the Family AIDS Network, did not mention that she was negotiating a contract with J & J to provide it with assistance in compiling its referral list. And almost all the other speakers noted that they had been flown to the meeting at J & J's expense.

"I am concerned that there is extreme bias in the people that we have heard," one FDA committee member said after the public testimony ended. "I think even though their testimony was heartfelt, I don't know the number or the opinions of people who might have had contrary opinions . . . I don't know how representative the samples of all the people who had their fares paid."

Other advisory board members scoffed at testimony that suggested that the home test would benefit those who most needed testing: the poor. "I was very concerned to hear examples of migrant workers and others being put forward when I can't imagine migrant workers having fifty dollars to pay for these tests," one said. Another went even further: "I think getting your test results over the phone is also a little problematic, especially if you don't have a phone. Getting your test results over a pay phone I don't think is a solution."

The idea that rural Americans would benefit from the confidentiality of a home test kit was similarly derided. In small town America, clerks in the pharmacies where such kits would be sold are hardly likely to be strangers.

Committee members stayed with the issue until 7:35 that night, voicing their concerns about counseling being controlled by a for-profit company. They were skeptical about permitting the release of a product they all knew would be used predominantly by the "worried well," those people least likely to test positive. The members were not asked to vote, but the clear majority said they favored requiring Johnson & Johnson to conduct some sort of pilot study prior to approval.

In the months that followed, the debate heated up as Strub used *POZ* to push forcefully for immediate approval of the test kit. He insisted his payments from J & J were for consulting, not for editorial support, but the company got it — in spades. But in the October-November 1994 issue, Strub printed a joint statement from the same group Decker represented at the hearing, along with form postcards addressed to President Clinton and the assistant secretary of the Department of Health and Human Services. The return address contained a play on ACT UP's tag line: "Delay = Death."

Although Strub painted the opposition as a band of right-wing epidemiologists, the primary opponents of the home test kit were members of the National Alliance of Gay and Lesbian Health Clinics. "The potential for catastrophic impact on individuals using such a home test product far outweighs the intended advantages," Michael Savage, representing the eleven-clinic group, wrote to the FDA. "Comparisons to home pregnancy test kits or home cholesterol tests do not stand; neither of those is perceived to be the detection of a life threatening sexually transmitted disease for which there is yet no known cure." A few days after that letter was made public, Johnson & Johnson retaliated by withdrawing a $5,000 gift it had promised a member clinic.

Soon the White House became involved when Chief of Staff Leon Panetta wrote to FDA Commissioner David Kessler inquiring about the status of home testing approval. "First of all, let me assure you that FDA continues to give the highest priority to the review of products related to the prevention, diagnosis and treatment of HIV infection," Kessler replied. By then, the application for the approval of OraSure had been with the FDA for thirty months. "There are no policy impediments to the approval of a home use HIV test kit. Any remaining concerns about impact of product approval on the public health will be examined through post-approval studies."

Opponents of home testing were stunned at this reversal of the FDA's position and its seeming disregard for its advisory committee's recommendation for premarket testing. The National Alliance clinics, supported by the National Association of People with AIDS and Americans for a Sound AIDS policy, demanded that the FDA investigate Johnson & Johnson for buying influence and for illegally promoting an unapproved product. No one could deny that J & J, like most such companies, bought what access it could. The company not only had Koop on its payroll but had also hired Gary Noble, the former associate director for AIDS at the Centers for Disease Control. Johnson & Johnson had also promised its community advisory board a donation of twenty-five cents for every test kit sold, to be distributed to community groups counseling HIV-positive people. "We will have five to ten million dollars a year to distribute," said Bruce Decker, "but we're not advertising that because we don't want people to think that we're paying groups off."

The more serious charge was the promotional issue, since FDA regulations specifically prohibit promotion of unapproved products. Epitope, for example, had been strongly chastised for distributing information on OraSure at a meeting of the American Dental Association in October 1991. Small pharmaceutical companies like ICN had been virtually cut off by the agency for touting the worth of their drugs to physicians. But Johnson & Johnson denied that Strub's crusade was promotion. Nor, they said, was C. Everett Koop's appearance on the *Today* show when he demonstrated the use of Confide.

J & J and its supporters knew how to use their muscle. In late November 1994, Chris Bull, the Washington correspondent for *The Advocate,* a gay news magazine, began work on an article about the dispute. After his interview with Sean Strub, Strub's attorney called the reporter. "He said that he wanted to make sure that I was going to be fair to Sean and that he had the feeling that *The Advocate* was out to get Sean," Bull recalls. The attorney then phoned Bull's editor in California, to reiterate his concerns and remind him about libel law.

Meanwhile, the reality of the Republican Congress had already sunk in at Johnson & Johnson. New allies were needed for the new era. House Speaker Newt Gingrich's Progress and Freedom Foundation received a $5,000 check from Johnson & Johnson. And in December a voice hardly associated with AIDS entered the debate. Paul Weyrich, the president of the conservative Free Congress Foundation and a founder of National Empowerment Television, called a news conference and said, "The FDA now for seven years has sat on a proposal for home-access HIV testing and counseling. We are not going to tolerate this unconscionable delay any longer, and if they persist we will seek a legislative remedy, which I think is now very possible given the new political realities in Washington."

Weyrich was joined by William Mellor III, the president of the conservative Institute for Justice, who added that his group was exploring options to force the FDA to speed up its procedures. "In this case, delay means death," Mellor said.

He sounded suspiciously like Sean Strub.

ELEVEN

The Enemies of
the People

In the Henrik Ibsen play An Enemy of the People, *a provincial physician discovers that his town's healing baths are polluted and that typhoid threatens visitors to the town's only attraction. No one wants to believe him, because closing the baths will bankrupt the community. The newspaper refuses to print his warning. The denial turns to anger, directed at the physician. He is fired and reviled as a villain of the common good. "Any man who wants to destroy a whole community must be a public enemy," one character says. The crowd shouts, "Yes! Yes! He's an enemy of the people."*

Stephen Joseph arrived in New York City in 1986 scarred by decades of public health battles. He'd worked for the Agency for International Development in Cameroon, trying to keep children alive, and wound up in the crossfire of controversy over the distribution of infant formula in Third World countries where the water supply is usually polluted. When the Reagan administration refused to put babies' lives above the interests of Nestlé, Joseph, the highest-ranking medical professional in the AID, quit. He knew about becoming an enemy of at least some of the people.

Even in the quietest of times, though, Third World politics are child's play compared to the constant guerrilla warfare of public health in New York City. And Steve Joseph did not become commissioner of public health in the quietest of times.

When he arrived in the city, more than seven thousand New Yorkers had been reported with AIDS; half of them were already dead. New York had no money to cope with the epidemic and had no coherent strategy for combating it. Should the city require, or at least encourage, New Yorkers to be tested? How could the results be kept confidential? Should people who tested positive be asked for the names of their sexual partners so that they could be warned? How could the infected be protected from discrimination? Should they be quarantined? Tattooed? Sent to deserted islands? Should condoms be passed out in schools and intravenous drug users be given clean needles? Should gay bathhouses be closed?

The city, like the nation, faced a thousand complex questions about a disease whose complexities were barely unraveled. Answers were being forged amid vituperative battles at public hearings and at demonstrations, in the headlines of the city's hysterical tabloids, in courtrooms, in backrooms where politicians count votes before lives, in gay bars and community centers — but rarely in the offices of public health professionals.

Those professionals knew what measures would best contain the epidemic. It was Public Health 101. Routine testing was essential — when a person checked into a hospital, when a person visiting his or her physician displayed any hint of HIV infection or risk behavior, when a woman became pregnant. A system had to be created to inform the sexual partners of those who turned up positive. Those who were infected needed to be counseled by physicians and told, point blank, to stop having unsafe sex or sharing syringes. Every measure that would help reduce transmission — from testing of the blood supply to condom distribution — had to be encouraged throughout society.

These were the policies employed to fight tuberculosis, infectious hepatitis and syphilis. First, testing and contact tracing. Then, with tuberculosis, slum clearance projects and the installation of ultraviolet lights in health care settings. With infectious hepatitis, the screening of the blood supply and the use of gloves and masks in hospitals and clinics. These precautions worked. The epidemics of syphilis and tuberculosis, which had killed thousands of Americans, were stopped. Infectious hepatitis was brought under control. Once the population felt safe, the stigma surrounding these diseases disappeared.

But Joseph stepped on a land mine every time he tried to institute these policies for HIV. The first one exploded at his inaugural press conference, when he was asked his opinion of needle exchange programs and responded calmly that he supported any program that could reduce HIV transmission among the city's quarter-million intravenous drug users. AIDS activists cheered. They were the only ones.

"Free Needles and Condoms? It's Madness," blared the *New York Daily News*. "It's genocide, pure and simple," said City Councilman

Hilton Clark, who represented central Harlem. "When the first needle is given out by Dr. Joseph, he ought to be indicted and arrested for murder and drug distribution."

Archbishop Joseph Cardinal O'Connor sermonized, "It drags down the standards of all society." City Council minority caucus member Wendell Foster called the program "planned assassination in the black community."

A year later, Joseph touched off a latex battle when he announced plans to distribute a million condoms as the city's frontline weapon against AIDS. "Everyone needs to be a condom expert, or condom comfortable," he told 250 public health experts at a condom conference in February 1987. And he meant it. He encouraged pharmacists to put condom displays right out front in their stores and oversaw a massive condom campaign on radio and television targeting gay men and heterosexual women. Again, AIDS activists applauded their free-thinking health commissioner.

But not everyone agreed. Brooklyn councilman Noach Dear pronounced the ads "disgusting."

"We think the ads are an implicit endorsement of sexual promiscuity," said Joseph Zwilling, a spokesman for Cardinal O'Connor. The condom campaign could "mislead people into thinking there is something called safe sex."

Even feminists blasted the commissioner, who was one of the first public health officials in the country to warn of the dangers of AIDS to women. One of the city's condom ads showed a couple kissing. "He'll tell you just what you want to hear," the voice-over said. "But what he can't tell you is if he's got the AIDS virus. So protect yourself. Use a condom . . . And if he says no, so can you." One feminist's response: "We are not happy that . . . women do seem to be given the brunt of the responsibility for safe sex, as they have for contraception," said Kelli Conlin, president of the New York City chapter of the National Organization for Women.

Then, on June 5, 1989, from the podium at the International Conference on AIDS in Montreal, Joseph became the target of attacks from the other side for suggesting the creation of a government registry of infected individuals so their sex partners could be warned of the risk. Contact tracing, a standard public health procedure, had been used for decades to combat tuberculosis, syphilis and hepatitis. But this was AIDS, the most politicized disease in human history. The idea of a central registry raised the specter of being put on a list for deportation to a quarantine camp. Informing sex partners violated the privacy protections that AIDS patients had won.

A near riot broke out in the convention hall as activists attacked Joseph's proposal. The next day, in New York, two hundred AIDS demonstrators blocked traffic on the Brooklyn Bridge and shut down the health department, shouting, "First you don't exist, now you're on this list."

Mayor Ed Koch, the New York State health commissioner and most other health officials in the state abandoned Joseph on the issue. Okay, Joseph said, then what about asking physicians to encourage patients testing positive to inform their sexual partners, and asking doctors to notify them directly if patients refused? That, too, crossed the line into political incorrectness in a disease where the risk to the uninfected must be ignored in order to protect the rights of the infected.

Sometimes Joseph managed to infuriate both conservatives and AIDS activists simultaneously. When the media became enamored of the much-feared "heterosexual breakout" story, Joseph declared that AIDS posed little risk to white suburbanites. He predicted, quite accurately, that heterosexual AIDS would afflict mostly the poor in the city. As if foreshadowing the coming of Mary Fisher, he said, "The relatively uncommon case of the Park Avenue socialite infected by a bisexual former boyfriend, which receives such media attention, is multiplied several thousandfold among her black and Hispanic counterparts, who receive considerably less public concern and who, being at much higher risk, deserve far more intensive health protection."

It was irrelevant that his statement was correct. Gay activists plastered the city with posters branding Joseph a pig for uttering a truth that might breed public indifference to AIDS. Conservatives were equally incensed. Fear of AIDS had been their new strategy for the promotion of chastity.

Joseph wasn't naive. He knew needles and condoms and risk categories were hot buttons. "The politics of AIDS defined AIDS well before any detailed medical definition took hold," he wrote in his book, *Dragon Within the Gates*. "AIDS is the first major public health issue in this century for which political values rather than health requirements set the agenda."

But the one act that generated the greatest controversy caught him entirely off guard: the battle of the numbers.

From the moment HIV was discovered, public health officials faced the challenge of estimating how many Americans might be infected. It wasn't an academic exercise; they needed to plan for adequate hospital beds and emergency funding. Any reasonable estimate needed to calculate the number of gay and bisexual men in the population, the number of drug users, hemophiliacs, transfusion recipients, women and children at risk. Epidemiologists then had to come up with a ratio between the number of AIDS cases and the number of infections.

None of that was easy. No one knew in 1984 or 1985 how long HIV infection lasted before developing into AIDS. No one was sure how many intravenous drug users lived in New York City or how many sexual partners each had. No one had any idea how many gay men lived in Greenwich Village, Harlem, Queens. The health department used the only available figure, Kinsey's 1948 estimate that 10 percent of American men are more or less exclusively homosexual. That estimate was forty years old and had never been validated, but it was the best that anyone had.

The officials estimated a population of 500,000 gay and bisexual men and 250,000 intravenous drug users in the city, then sampled each group to come up with an infection rate. Their final estimate was that New York had 500,000 HIV-positive residents — 250,000 men infected through sex with other men, 150,000 infected through intravenous drug use, 50,000 through heterosexual sex and the remainder through blood products. With the national estimate at between 1 and 1.5 million infected, and one-third of the nation's AIDS cases already reported in New York, the figure seemed realistic in 1985.

A year later, however, it seemed less reliable. If 500,000 people were infected, and if only 100,000 had been infected as early as 1980, the city should have had 20,000 AIDS cases by 1986. Only 8,300 had been reported.

When he arrived in the city, Joseph asked, Where were the rest? His staff went looking to see if physicians and hospitals were just not reporting. When these investigators came up empty-handed, Joseph ordered a recalculation of the projected figures. By then he had more solid numbers from San Francisco, a city with a better fix on its gay population. New York's health department reworked the San Francisco calculations to apply to the city, and wound up cutting the estimated number of infected New York residents in half.

When Joseph announced the new figures in the spring of 1988, he expected a celebration, especially among gay New Yorkers. Fewer corpses, fewer funerals.

Fat chance. AIDS activists accused Joseph of massaging the data to downplay the epidemic and justify the city's lack of funding for AIDS. Gay activists ranted that he was plotting to diminish the size and importance of their community.

The commissioner tried to reassure them that the new estimate could not possibly diminish the city's investment in AIDS. Even with the new numbers, he still expected 43,000 AIDS cases by the end of 1991.

No one would listen. As it turned out, even his revised estimate proved to be too high.

Posters began to appear on every available wall and lamppost, reading "The AIDS Estimates Are a Lethal Lie" and "Stephen Joseph Has Blood on His Hands" superimposed over a crimson hand print.

The health department was hit by a series of phone zaps — organized call-ins meant to tie up telephone lines. Joseph was hounded wherever he went. He received harassing calls at home in the middle of the night: "We'll crush you if you don't resign." Hate mail arrived almost daily.

One postcard with a photograph of the Lincoln Memorial in Washington was addressed to: Steven the Pig Jos., Commie of Health. "I fuck yo wife! No you idiot this is not the Steven Jos. Memorial but you could always drop dead."

The harassment of Joseph was part of a concerted effort dubbed "Surrender Dorothy." ACT UP was playing the Wicked Witch of the West.

Joseph left New York when David Dinkins became mayor. The needle exchange program was dissolved. A battle exploded over the so-called Rainbow Curriculum, a required part of the city's educational program designed to promote tolerance — which only made AIDS education more controversial.

"AIDS is one of those transcendent phenomena," says Joseph, who is now the assistant secretary of defense for health. "Everything that is America is in the epidemic, both the good things and the bad things. All the courageousness and cowardliness, all the tolerance and all the prejudiced bigotry, all the technological mastery and all the social stupidity. All the poles of everything that is our nation is in our epidemic.

"I worry, though, as part of that, that the dead hand of political correctness is creeping over the entire society. I'd like to hear some people who have some unorthodox ideas — wrong or right — out there in public, so we'd have people to shoot at. That's your damned job when you're a public official — to get shot at. And people aren't doing their jobs.

"Remember Ibsen's play *The Enemy of the People,* how the medical officer in that little town warned that the mineral baths they thought would revive the economy were actually polluted. They wouldn't listen to him. They tried to shut him up and run him out of the town. They finally declared him an enemy of the people.

"That's the job of a public health official. To be squeezed. Threats to the public health always involve vested interests, sometimes in a nefarious way, sometimes because of human fallibility. Sometimes it's just minor and sometimes, as it is in AIDS, it's more dramatic. But you have to be willing to be like Ibsen's character, an enemy of the people. That's what it means to work in public health."

AIDS is the most politically controversial epidemic in human history. Two charged forces, Gay America and the Christian Right, seized the epidemic as their battleground. Waging competing jihads, they both claimed the moral high ground, slinging blame and attempting to legislate their own versions of political correctness. Neither was willing to concede an inch or put aside their wider agendas long enough to deal realistically with a plague jeopardizing the lives of millions. When they faced off, rational discourse became impossible.

"No one talks about public health," says Don Francis. "When they talk about public health, they're usually talking about something else, about politics or their idea of morality or budgets. In my twenty years at the CDC, I have never witnessed science abandoned for political principles quite so thoroughly. A society that allows narrow political vision to guide public health policy is doomed to succumb to disease."

AIDS policy was doomed because it was caught between the demands of gay activists and Jesse Helms. The noise became deafening. The right supported tried-and-true public health measures, from mandatory testing and reporting to contact tracing of sexual partners of the infected. Gay America insisted that those measures were inappropriate to a plague that spread hysteria as well as disease. Conservatives used AIDS to promote their hatred of homosexuality; liberals used it as an excuse to declare war on bigotry.

The problem is not unique to AIDS, of course. National health policy on cigarettes has been caught between the tobacco lobby and the clean-air crowd. Christian Scientists have fought against required immunization of schoolchildren, and fundamentalist Christians have advocated anti-alcohol crusades.

And neither liberals nor conservatives have a monopoly on inconsistent positions on public health. Republican libertarians horrified at the notion of the federal government's banning assault weapons unabashedly demand mandatory testing for HIV, while liberals support stringent gun control but eschew testing as an assault on privacy.

Both sides insist that the problem is that AIDS has been politicized. Depoliticizing AIDS, however, is a code word for changing the underlying political assumptions, rather than for throwing assumptions out entirely.

Some of the arguments — like the condom wars or needle exchange — at least have serious implications. But too many are meaningless exercises in political correctness that have led to a public policy based on wishful thinking, political posturing and mental masturbation.

People with AIDS are the losers.

Jesse Helms never mentioned the word "homosexual" during most of his twenty-three years in the U.S. Senate. It's not that he approved of homosexuality. The senator from North Carolina was too busy battling communism, saving the Panama Canal and whipping up support for South African–backed guerrillas in Mozambique to worry about a few perverts.

Then came glasnost. Helms wasn't finished fighting the cold war, even though the rest of the world might have believed it was over. He never forgot for a second that Reds were in power just ninety miles from U.S. shores and that the hammer and sickle reigned supreme in China, North Korea and Vietnam. But without the Soviets, it just wasn't the same.

He lusted after new ideological combat, and there weren't enough commies left to keep him in practice. There were, however, plenty of homosexuals — and a high-profile epidemic in their midst. Most members of Congress saw AIDS as a new, potentially serious disease. They pulled together and handed funds over to the Centers for Disease Control to track the disease, to the National Institutes of Health to sort out its biology, and to scientists nationwide to search for a cure.

Not the senator from North Carolina. What was a disease to his colleagues became a political crusade — and an opportunity — for Jesse Helms.

His first foray into the untested political waters of AIDS was an attempt, in the summer of 1986, to overturn a District of Columbia law prohibiting insurance companies from denying coverage to the HIV infected. "The truth is the so-called homosexual rights crowd has

snookered the entire District of Columbia into footing the bill to provide special treatment for those who are at a health risk because of
AIDS," said Helms, adding that the law would lure scores of diseased
homosexuals into the nation's capital.

The tactic played like a charm. It made the front pages of the
Washington Post and the *Los Angeles Times*. Helms's biggest crusade
of the year before — banning tax exemptions for groups promoting Sa-
tanism and witchcraft — had merited hardly a line on the inside pages.

The Grand Old Man of the Far Right found his most fertile field for
combat since Mikhail Gorbachev ruined the fun.

Gay men barely noticed the first stirrings of Jesse Helms's homophobia; they were still too busy having their own fun.

After decades of repression — of cover marriages to satisfy the
family and cover dates to fool the guys on the job — they had begun to
discard all pretense in the 1970s. Farm boys from Kansas and lawyers
from Texas, doctors and hairdressers and artists from Idaho to Maine
had fled their hometown closets for self-imposed ghettos in San Francisco, New York and a dozen other cities. Twin Peaks, a gay bar in San
Francisco, installed plate-glass windows, refusing to shelter its patrons
from scrutiny. Gay fashion — the short hair, mustache, blue jeans and
leather jacket that defined the gay urban clone — went public in New
York's Greenwich Village. Freedom was declared.

Freedom, of course, meant sex — the more the better. The symbols
of liberation from the bourgeois norms of dreaded straight society
were bathhouses and adult bookstores, cruising spots and at-home
orgies. Gay America thrived on being everything Straight America
despised.

In San Francisco, Harvey Milk, the gay city supervisor, suggested
that freedom might have as much to do with coming out — with becoming visible and politically active — as with cumming. He was lionized, but his counsel was strangely ignored. A nascent gay political
movement hovered at the fringes at voter registration time. In 1984, its
leaders passed the hat to raise money to defeat Ronald Reagan. But the
party was too hot for any serious interruption. Even the news — carried in *The Advocate*, Gay America's answer to *Newsweek* — was sold
with a young stud on the cover.

When the *New York Times* reported on the rise of a new gay cancer,
Gay America responded with angry denial. Early warnings that sex
might be spreading the disease were met with hostile suspicion that the
"breeders," as straight people are less than affectionately called, were

plotting yet a new way to try to scare them straight. "AIDS comes from a government laboratory, not your lifestyle," declared stickers plastered all over Castro Street, the heart of gay San Francisco.

Gay physicians and activists who bucked the party line were branded as "sexual fascists" and traitors. When the gay journalist Randy Shilts suggested that the community needed to at least discuss its sexual practices, to talk about promiscuous sex in bathhouses and backrooms, he was ostracized and vilified. "There was a time during that period that I simply couldn't walk down the street in my own neighborhood without getting harassed," Shilts recalled shortly before his death in February 1994. "I was the target of the PC patrol, who behaved like lavender fascists." Things never got much better for Shilts. When gay journalists organized their first national conference, in 1992, Shilts was openly derided as the Dan Quayle of Gay America.

Reality crept in, inevitably, as the number of obituaries in local gay papers began to equal the number of personal ads. Gay men who'd juggled complex schedules of work, parties and bathhouse visits were soon replacing their noontime quickies with funerals and their evenings at the bars with visits to friends dying miserable and disfiguring deaths.

The lights had been turned up on the party, and Gay America saw the unanticipated destruction on the floor. "When I first heard about AIDS, I thought, Oh, God, they've finally found a disease for the diseased," said Bill Kraus, a congressional aide and San Francisco activist. "It rekindles in the psyche all the hateful propaganda that you are sick."

Gay men were sick, and in increasing numbers. Suddenly, life in the fast lane seemed perilous. Just as Helms and his kind were discovering gay male promiscuity, gay males were considering other options. "If there is anything positive about this horrible situation, assuming the great majority of us survive, it will have been a crisis that makes people stronger," Kraus said. "I see it detrivializing sex. I think that will be permanent. I think there's room in human society and gay society for people to be kinder and warmer to each other."

Kraus didn't live to discover that he was wrong on at least one count. As the epidemic became a part of daily life — as young gay men read the obituaries each morning and wondered whether to cross the names of deceased friends out in their address books — kindness and warmness gave way to anger and blame. Gay men were Americans in the 1980s, after all, and the eighties was the decade of the victim.

• • •

Jesse Helms didn't wait until the eighties to start playing the blame game; he practically invented the politics of blame. As a newspaper reporter, a television commentator and then as a U.S. senator, he dedicated himself to weeding out enemies, foreign and domestic, who he accused of undermining the moral strength of the nation. In his nightly commentaries on North Carolina's WRAL-TV in the 1960s, he portrayed decent, God-fearing Americans as innocent victims of long-haired college students, civil rights workers and Dr. Martin Luther King.

When the eighties arrived, with the civil rights movement buried along with Medgar Evers, King and Malcolm X, Helms had his new enemy, the "Sodomists" who were spreading disease and perversion and threatening God's promised land. "I may be the most radical person you've talked to about AIDS," Helms told Lesley Stahl on *Face the Nation,* pausing to make sure his position was engraved in the minds of the viewers. "But I think somewhere along the line that we're going to have to quarantine if we are really going to contain this disease."

His first move in that direction was to demand that Congress keep the lid on the number of perverts streaming into the country, to protect America from the danger of HIV spilling across the nation's borders from overseas. Never mind that by then AIDS was the only area of international trade in which the United States had a clear surplus. Helms seemed convinced that a Parisian who tested positive would throw his hands up and yell, "Mon Dieu, I must go to America, where there is no national health care plan," or that a Mexican peasant who discovered his ailment — probably when he was diagnosed with pneumonia or cancer — would crawl out of his hospital bed and across the Rio Grande.

So in 1987 Helms asked his fellow senators to add HIV infection to the list of infectious diseases that keep immigrants out. Helms's move worked. The Senate supported him. The media — even CBS, which he calls "Rather biased" — played up the story, and Helms's campaign coffers began filling with out-of-state contributions.

In Blame the Sodomites, Part II, Helms found his most winning issue, the single one with which he has been able to bash both Gay America and the public health establishment for nine years: the promotion of safe sex.

It began as a simple discussion of comic books, specifically *Safer Sex Comix,* an AIDS-prevention series produced by the Gay Men's

Health Crisis. Helms declared them lewd and lascivious and a violation of American morality. The comics were so obscene, Helms said, that when President Reagan saw them, he nearly wept. The comic books do not encourage the reader to change his "perverted sexual behavior," Helms said. "In fact, the comic book promotes sodomy and the homosexual life style as an acceptable alternative in American society . . . under the pretense of AIDS education."

According to Helms, the real villain was the Centers for Disease Control, which was undermining Christian values by funding the Gay Men's Health Crisis to produce such swill. Although GMHC did have grants from the CDC, none of that money had been used to produce *Safer Sex Comix*. So he turned his attention to GMHC's safer-sex workshops, events that were federally funded. He fulminated against using taxpayers' money for workshops to teach men about "asking· someone for his phone number, meeting someone new at a bar and letting him know you are interested in having safe sex, and negotiating a contract for safe sex, discussing your sexual limits."

Public health officials argued that the issue was not approval of homosexuality but education of gay men to stop the spread of a deadly disease. Producing materials dealing with the risks of specific homosexual practices doesn't cause homosexuality any more than fire-safety films cause pyromania.

Helms didn't buy it. He didn't want gay men to learn how to have safe sex; he didn't want them to have sex at all. The only prevention campaign he was willing to fund was a late night version of Nancy Reagan's Just Say No. Caught up in moral fervor, he refused to be convinced that his morality might be irrelevant to an epidemic. The majority of the Senate went along with him, approving, 94 to 2, his proposed ban on funding for AIDS prevention programs that might "encourage" homosexuality.

The prevention battle became something of an annual ritual. In 1988, with his paunch thrust forward like a latter-day Napoleon, Helms was back to the podium with a new proposal designed to "remove any question" that federal funds would be spent to condone homosexuality. "This subject matter is so obscene, so revolting, it is difficult for me to stand here and talk about it," said Helms. "I may throw up."

Somehow, he found a way to go on: "This senator will not allow one dollar of taxpayers' money to promote sodomy. This senator is not a goody-goody two-shoes. I've lived a long time . . . but every Christian ethic cries out for me to do something. I call a spade a spade, a perverted human being a perverted human being."

The Senate — with a third of its members facing reelection battles — indulged Helms once again. An anti-AIDS strategy that was little more than wishful thinking had enormous political appeal. Anyway, by then Helms had turned up the debate to such a fever pitch that moderate voices were drowned out. Lawmakers who clearly saw the extremism of Helms's positions nonetheless gave in to them. It was a moment in American politics when the word "liberal" had acquired a nasty taint, and to do anything that seemed indulgent of homosexuality was to be accused of the utmost liberalism.

The fruits of Helms's hateful rhetoric: hospitalized AIDS patients were left lying in their own vomit because nurse's aides refused to come near them; surgeons refused to operate on them; X-ray technicians donned spacesuits to wheel patients to and from their rooms. In Miami, morticians dumped the corpses of AIDS patients in public landfills. When a Hispanic AIDS group tried to move into an office building near downtown, an African American member of the county council threatened to bring in "the brothers" to burn them out.

It was not just the sick who suffered. As the rhetoric around AIDS obliterated the realities, gay men became the nation's modern lepers. Diners refused to be served by gay waiters, healthy or not. Jurors refused to serve on panels with gay men. In Queens, New York, the widow of an AIDS patient received a letter from her neighbors suggesting that she move. HIV-infected children were barred from schools.

The fear and hostility were not simple human reactions to a terrifying disease. They were whipped up by crusading religious figures and politicians who saw AIDS as an opportunity. Ministers like the Reverend Billy Graham who declared that AIDS was God's way of punishing sodomites and junkies saw their collection plates overflow. Hatred was good business.

The CEO of this enterprise was Jesse Helms, who insisted that the impending plague was a homosexual conspiracy that posed no real threat to God-fearing Americans. "Let me tell you something about this AIDS epidemic. There is not one single case of AIDS reported in this country that cannot be traced in origin to sodomy," he said during a debate in October 1988 on a sweeping AIDS research and testing bill that guaranteed confidentiality for those testing positive for HIV. Helms didn't want any guarantees — of confidentiality or anything else — for sodomites. The fact that at that moment almost four thousand women and six hundred children had AIDS didn't faze him. He was concerned with a larger truth, and he played the Bible-belt purist jousting with the fancy-pants urban moral relativists as he stopped the Senate dead in its tracks during a Senate-House conference to resolve minor differences in the AIDS bills. He staged a one-man filibuster and forced the bills' sponsors to reduce funding for AIDS prevention and water down confidentiality provisions in order to pass the bill into law.

Helms seemed to revel in the fantasy that if the nation would just ignore the epidemic, it would disappear — along with the dreaded sodomites. So, unlike virtually every other member of Congress, from Orrin Hatch to Teddy Kennedy, he added the AIDS research budget to his long list of targets.

In October 1990 he tried the direct approach, introducing an amendment to cut $441 million from the 1992 AIDS research budget. It failed miserably, so he switched tactics. "Many Americans will die because of the politically directed priorities of the AIDS lobby," he said, proposing an amendment to transfer $120 million from AIDS research into programs to combat Alzheimer's and infant mortality. Helms railed against the government for spending more than a third of its health research and education budget on AIDS when AIDS accounted for only 1.3 percent of the deaths in the country. "These funds are being allocated to fund research and treatment of AIDS not because of its threat to society, but on the basis of media hype and who can make the loudest noise in the halls of Congress," he said.

Playing one disease against another didn't work. Most legislators and their constituents understood that the infectious epidemic posed a unique threat to the nation. Most legislators also knew that Jesse Helms had a wider agenda. After all, he had never lobbied for taking money from B-1 bombers or Minuteman missiles to find a cure for Alzheimer's disease. Helms wasn't well known for his compassion. He was the only senator to vote against a 1987 school aid bill designed to boost elementary and secondary education, and one of four senators to oppose an increase in the 1988 budget for a federal program to improve the health of poor pregnant women and their infants. He'd voted against the Fair Housing Act, funding for child care, food stamps and an increase in the minimum wage.

Despite his defeat on research funding in 1990, Helms continued his battle against AIDS year after year. The following July, he defended innocent virgins like Kimberly Bergalis by pushing a bill through the

Senate that mandated ten-year prison sentences for HIV-infected surgeons who operate without warning their patients. "None of these
should be treated any different than the criminal who guns down
helpless victims in the street," he bellowed on the Senate floor. "I've
got some grandchildren I'm very fond of. If some suck-egg mule did
that to them, I don't know if I'd be out of prison myself."

That September he targeted a planned survey of adult sexual behavior that public health professionals believed was essential to scientific planning of AIDS prevention programs. Scientific? asked Helms.
No way. The survey was designed to provide evidence "to legitimize
homosexual lifestyles," he said. "It's a clear choice between support
for sexual restraint among our young people or, on the other hand,
support for homosexuality and sexual decadence." The $10.1 mil-
lion was switched into a program to provide abstinence counseling to
teens.

Then Helms's health began to fail. In 1991, the senator was treated
with radiation for prostate cancer, and his wife of fifty-one years had
surgery for colon cancer. At the end of 1992 he wound up in the
hospital for quadruple-bypass heart surgery and began treatment for
Paget's disease, a bone disorder. If Helms was weakened by his medical
ordeals, he found the perfect tonic when the newly inaugurated president moved to lift the ban on gays in the military. Helms raced around
the Dirksen Senate Office Building, organizing Republicans to tie up
the Senate with a bill to lay the ban in legislative cement.

When President Bill Clinton backpedaled, announcing that the
Pentagon would just suspend enforcement of the ban, Helms resolved
any lingering doubts that his heart surgery had taken the bite out of the
Republican maverick.

"President Clinton obviously is attempting a strategic retreat," he
said. "But the truth is, Mr. Clinton's tail feathers are on fire, and he is
now trying to douse the flames which he himself deliberately set. Perhaps it will teach him the hazards of playing with matches to satisfy his
militant 1992 supporters."

By the end of his first week of Clinton bashing, it was clear that
Jesse Helms was looking forward to four more years . . . of fun.

Gay America joined its worst enemy in the assault on the new president. A month before Bill Clinton's inauguration, AIDS activists presented their demands to the president-elect. "AIDS is a national health
care emergency, if not a natural disaster, which deserves the kind of

financial attention that has been given the Florida hurricane, the S & L crisis, the Persian Gulf War, and the Chicago sewer system," Daniel T. Bross, then the chairman of National Organizations Responding to AIDS, told Clinton's representative Tim Westmoreland at a meeting called to discuss the new president's AIDS agenda.

The price tag the delegation attached to that health care emergency was $3 billion in research, housing, prevention and education, a 50 percent increase over the then-current level of spending. They also demanded an end to the ban on HIV-positive immigrants, the vigorous enforcement of the Americans with Disabilities Act and the dissemination of educational materials and public service announcements that were explicit and specific. Those demands were in addition to earlier ones for a "Manhattan Project" for AIDS, clean needles for junkies and the appointment of an AIDS czar.

Clinton wasn't in the White House five months before AIDS activists declared him to be a failure. ACT UP/Presidential Project began handing out bumper stickers: "25,000 Dead Since Jan. 20, Thanks for Nothing Bill." In early June, at the Ninth International Conference on AIDS, Aldyn McKean of ACT UP, who introduced himself as "a proud queer, an AIDS activist and a person with AIDS," reiterated the president's campaign promises on AIDS and told the fifteen thousand delegates from across the planet: "Sadly, I have to report to you that absolutely none of that has been done."

On computer bulletin boards where AIDS patients and activists shared information about treatments and complaints about public policy, Clinton took a drubbing. "Bill Clinton and his clone, Al Gore, are cut from the same political cloth and could not give a damn about anything but their own self-gratification," Ed Davis wrote in August 1994. "Please, quit listening to their pretty words and start looking at what they are really doing." There were occasional voices of support for Clinton. During a heated bulletin board discussion of the "rudderless president," Mary Elizabeth, who runs the most widely used electronic AIDS network, wrote, "Why blame Clinton all the time? He is one man who has tried . . . Why not direct some anger towards the real villains, Helms, Dole, Nunn, Hatch, etc. that seem to oppose everything he tries to do."

But nobody listened. In the gay community — as in the U.S. Senate — reasoned voices were drowned out, or caught up in the rhetoric.

At the Tenth International Conference on AIDS in Tokyo, in August 1994, representatives of ACT UP/NY handed out Clinton's first

AIDS report card. He flunked. An F for research. An F for failing to collaborate with other heads of state to create a global response. An F for not taking a stand against travel and immigration restrictions. He received only one passing grade, a D for prevention efforts.

The poor grades ignored the fact that within six months of his inauguration, Clinton had asked Congress to increase funding for AIDS research and treatment by 28 percent, that he'd appointed a Nobel Prize–winning immunologist to direct NIH, that he had lifted the ban on fetal tissue research. That his administration went on to streamline disability regulations to help women and children with AIDS and to create state and local prevention councils to involve activists directly in the planning of AIDS education. That prominent gay figures like Victor Zonana, a reporter for the *Los Angeles Times,* and Nan Hunter, the former director of the Lesbian and Gay Rights Project at the ACLU, were appointed to senior positions at the Department of Health and Human Services, or that people with AIDS were regularly consulted on AIDS-related decisions.

Clinton was criticized for not lifting the ban on visas for HIV-positive foreigners — although the minute his secretary of Health and Human Services mentioned doing so, the ban had passed into law, negating the president's authority in the matter. He was reviled for being slow to appoint an AIDS czar, never mind that no one had ever delineated what this newly minted figurehead would really do. He was berated for not authorizing a national AIDS research program along the lines of the Manhattan Project, which accelerated the development of the atomic bomb, although such a project for AIDS has been condemned by scientists and many activists as well.

Do more, activists demanded. Use the White House as a bully pulpit — as if lecturing the nation nightly on the scourge sweeping across the land would have magical effects. Activists had a willfully naive level of faith in the power of politicians that few Americans retained by the late twentieth century, an almost visceral belief that firm leadership could command anything, even a virus. "We demand a cure," they chanted, turning it into a mantra. The only kind of president who would satisfy them was one who, hours after moving into the White House, walked back out onto Pennsylvania Avenue toting sacks of pills that would halt the epidemic by the next day.

Clinton was added to the lengthy roster of individuals and groups that didn't do enough about AIDS. That was hardly surprising. In confronting the epidemic, gay men followed a script right out of a handbook on how to become a successful victim: We've been beaten by gay bashers, kicked out of our homes and churches by homophobes, ignored or defamed by the media. Now we're dying, and nobody cares because we're faggots.

They were wrong, for the most part. Ronald Reagan's refusal to confront the epidemic was not just a conspiracy of indifference to the fate of gay Americans. It simply did not fit America's emerging self-concept. The 1980s were the quintessential feel-good era. In that "morning in America," wars were to be short and successful, with all but the victorious moments hidden from the press. AIDS was hopelessly out of synch with the times.

After all, it's not easy to maintain the illusion that happy days are here again while talking frankly about an impending plague.

In fact, it wasn't just a question of political posturing, or even political will. The deeper problem was that America had become a notably uncaring society. Ever since John F. Kennedy challenged Americans to ask themselves what they could do for their country, they had cared deeply, passionately and persistently — yet the social problems refused to go away. When they elected Ronald Reagan, they were granting themselves a vacation from caring. AIDS asked them to return to work, with a vengeance. They weren't so inclined.

Gay America was little different. If relative indifference to AIDS is a sign of American homophobia, African Americans might legitimately ask gay leaders if their indifference to sickle-cell anemia or systematic racial discrimination is a sign of racism. Women might suggest that the gay community's failure to mobilize around abortion rights or the crisis in breast cancer is a sign of its sexism. And poor people might wonder why Gay America didn't discover health care inequities until AIDS. Everyone might be right. But even those truths are subsumed in the larger reality of public indifference, fed by an overwhelming sense of public helplessness.

Perhaps if the first young men with odd cancers had turned up in doctors' offices when America still maintained its innocence, its belief in its ability to solve all the great problems, the history of the epidemic would have been different. That is what happened with polio, after all. In the 1950s, Americans still had faith in their abilities to solve even the most overwhelming problems. American science and technology had just won a long global war. Turning their attention to a dreaded disease, they were convinced they could find yet another technological fix to save tens of thousands of children from paralysis and death. And Americans did it — not their government, but ordinary Americans in Kansas and Idaho and Maine who sent their coins to the March of

Dimes because nobody yet believed that the government was responsible for solving all ills.

AIDS, however, swept through the population just as the nation reached a historic low in its ability — or at least its stamina — for problem solving. Ordinary Americans, the same people whose charity and volunteerism had forged a vaccine for polio, had become passive, convinced of their own powerlessness, reliant on government solutions to a staggering, and growing, number of social problems.

AIDS wasn't ignored because no one cared whether gay men died. Gay men were parts of families and churches and workplaces that embraced and supported the sick more frequently than they rejected them. The federal budget for AIDS research and treatment increased fiftyfold — 5,000 percent — in the first decade of the epidemic.

AIDS, however, demands not just an acknowledgment of a massive new medical crisis, but an admission that the nation's deepest problems — from racism to a crumbling health care system, from the corrupt relationship between corporations and researchers to teen alcoholism — still have not been solved. AIDS unmasks all of America's illusions about itself as modern, sophisticated, tolerant, even competent. The challenge of AIDS exceeds the national attention span and overloads the national capacity for self-reflection.

That there was no special conspiracy to let gays die is pointed up by the fact that the single social problem on which America made the most remarkable progress during the worst of the epidemic was discrimination against gays. By 1994 three openly gay men were serving in the U.S. Congress. The Senate majority leader in Minnesota was a gay man, and there were lesbian and gay state representatives in Wisconsin and Maine. Despite the conservative landslide in the midterm elections, lesbians and gays were elected to the legislatures of six states, including, for the first time, California. Seventy cities across the country have now passed gay and lesbian civil rights statutes or hate-crimes bills. Domestic partnership — a kind of same-sex marriage — is a reality not just in San Francisco and New York City, but in Hartford and Honolulu.

Newspapers and television stations have hired openly gay and lesbian reporters to cover the gay community as news, not as a freak show. Movies and television programs portray lesbian and gay children and parents and friends in ordinary jobs and ordinary relationships. Tom Hanks won the 1994 Oscar for playing a gay man with AIDS in *Philadelphia,* a movie that became a huge box-office hit and even boosted Hanks's star status.

Discrimination thrives in some families and workplaces, but the closet door has swung wide open and tens of thousands of gay men and lesbians have come out — for the most part without losing their jobs. And when young men fall ill, their families from small towns in Ohio and cities in California meet their sons' gay friends and embrace them in remarkable numbers.

Although the number of violent crimes against lesbians and gays appears to be rising, it might well be because the police and the FBI are, for the first time, keeping records of such acts. Congress has declared these to be hate crimes, crimes beyond the pale with concomitantly stiffer sentences.

Reality — political, scientific and social — has gotten lost in the rhetoric, just as it evaded the rhetoric of Jesse Helms. Most straight Americans don't spend even twenty minutes a year hating gays. Clinton has shown more leadership on AIDS than either of his two predecessors. A president's power is limited; the budget is always tight and a dozen other serious, immediate problems overflow the political plate. On top of everything else, scientists are confronting dilemmas — how to kill a virus and how to regulate the immune system — that have eluded them for decades.

The reality also is that Gay America bears some responsibility for the epidemic's continuing toll, and has been notably unwilling to accept it. While the community deserved and received tremendous kudos for its early efforts in AIDS education and prevention, safe sex never became universally ingrained in gay male culture. In fact, it has never been clear whether those efforts to encourage safe sex — all those posters of sweaty, muscled young men locked in embrace, holding condoms — were responsible for the early rise of safer practices or whether the deaths of so many gay men drove the message home. What is clear is that as younger men become sexually active, they avoid safe-sex messages — and that as the epidemic continues, gay Americans of all ages are abstaining from safe sex to a terrifying extent.

"In what often seems like a stroke of PR brilliance, the lesbian and gay movement has convinced many that we have brought the rate of HIV infection to a standstill through safer sex," wrote Michelangelo Signorile, a founder of the "bad boy" school of gay journalism. "Soon enough the world will realize that safer sex has broken down substantially . . . and that HIV infection is exploding in our community. How can we continue to point fingers at the media, government, and an uncaring public when we appear so grossly irresponsible?"

Signorile was not engaging in wanton hyperbole. Men who have been HIV negative for years are suddenly turning up positive — and admitting to those nights when they just couldn't face life with latex, when drugs or alcohol left them too foggy to remember to put on a rubber, or when the guy next to them in bed was too hot to turn away. A 1991 survey by the San Francisco Department of Public Health found that 43 percent of gay men between the ages of seventeen and nineteen, and 52 percent of African American gay men in that age group, were having anal intercourse without condoms. The statistics from other cities weren't much more encouraging. A study of gay and bisexual men in sixteen small cities reported that about one-third were engaging in unprotected anal sex. In 1994, the new infection rate among twenty-year-old gay men was 3 percent per year — roughly equivalent to the infection rate in the same age group a decade earlier.

Blaming Jesse Helms for those chilling statistics might be satisfying, but it isn't true. Despite his best efforts, gay men in San Francisco have been exposed to a decade of explicit safe-sex advertisements on buses, taxicabs, billboards, radio and television. They have received a barrage of explicit instructions on how to suck, fuck, lick and whip safely.

A substantial percentage of them seem impervious to the message.

Unless something changes drastically, the majority of today's gay urban twenty-year-olds could eventually become infected. And there is no reason to believe that more flavored or colored condoms, hotter bodies on AIDS awareness posters or X-rated messages about the properties of semen will change that reality.

Nobody wants to talk about the realities of prevention because the admission that prevention doesn't work — an admission of powerlessness against nature, both human and viral — is simply too terrifying.

Yet everyone knows that twenty-eight years of explicit warnings and advertising on the dangers of smoking has not sent cigarette manufacturers into bankruptcy, and that more than a decade of explicit warnings and advertising — not to mention legal sanctions — has not gotten Americans to buckle up.

Activists continue to insist that it must be someone's fault that young people — teenagers and college students, who are at the age when they are certain they're invulnerable — don't wear condoms. It must be someone's fault that junkies — men and women who spend their days sticking needles into their arms and injecting heroin and cocaine into their veins — are not making carefully calculated, rational decisions about their sexual partners and practices.

The blame does not belong only to what David Kirp, a gay faculty member at the University of California, calls "the AIDS dishonor role — Jesse Helms, Robert Gallo, William Dannemeyer, George Bush, above all Ronald Reagan. The tempter in our own bedrooms represents a much bigger threat than the meanest homophobe," he wrote in *The Nation*.

But the discussion rarely goes much further. When it does, the train inevitably leads back to blaming straight America. Young gay men don't value their lives because homophobia has taught them self-hate, the argument goes. They practice unsafe sex because they want to die. This argument is not only whiny but absurd. Is self-hatred responsible for cigarette smoking and drunk driving? for indulgence in junk food? for addiction to fast cars and skydiving?

The reasons for the resistance to safe sex are complicated — the subject of a growing number of psychological treatises. No one, however, seems willing to consider that the messages Gay America sends out on AIDS might be one lethal reason. For more than a decade, community leaders have declared that the party can remain steamy even in the face of a sexually transmitted plague. It's not the number of sexual partners you have but the kind of sex you practice that puts you at risk, they explain with the seriousness of consultants for the CDC. So keep it hot, just keep it safe, they've advertised on dozens of erotic safe-sex posters and in hundreds of seminars on how to enjoy yourself during an epidemic. Their adherence to the technical truth of HIV transmission has belied the deeper reality of human behavior. Hot parties are about loss of control; drugs and alcohol are part of the fabric of that scene. Neither the heat of unbridled passion nor the effects of drugs and alcohol fosters sexual responsibility.

And it gets worse. Activists have helped sow a community ethic that demands that the uninfected assume full responsibility for self-protection. There is no social pressure on HIV-positive men to acknowledge their infections before engaging in sex, to keep their partners from risk. The message is not Do Not Harm; it is Every Man for Himself. It is hardly surprising, then, that researchers have found almost no correlation between close links to the gay community and responsible sexual behavior by HIV-positive men. Even those who are part of support groups and training seminars adhere to this dangerous dogma and seem content to let their partners decide whether or not to use condoms. Finally gay men, particularly young gay men, open *Out* magazine and *The Advocate* and see advertisements from nutritional supplement companies, pharmaceutical companies, AIDS service organizations and public health groups that feature photographs of healthy, husky and handsome young men who are "learning to live with HIV." They watch long-term survivors of AIDS talk about their full lives. They meet dozens of happy, productive and handsome people with AIDS in *POZ,* the magazine for the HIV positive.

Such messages offer hope to infected men who've been warned of impending demise. But to the uninfected, the message is that HIV isn't so disastrous, and it breeds a false sense of security. How many twenty-year-olds are likely to protect themselves against infection if they believe they might live twenty or thirty sexually happy years with HIV without being sick?

Almost as disturbing as the reality of the relapse from safe sex is the absence of any serious discussion of it. For more than a decade, Gay America has prevented such essential candor by silencing those who dare suggest that the community's sexual mores might need reconsideration. Before most Americans even knew an epidemic was seeping into the nation — before anyone was sure an infectious agent was even involved — a campy singer named Michael Callen and a former hustler, Richard Berkowitz, tried bucking the popular line of the day that gay male promiscuity had nothing to do with AIDS. In their political tract "We Know Who We Are," they called for the closing of the bathhouses. "If going to the baths is really a game of Russian roulette, then the advice must be to throw the gun away, not merely to play less often."

Hogwash, the community responded. There's no evidence that sex is making us sick. Maybe it's a government plot. Maybe it was a bad batch of drugs. Prophets of doom like Callen and Berkowitz were accused of being "sexual Carry Nations."

The same scenario was played out on the West Coast. In March 1983, at a meeting to mobilize gay men around the new disease, San Francisco Supervisor Carol Ruth Silver mentioned the possibility of asking the public health department to close down the bathhouses there. She was booed, hissed, heckled and cowed into silence, as were journalists, public health officials and other political leaders who supported her position.

Twelve years later, little has changed. Few men any longer deny that AIDS is sexually transmitted, but promiscuity is still celebrated as a proud tradition and as an inalienable right. "Safe Sex Is Hot Sex" is the mantra. Gay Men might be using condoms, but most still treat any suggestion that bathhouses and backrooms might be dangerous as a plot against the Queer Nation. And the tone of public discussions of anonymous sex and bathhouses is eerily familiar, even though death has silenced most of the earlier voices.

After years when the specter of death kept the party sedate, by the mid-1990s it was business as usual in bars, backrooms and bathhouses. Dozens of new sex clubs were opening in cities all across the country. Within weeks of its opening in March 1995, the Crew Club in Washington, D.C., had more than three hundred members. They were flocking to a gay men's social club, the club's owner explained to a reporter from the Washington Post, a "safe space" where the primary attractions were weightlifting, shooting pool, tanning and sipping sodas. He seemed hesitant to discuss the bank of tall, open-sided cages made of chain-link fencing which patrons used to exhibit their sexual prowess — at least before local health department officials forced their removal. Traveling sex parties on Miami's South Beach and new bars like Risk (which calls its gay party night Uranus and advertises it with the phrase "Put Uranus at Risk") were creating a potentially lethal environment. Despite health department regulations prohibiting most types of sex in commercial establishments, no bathhouse or sex club had been closed in New York City. City officials in Los Angeles tried, suing to close two bathhouses on public health grounds. The community reaction was so violent that they settled out of court when the clubs agreed to "safe sex rules."

A small group of men tried to sound the warning, as had others a decade earlier. Freddie Rodriguez of Health Crisis Network in Miami attacked the owners of Risk for sending the message that risk-taking was sexy. In New York, Dennis DeLeon of the Latino Commission on AIDS suggested that latex parties and other stunts designed to eroticize safe sex simply weren't working. A few activists even dared suggest that the celebration of gay male promiscuity itself might be undermining any meaningful AIDS prevention work.

Their voices were almost hushed until early 1995, when a new organization in New York, the Gay and Lesbian Prevention Activists, declared war on the bathhouses and other commercial sex establishments. They served their owners with demands for the removal of the doors on cubicles where men have sex, regular monitoring of their patrons' sexual activities and full compliance with health department regulations. They threatened to expose noncompliant owners to city authorities and to the press. As if to drive that reality home, they dressed a female reporter in male drag and took her on a tour of Zone DK, a sex club where city inspectors observed unsafe sex on virtually every visit.

"I'm no longer willing to hold gay men hostage to a public relations agenda," declared Duncan Osborne, a gay writer who was vilified for taking the reporter to the sex club. "It's more important to save lives than for us to look pretty."

Osborne and crew became the new villains in the Battle over the Bathhouses, Act II. Their opponents accused them of every conceivable sin, from being self-hating homosexuals to purposefully attempting "to draw down punitive action from city and state government." They predicted dire consequences for gay men if the new prevention activists continued their crusade. Today the bathhouses, tomorrow your bedrooms, warned the signers of a "consensus statement," which argued that regulation of gay sexual activity in public places would lead inevitably to regulation of gay sexual activity in private. "I hear Jesse Helms knocking at my door with police in tow already," one man wrote on an electronic bulletin board.

"The possibility of homosexuality being again classified as a 'disease' is very real, and the claim of protecting the 'public health' by stamping out the 'disease' seems very, very possible," argued Dave Hatunen of Daly City, California, in another electronic posting. Lest his readers think him paranoid, Hatunen reminded them that "public health" rationales have been used to justify atrocities throughout human history, citing the eugenic practices of the Third Reich as but one example.

Instead of closing the bathhouses, the consensus statement signers suggested a sort of marathon community consciousness-raising session. "Discussing our attitudes and feelings about the kinds of sex we have and about how we deal with the ever-present risk of HIV infection is the most important thing we can do to stop the spread of HIV."

The new prevention activists were neither impressed with the suggestion nor deterred by the vitriol from speaking frankly about what was happening in the community. "No one, from street radicals to professional AIDS educators, is willing to speak up about it, afraid that doing so will be 'sex negative' — as if death is 'sex positive,'" wrote Michelangelo Signorile. "Undoubtedly many will charge that this or any critique of how we conduct ourselves sexually is not 'sex positive.' But it is time to turn this hackneyed phrase around. 'Sex positive' does not mean taking crystal meth and heading to a sex club to become someone's repository as a way to fill that empty feeling you may have inside."

If the PC police make serious discussion of the decline of safe sex difficult, they make any mention of the dangers of unprotected oral sex impossible. The party line is that oral sex without a condom is risk-free for the performer and practically risk-free for the receiver, especially if the recipient does not ejaculate into his partner's mouth. When San Francisco researcher Michael Samuel used a survey of eighty-two HIV-positive men to show that the dogma was flawed, his study was attacked as unscientific, the participants were branded as liars and the researcher himself denounced as a homophobe trying to force gay men to abstain.

Yet the first case of HIV transmission through oral sex was reported in *The Lancet* in 1986. Dutch researchers reported in 1992 that 9 percent of the subjects in their study of HIV-positive gay men claimed oral sex as their only risk factor. Even the American Association of Physicians for Human Rights, a lesbian and gay doctors' group, changed their 1983 guidelines on safe sexual practice. They warned that "oral sex can result in HIV infection" and cautioned that partners should avoid both "pre-cum" — the fluid that flows from a man's penis prior to ejaculation — and ejaculates.

But the truth won't sink in. Come on, men say, there's hardly any virus in pre-cum. It's just the opposite, according to Deborah Anderson of Harvard University Medical School. While HIV can be detected in only 30 percent of semen samples, it can be found in 52 percent of pre-ejaculate samples. Self-styled "oral advocates" — whose favorite button is "Safe Sex Sucks" — claim that oral sex is dangerous only if you have open cuts in your mouth. But more than two years ago, researchers reported that HIV can enter the mucosal lining of the mouth, or the rectum, through the long arms of dendritic cells that pick up foreign microbes and cells without any tears or breaks.

The problem is that nobody wants to suck latex, and flavored condoms are a poor substitute even for cherry Life Savers. Gay men so desperately want to feel free to engage in some sort of sex without any barriers that they discount the studies as flawed or biased or downright bigoted.

Activists, and even medical practitioners, have done little to force them to face reality. In fact, many have done the opposite, straining all logic to justify misleading their constituency. "Sex negativity is the problem," says Steve Michael of ACT UP/D.C. "If we tell people to say no to too many things, they'll just say fuck it, why bother, and say no to nothing. After all, it's not like oral sex is as dangerous as other things."

Michael finds support from psychologists and other professionals who reiterate his comments in more "acceptable" jargon: ". . . the belief that urogenital sex carries a high risk of transmission yields an increase in unprotected anal sex."

The only major gay voice to refuse to follow that party line is journalist Gabriel Rotello, whose attacks on the manipulation of risk statistics infuriated community leaders. In fact, the level of risk Rotello gave in a review of the subject for *Out* magazine — between 0.5 and 1 percent per partner, which translates into between 1 in 100 and 1 in 200 — is more than twice as high as the risk estimated for women who engage in unprotected vaginal intercourse with infected men.

The gay movement in America has failed its own not just with easy blame and dangerous denial, but with a lack of political sophistication that has pained even many of its firmest allies on Capitol Hill.

"Whose fault is this?" asked Theo Smart, a New York AIDS activist. "Partly ours," he answered, "because we don't know how the system works . . . Clinton still represents a Yield sign — we can get somewhere, we just have to gun it. We can't expect him to fight our fight for us; he won't, but we will never find a politician who will. Frankly, we won't achieve our goals by scapegoating this politician."

Gay activists cannot claim that they don't know how the system works. Their number includes too many lawyers and political organizers, writers, intellectuals and editors to sustain such a pretense. They know. They just refuse to listen. Massachusetts Congressman Barney Frank, who is openly gay, has explained it to them time and time again. Whenever ACT UP holds another die-in, in which activists fall on the ground and pretend to be corpses, he asks: When was the last time the American Association for Retired Persons had a die-in? Does the National Rifle Association have shoot-ins? "We're here, everyone knows we're here," he tells organizers repeatedly. "That's not the point. The point is to forge an effective political force."

Frank is not opposed to demonstrations and militant actions, but he suggests that the community needs to choreograph those activities with the tactics used by the NRA and the AARP, two of the most effective political forces in the nation: dressing up in ties and jackets, organizing, pooling of money, playing the game and disavowing crazies.

Congressional aides to a broad range of legislators from both parties agree that AIDS activists have been miserable organizers. "They show up at the last minute when they want a lot of money," says James Guyton, Frank's aide on health policy. "They refuse to play by the rules of the game and insist they want to change them. That's fine, but not if your goal is to win votes to counter an epidemic. They have to decide what their real goal is."

In the first months of the Clinton presidency — a real opportunity for influence and change — the community almost willfully insisted that *all* its goals be met. The list of demands was so long and diverse that it seemed gay leaders had decided that Clinton was the president of Gay America. The possibility of picking the best — or most crucial — shots didn't seem to occur even to responsible leaders, who spent millions of dollars, and almost all their political capital, on the gays-in-the-military fiasco. The backlash was predictable, and swift. Clinton got the message loud and clear: stay away from gay issues.

When he backed off, the crazies hit the streets, and instead of disavowing them — as Jewish leaders did when Meir Kahane threatened to defend Jewish New Yorkers with guns or as black leaders did when Louis Farrakhan's minions spouted anti-Semitic ravings — the community embraced or at least indulged them. No one condemned Luke Sissifag, né Luke Christian Michael Montgomery, who supported himself as a male hustler and proudly flashed business cards imprinted with his likeness with a gun. He was hailed as a hero when he attacked Clinton during his first major address on AIDS.

When activists attended a 1994 meeting of federally funded AIDS researchers and saw fliers from the PWA Army ("We've been too nice for too long"), they seemed neither horrified nor alarmed, although the flier announced in bold print: "You've fucked US long enough — Now WE'RE gonna fuck you and your sons and your daughters." No one seemed worried by the flier's direct threat: "The PWA Army is a group of people with AIDS and HIV who are willing to sacrifice their lives to save the lives of current and future PWA's. Beginning October 1, 1994, we will EACH infect at least two HIV-negative people per day if the following demand is not met." The demand was for a cabinet-level AIDS coordinator.

In 1993, instead of organizing a political demonstration along the lines of the 1963 civil rights March on Washington, Gay America planned a party. Barney Frank asked: Why are you bringing a quarter of a million people to Washington on Sunday, when Congress is off playing golf? He looked at the list of speakers and reminded organizers that civil rights leaders brought Roy Wilkins, Martin Luther King and union leader John L. Lewis to the podium, not Moms Mabley or Redd Foxx. Why do we have to have a lesbian stand-up comic and a bunch of drag queens? Frank asked.

Instead of being listened to as a seasoned political pro, Frank has been mocked and dismissed as an Uncle Tom who is ashamed of gay culture. The community is still too suspicious of people who try to play by the rules — since those rules were hardly written by or for Gay America. Besides, after decades of cowering in the closet, in-your-face politics is more fun.

Activists deemed no one pure enough. No sin was forgiven, even if it was committed by a lawmaker sympathetic to gay concerns. Witness the evolution of activists' relationship with former California Senator Alan Cranston.

He was the first senator to address a Gay Freedom Day audience in San Francisco and one of the first to push for congressional hearings on AIDS — in 1983. But in 1987 Cranston fell from grace after a single vote, when he joined ninety-three other senators in supporting a Helms bill that denied AIDS education funding to any group that might "promote or encourage" homosexuality. Activists organized a demonstration at Cranston's next public appearance, a fundraising dinner. His aides canceled the event rather than allow the senator to be publicly humiliated by the gay community.

New York Governor Mario Cuomo fared no better. His record on AIDS was not perfect, but he was an AIDS saint compared to most of the nation's governors. Even rabid Cuomophobes had to admit that he was more friendly to gays than George Pataki, his opponent in the 1994 election campaign. So in the fall of 1994, the Empire State Pride Committee, a group of moderate gay activists, asked Cuomo to chair a dinner honoring another elected official. A small group of activists held a press conference denouncing the Pride Committee and set up a picket line outside the dinner. "We're going to hold Cuomo's feet to the fire," said Michael Petrelis, who organized the protest. "He's been lousy on AIDS."

The problem is a dangerous, self-indulgent and woefully immature political style that calls attention to AIDS, and is fun, but is less about AIDS than about proving that Gay America is Out and Proud. The governing zeitgeist — We scream, therefore we are — is incongruent with saving the dying.

TWELVE

Strike a Pose

By *1990, ACT UP had the hottest brand name in the history of American activism. SDS — Students for a Democratic Society — might have kidnapped a few university deans back in the sixties, but they didn't have their own weekly television show. The Black Panthers redefined the ghetto concept of bad, but they didn't see any profit from it.*

The ACT UP boys flaunted style and flair in the Doc Martens boots and cropped hair that became all the rage from the East Village to the Castro; they were packaged by the same advertising executives who spent their days tending to the corporate images of CitiBank and IBM; they were financed by trademark T-shirts with designs willed to them by graffiti artist Keith Haring; they marketed a sensual anger that became Gay America's new aphrodisiac.

By 6:30 p.m. on any Monday night in New York, the square around Cooper Union, where Abraham Lincoln once spoke, was filled with self-styled faggots with an attitude. Hundreds entered the Great Hall. Hundreds more loitered outside. ACT UP was the center of activism, but it was also the heart of the city's best cruising. Few men who weren't at least minimally attractive dared show up.

ACT UP glowed with a sense of its own radicalism, but the bad boys of the late eighties and nineties were never radicals in any meaningful sense of the word. They never challenged the structures of government; they simply wanted government to respond to their crisis.

For the most part, ACT UP was a group of well-educated white men who discovered that America was a flawed paradise only when a plague struck their community and sex became deadly. Suddenly yuppies who had purchased East Side co-ops with profits from junk bond deals were outraged at the lack of access to health care. Corporate lawyers and accountants were livid about overpricing. Gay Republicans were incensed at government indifference and ineptitude. They saw themselves not just as victims of a virus but as moral outcasts. They found anger, anger imbued with a magical quality. It vanquished fear. It was the only way men too young to begin the day reading the obituaries could hold doom at bay.

"I'll be damned if I'm going to die just because the Centers for Disease Control, the National Institutes of Health and the Food and Drug Administration say I have a fatal illness," screamed John Fisher of ACT UP/Fort Lauderdale. But Fisher's anger could not stop cytomegalovirus from infecting his eyes. He died eighteen months after he uttered those words, not by decree of any government agency but from a brain infection.

Michael Petrelis and Larry Kramer shrieked that the infected should take to the streets, in emulation of Jewish guerrilla groups in the years before the creation of Israel. Throw bombs, start fires, kidnap, plan assassinations, Kramer and Petrelis urged. Their justification was pragmatic: "They won."

But no bombs or fires, kidnappings or assassinations could stop the disease that filled their calendars with funerals and memorial services.

ACT UP succeeded in forcing AIDS onto television, into homes across America, into a commanding position on the national agenda. With the naiveté of the privileged, its members believed that would be enough. They endowed the U.S. government with a power over the virus it just did not have. They questioned the sincerity of the government rather than its competence. They challenged the priorities of scientists rather than their research. When the death toll continued to rise geometrically, they acted out in fury, declaring even their friends to be enemies, and their enemies to be Hitler.

Five hundred young men and women stormed the lobby of the Marriott Hotel like marines securing a beachhead. "Say hello to all the rich scientists," one yelled as the horde rallied — frolicked, actually — at the fountain inside the headquarters hotel for the Sixth International Conference on AIDS. It was June 19, 1990, and specialists from 121 nations were pouring into San Francisco for the annual meeting of the international AIDS establishment — the largest scientific three-ring circus in medical history.

A small group formed a circle on the floor of the lobby and began chanting, "It's our conference too!" Someone scurried off to hand out a press release explaining ACT UP's intention to remain right there until more free passes were provided to people with AIDS. Few activists understood much of the scientific mumbojumbo that was the lingua franca of the meeting. Fewer still were interested in the endless sessions on the acceptance rates of lubricated versus nonlubricated condoms among Ugandan truck drivers. They were making their stand on principle: how dare scientists hold a conference on AIDS without inviting people with AIDS to attend.

Young men with bleached white hair sported buttons reading, "It's *Mr.* Faggot to You." Baby dykes adorned themselves with stickers declaring, "Sister Vicious Power Hungry Bitch" and "Queers Against Profiteers." They swaggered in black leather jackets designed to convey maximum attitude. To the new generation of "in-your-face queers," as they called themselves, black leather was what tie-dye had been to rebels of an earlier era.

Two young men sat on a sofa underneath the faux palm trees by the front desk, kissing passionately, playing both to the crowd and to dozens of news photographers and cameramen from ten countries. ACT UP's media contacts, wearing green arm bands, ran around with portable telephones, doing spin control. AIDS researchers from Bulgaria and Romania, Rwanda and Cuba wandered through the crowd unclear as to what, precisely, was going on in America.

Five hours later, the guests regained the hotel. There were no broken chairs, no defaced mirrors, no trash on the floor. The lobby was pin neat.

This was not the 1960s. This was ACT UP.

"They really just are yuppies with a cause," said Jean Jackson, a New York social worker and an ACT UP member. "They aren't trying to smash private property, they just want to make sure they are around to enjoy it."

Every word, every move, was recorded by hundreds of video cameras, tape recorders, photographers and print reporters with pads in their hands. ACT UP was a well-oiled machine determined to seize center stage during the conference — and its members succeeded in dictating what the world would see and think about AIDS for six days.

ACT UP Los Angeles trucked in two fax machines, twelve cellular phones, ten pagers, seven computers and three printers. ACT UP San

Francisco supplied nine televisions and video recorders and a laser printer for press releases. ACT UP New York brought the cash. Its coffers were overflowing from a benefit art auction: $350,000 in one night. The chapter was clearing an average of $17,500 a month in T-shirt sales alone. Its budget for the week was $83,000. It wound up spending $22,000 in photocopying.

All without anyone in charge. In an anarchist organization no one gives orders, and no one has ever accused ACT UP of being anything but anarchic. ACT UP was never so much an organization as a state of mind, an amorphous collection of chapters and individuals who launched a holy war against what they saw as the aloofness of science and medicine and government to AIDS.

Command central for the San Francisco conference was a suite in a Best Western motel, where six phones rang day and night as five media czars matched up reporters from across the world with activists who could be interviewed in half a dozen languages. Amid a mass of half-eaten doughnuts and overflowing ashtrays — under a sign declaring, "You Sleep, We'll Fight AIDS" — two fax machines spewed out the week's schedule.

"This is the only revolutionary organization in history that has its own spin doctors," said Steve Sternberg, a reporter with the *Atlanta Constitution*.

The international media — 1,400 strong — had a week-long love affair with AIDS activism. Inside the convention hall there was little news to report: no major medical advances, no new understanding of how HIV caused AIDS, no promising vaccine on the horizon. But the streets of San Francisco were filled with a new phenomenon in American society: street activism aimed not at changing government military policy or social spending, but at demanding a cure for a fatal ailment. The international press could not resist its allure.

AIDS activism wasn't a single, unified movement. The Sisters of Perpetual Indulgence — part campy theatrical troupe, part political shock troop, and the heralds of every party — had been vamping around San Francisco for years, sounding the call for safe sex. Upper-middle-class white men found something in common with the homeless and devoted themselves to creating housing for people with AIDS dying on the streets. Policy wonks donned suits and ties to negotiate funding with governors and mayors and members of Congress.

But in the eyes of the nation, AIDS activism was that bold energy behind banners proclaiming "Silence = Death" in graphics that obliterated any possibility of fear, grief or shame. ACT UP defined AIDS activism, and the San Francisco meeting was its defining moment. Bartenders from New York and writers from Minneapolis, L.A. lawyers, Texas physicians, Florida social workers and students and teachers descended on the city, waiting to yell and scream, to be filmed and interviewed — for the chance to change the hearts and minds of America in one monumental burst of fury and fantasy.

As she ran through the streets screaming the sound bite of the day, Doris Feinberg breathed in the air of anger like a drowning woman. For five years she had been submerged in grief. First there was Lenny, whom she'd buried in September 1987. Doris and her husband had bankrupted themselves trying to keep their eldest son alive. She'd camped out on the doorsteps of physicians in Israel and harassed scientists in Germany. She'd flown back and forth to England in a day looking for drugs, any drugs. Looking for hope.

Not three years later, she'd held on to her younger son, Jeffrey, when he, too, died of AIDS. Lenny had died in his arms when they were both in Munich searching for treatments. For two years, Doris and Jeffrey had worked to make Lenny's dream of a community resource center for people with AIDS into a reality. Body Positive was the heart and soul of Miami's AIDS community, and Doris was its den mother.

Everyone glanced at the elegant woman, almost as beautiful as she'd been when she worked as a showgirl, swimming in an oversized champagne glass in a casino in Havana. There were scores of other black leather jackets in the crowd; hers was the only one from Saks.

After all those years of grief and caretaking, San Francisco was Doris Feinberg's first moment of release. "George Bush, you can't hide, we charge you with genocide!" she screamed in solidarity with a crowd half her age. By then, she was used to hanging out with the kids — no one else seemed to understand. Other mothers in Miami bore the same scars. Several had also lost two sons. A few met in quiet support groups, sharing their grief. But most were Cuban or Haitian. The former exchanged knowing glances at social functions but kept up appearances by explaining their sons had succumbed to cancer. The latter lived in a world apart. Doris didn't want a support group. She didn't want to grieve.

"ACT UP, fight back, fight AIDS!"

Jon Greenberg had already been yelling for two years. He loved the naughtiness of ACT UP, but he was tired. Too many fights, too little progress. He rarely talked about the fact that he was infected with HIV. He never watched the clock ticking. Unlike most of the other HIV-positive men in ACT UP, he refused to make regular trips to the doctor or obsess about every rise and fall in his T-cell count. He went to the acupuncturist, read up on roots and Chinese herbs and figured out how to take care of himself.

His allegiance to alternative therapies gave him an anomalous place in his own activist world. Jon was impatient with the insistent activist "Drugs into Bodies" drumbeat, which presupposed that some scientist in Washington would find a healing potion on his shelf. Jon wanted to look beyond the storerooms and labs of pharmaceutical companies.

He had no ideological commitment to the Natural, the Whole, the Pure. He was simply convinced that science — establishment science — was refusing to test alternative treatments, traditional home remedies, roots and herbs that didn't make money for anyone. Medicine had been destroyed by the profit motive, in his view, and Jon wasn't about to go down with the sinking ship.

"All people with AIDS should be their own doctors," he kept saying, and Jon delighted in trumping his. Others believed in Better Living Through Modern Medical Science; Jon believed in casting his net well beyond the prejudices of the AIDS establishment in his quest for health.

A gentle young man from Minneapolis, Jon had worked as a translator in Italy, moved on to Portugal and then taught in New York City. Despite his travels and his Phi Beta Kappa key from Columbia University, he'd seemed lost until he was faced with AIDS. He'd shot up drugs, had no direction in life and was, in his own eyes, a nasty and awful person. "Jon was happier after he got AIDS," his brother Neil once said. "It helped him slay the dragons. He found the freedom to become himself."

In San Francisco, Jon joined the daily demonstrations. But behind the scenes he was lobbying to get alternative treatments onto the agenda of the international AIDS establishment. It was a lonely pursuit.

The activist face the world saw most clearly in San Francisco was the boyishly handsome visage of Peter Staley, a former Wall Street bond trader who'd long planned to stand before cheering crowds as a congressional candidate. His was the activist voice that echoed across the auditorium at the opening ceremony of the conference. His constituency was a motley group of AIDS activists who melted out of the audience to line the stage as Peter, well dressed and polite as ever, rose to the podium and issued an invitation to the twelve thousand besuited health professionals gathered in the cavernous auditorium: "Join us in a chant against the man who chose to show his commitment to AIDS by refusing to be here today." Peter then yelled, "Three hundred thousand dead from AIDS. Where is George?" Members of ACT UP, who'd sneaked in with forged credentials, echoed him. Zairan physicians and Korean social workers seemed confused but felt politeness dictated joining in. "President Bush, we're watching your actions, not your words. Your actions are killing us. Your words are lies."

It was hardly the campaign speech Peter Staley had planned. In 1983 he had gone from Oberlin College to Morgan Guaranty Trust. In that heyday of Reaganomics and junk bonds, Peter was a classic yuppie who planned to make his fortune before he hit thirty and then emulate his grandfather — Eisenhower's missile czar — by entering politics.

Peter had all the polish inherited by young men who grow up on Philadelphia's Main Line, study at a fine liberal arts college and spend the obligatory junior year abroad, in his case at the London School of Economics. The only thing standing in the way of his career plans was his sexual orientation. But a firmly locked closet door created the illusion that even that was not a problem. He built a comfortable double life — bond trader by day, barhopper and bathhouse sybarite by night. When the other traders, part of a quintessential boys' club, swapped the obligatory locker room homophobic jokes, Peter just grinned and bore it.

Then AIDS got in the way. When Peter tested positive for HIV in October 1985, he told his family members — one at a time. He confided in a few friends. Then he huddled in yet another closet.

Larry Kramer was fed up. For nearly five years the gruff-voiced playwright — who'd achieved far more fame for his fury than for his dialogue — had been using the telephone in his Fifth Avenue apartment to scream at whoever would listen to his diatribes about AIDS as a holocaust, as genocide by straight America against the despised faggots in its midst. Kramer was on a constant tear, desperate to cut through the indifference of New York. He'd blasted the *New York Times* for not whipping the nation into a frenzy about AIDS. He'd denounced scientists at the National Institutes of Health who seemed unable, perhaps unwilling, to stop the dying.

On March 10, 1987, Kramer stood in the old school auditorium at the Gay and Lesbian Community Center in New York as the monthly celebrity in the Second Tuesdays speakers' series. He was a last-minute replacement for the writer Nora Ephron and was not about to give the kind of witty and chatty literary talk she'd been expected to deliver. "Two-thirds of this room will be dead in less than five years," he declared. "How long does it take before you get angry and fight back?

"Our continued existence as gay men upon the face of this earth is at stake. Unless we fight for our lives, we shall die." Kramer's proposed weapons were protests, pickets and arrests, and he was looking for a few good men to join up. Inspired by the rage — an invigorating antidote to the gloom of doctors' visits and funerals — almost 70 signed on. Within two days, when the first formal meeting of the new group was held, 250 more had enlisted.

Two weeks later, scores of men and a scattering of women tied up traffic for hours on Wall Street, demanding that the Food and Drug Administration release a half-dozen drugs waiting in the pipeline. The cure had to be in there somewhere, the activists figured. The FDA, with its arcane ways and nine-year approval process, was keeping it from dying men. They hanged FDA Commissioner Frank Young in effigy — a figure made in the workshops of the producer Joseph Papp.

ACT UP — the AIDS Coalition to Unleash Power — had come out.

On Miami Beach, Doris Feinberg didn't hear about ACT UP. Despite the mounting death toll, Miami was still pretending there was no plague sweeping across town. Even on trips to New York and Europe in her peripatetic search for a cure, she heard no mention of the magic of anger. She didn't hear about much of anything in those last months before the death of her son Lenny.

Jon Greenberg couldn't avoid finding out about the hottest new trend to hit Gay America since disco. You opened a gay paper and there was ACT UP looking bold and bad. You turned on the television and there was ACT UP pointing a finger at the president, the mayor, the governor, the cardinal and anyone else remotely connected with power. You walked into a bar and there was ACT UP emblazoned on form-fitting T-shirts that proclaimed their wearers proud queers.

They were out and loud at the massive March on Washington for Lesbian and Gay Rights in 1987, carrying a serpentine sequence of graphic images — the AIDS version of a Chinese new year's dragon. They were handing out condoms at Shea Stadium and rallying in Rockefeller Center.

The revolution had begun, in quotable sound bites and riveting graphics that were ubiquitous on the streets of New York.

On education: "You Say Don't Fuck, We Say Fuck You."

On prevention: "Men Use Condoms or Beat It."

On treatment: "Time isn't the only thing the FDA is killing."

On profits: "Fuck Your Profiteering. People are dying while you play business."

On politics: "The Government Has Blood on Its Hands."

Peter Staley discovered ACT UP on March 24, 1987, when he walked through the group's first demonstration on Wall Street. Someone thrust a leaflet into his hand. "No More Business as Usual," it read. "AIDS is Everybody's Business Now." Morgan Guaranty's lead trader had also been accosted on the street. "The government shouldn't spend a dime on AIDS research," he mumbled to Peter. "They should die because they took it up the butt."

Peter had been too cowed to defend himself. But that night he rushed home to watch the demonstration as described by Dan Rather. He was enthralled by the possibility of a new type of power. The next Monday night, he headed over to the community center for his first meeting of ACT UP. Over the following months, he moved from protest to protest, carefully disguising himself with sunglasses.

A year later, when ACT UP returned to Wall Street to celebrate its first anniversary, Peter was among the first to sit down in the street and demand to be arrested. That afternoon he got his first glimpse of jail. That night his face appeared for the first time on local news in New York, with the caption "Peter Staley, AIDS Victim."

As the death toll mounted in the late 1980s, ACT UP members became marauding raiders, hitting target after target across New York City and around the country. On April 15, 1987, they struck at the general post office in Manhattan just as thousands of late tax filers raced to beat the midnight deadline. "How much longer must we wait?" they asked, for a national policy on AIDS, for the release of promising drugs, for national AIDS education and a firm stand against discrimination. In June they converged on the White House just as President Reagan was uttering the word "AIDS" in public for the first time. When police put on bright yellow rubber gloves, the activists —

dressed in conservative business clothes — began chanting, "Your gloves don't match your shoes! You'll see it on the news!"

In July they staged a four-day, round-the-clock sit-in at New York's Memorial Sloan-Kettering Hospital, demanding that the number of drugs tested against HIV be increased. In August it was a demonstration against Northwest Airlines, for refusing passage to a man with AIDS; in January 1988, an invasion of the editorial offices of *Cosmopolitan,* to protest an article claiming that most women were not at risk for AIDS.

No one ever knew where or how ACT UP would strike. The only thing clear was that each time their protest would be bigger, bolder, badder. One week it was a phone zap — a calling campaign that overwhelmed the switchboards of more than one public or corporate office — the next it was an invasion of a meeting or headquarters. Passes were rarely a problem; ACT UP quickly became expert at forgery.

By the time the group returned to Wall Street, in March 1988, it was a professional operation. Those planning to be arrested went through civil-disobedience training. A former network news producer taught them how to give TV reporters the perfect sound bite. Attorneys were on call. And affinity groups — small bands of activists staging their own miniactions within a larger demonstration — learned how to snarl traffic and break into buildings. Grand Fury, the design collective that created ACT UP's image, churned out the perfect look with the perfect quip. For Wall Street it was fake ten-, fifty- and hundred-dollar bills reading, "White Heterosexual Men Can't Get AIDS . . . Don't Bank on It." For a concurrent attempt to embarrass the *New York Times,* it was the production of "New York Crimes" — ACT UP's version of the paper, which was wrapped around copies of the paper in coin boxes.

By April 1988 ACT UP had franchises in practically every city. All summer, demonstrators followed presidential candidates around the nation, hoping to force them to confront the reality of AIDS. In October they descended on Washington, a thousand strong, to invade the Food and Drug Administration. The demonstrators were well versed in the intricacies of FDA regulations; their Treatment and Data Committee had prepared a forty-page FDA Action Handbook and run a series of teach-ins. The action was marketed in advance to a willing press corps. That night, ACT UP led the network news. Their antics were translated into French and German and beamed to Europe.

There was never just one ACT UP, or even an educated guess as to how many activists belonged; it varied from week to week, from action to action. In any given year, probably half the people who thought of themselves as part of the group had never been to a meeting.

ACT UP was an exercise in radical democracy. There was no structure, no elected leaders, no appointed spokesmen. Everyone, and no one, had the right to speak for the group. Dozens of people brought in wider agendas. Feminism, racial justice, holistic healing and gay liberation fought it out in the context of AIDS. The Floor — the collection of individuals who happened to be at one of the marathon Monday night meetings — ruled.

The anarchy was fueled by the millions of dollars that flowed into the group. Entertainers like Grace Jones offered their services for benefits. David Hockney, Christo, Annie Leibovitz, Robert Rauschenberg and ACT UP member Keith Haring donated works of art for benefit auctions. After all, ACT UP was radical chic. On occasion Susan Sarandon dropped in on meetings.

The money financed the work of dozens of committees fighting the medical and social scourge that was AIDS. The heart of ACT UP was a collective commitment to "Drugs into Bodies" — fighting the Food and Drug Administration, the National Institutes of Health, and pharmaceutical companies for medicines to stave off immune deterioration and a dozen infections that take advantage of it. Command central for the actions was the Treatment and Data Committee, a crew of young men with degrees from the nation's finest institutions. They were serious about their work, churning out studies and reports on neglected drugs and archaic regulations. They were oblivious to the fact that they had begun reinventing the wheel. That would come later.

Housing committees turned rhetoric into reality as they worked the streets and city halls across the country demanding adequate shelter for homeless men and women with AIDS. "We have a greater responsibility than just saving our rich, lily-white male asses," housing advocate Eric Sawyer reminded the group. Needle exchange advocates risked arrest month after month as they flouted the law and handed out clean syringes in the Bronx and Harlem, Watts and San Francisco. Women's committees tried to force the government to spend more energy, and money, on female AIDS patients. Youth brigades descended on high schools to warn teens of the dangers of HIV.

ACT UP made at least a token effort to be more than a group of white boys trying to save their own lives. In New York, the Outreach Committee tried to form coalitions with minority AIDS organizations,

326 ———————— THE GRAVEST SHOW ON EARTH ———————

without much success; the cultural distance between the ghetto and Greenwich Village was too great. A small group of African Americans and Latinos formed the Majority Actions Committee to remind the white group of the color of most faces of AIDS. It wasn't easy, as Raan Medley explained in an ACT UP newsletter. "How to be Black in ACT UP?" he asked. "Number 1: If you're going to be Black and in ACT UP, make up your mind now that you either like white people or can at least stand being in very close quarters with them because you will be doing a lot of that from now on . . . We are incredibly stressed out. You would be too if you were caught up as I was with being an Authentic Black Voice."

In New York, the Latinos essentially seceded, forming their own chapter. The few black people who stuck it out got token respect. But the boys from Treatment and Data, and the all-powerful Fund Raising Committee, were openly contemptuous of the lesbians from the Women's Issues Committee — dubbed the "ladies' auxiliary" — when they began stressing the importance of dental dams. It was the perfect time to smoke a cigarette or check out who was outside.

Doris knew that her second son, Jeffrey, was on his last legs. He was wasting away from constant diarrhea. He could barely get up and around. Everyone at Body Positive seemed to be sick, and Doris was growing increasingly brittle. She had no choice but to persevere. Up early every morning to take care of Jeffrey, off to Body Positive for ten-hour days of fundraising and organizing. She was always driving people to appointments and picking up medications, visiting friends in the hospital and taking everyone out for lunch. Community, that's what Lenny had wanted. That was what Doris was intent on creating.

Reports from the Holocaust fell into her lap like a shot of pure adrenaline. Larry Kramer had collected a decade of his writings and rantings on AIDS and Gay America into a slim volume that chronicled his evolution from a movie studio executive and screenwriter to Old Testament prophet. Many Jews were offended by Kramer's comparison between Nazi genocide and AIDS. Not Doris Feinberg. The public indifference to the dying reminded her of the willful blindness of Christian Germans during the war. Reagan's refusal to acknowledge the deaths of young men like her son reeked of intentional mass murder.

Who was Larry Kramer? Doris had to know. She called New York information, never expecting he'd be listed. When he was, she dialed the phone number, never expecting that he'd answer. When he did, his anger gave her a new outlet for grief, a path other than the one to the hospital and to the morgue.

Doris was an unlikely radical — but that hardly set her apart in ACT UP. She and her husband, David, had bought a luxurious house in Miami Beach by running a posh private club. They were members of the Volvo and Mercedes crowd. Beautiful clothes, lovely home, exquisite art. Three gorgeous children.

And then there was one. Radicalism didn't seem such a remote possibility.

In the year before San Francisco, Jon Greenberg was busy teaching, ignoring his health and looking for new ways to bring alternative treatments into the mainstream. ACT UP's Treatment and Data Committee virtually dismissed him, as if he were plotting a coup against the National Institutes of Health and Western medicine. Jon thought of the committee as a bunch of privileged brats who couldn't conceive of the possibility that capitalism and science might let them down.

But he was no more comfortable with most of the "alternative types" on ACT UP's Alternative and Holistic Treatments Committee. They were anti-establishment zealots bringing a wider agenda to AIDS. Essentially anti-scientific, distrustful of research and convinced of the mystical healing powers of ancient roots and urine, they were also almost all HIV negative.

Jon was impatient with the shaky claims of alternative healers; he didn't want to trade one authoritarian system for another. His idea was to liberate medicine from dogmatism, establishment or anti-establishment. He believed in science: if AZT was a lifesaving drug, prove it; if acupuncture, herbs and drinking urine were beneficial, prove that as well.

Jon spent most of 1989 trying to make sense of the conflicting claims of healers, gathering information into the same kind of compendium that other AIDS groups prepared on prescription drugs. He helped organize teach-ins and seminars where physicians and nurses, patients and acupuncturists could discuss their experiences and offer advice. Not particularly sexy stuff, but people with AIDS needed information, not rumors. Activism wasn't all frolicking through the streets.

Peter Staley's bailiwick was the fun part. Early on the bright, sunny morning of September 14, 1989, he and six friends, donned corporate drag with fake ID tags and strode toward the New York Stock Exchange just like the downtown traders they were emulating. The fake badges were courtesy of a Greenwich Village novelty shop, which happily copied them off a video Peter had provided.

The small group had no trouble crossing the portal of this bastion of American capitalism. Peter knew his way around from his years as a bond trader. He'd warned his friends to adopt a preppy but not overly formal look — and to fill their shirt pockets with pads of paper and pencils.

Just before 9 A.M., when the bell rang to open the day's trading, they climbed to the VIP balcony, twenty feet above the trading floor, and hoisted a banner over the rail: SELL WELLCOME, it read, referring to Burroughs Wellcome, the British pharmaceutical company that produced AZT.

AZT had been released twenty-nine months earlier for the treatment of full-blown AIDS — with a price tag of $10,000 for a single year's supply. That might have been acceptable to a good capitalist kid like Peter at a different point in his life. But in August 1989, when researchers declared AZT effective against HIV infection as well as full-blown AIDS — opening the drug's market to millions worldwide and sending Burroughs Wellcome's stock on a dizzying rise — the young man suddenly lost his taste for profit making.

Peter wasn't trying to shake the foundations of American capitalism. First he tried to reason with Burroughs Wellcome, flying to North Carolina to meet with corporate executives. His father was the CEO of a chemical company, so he was hardly intimidated by business honchos.

When he was ignored, Peter upped the ante. He and a small affinity group packed battery-powered drills, walkie-talkies and metal plates into their suitcases and returned to North Carolina. At Peter's insistence, the men with him shed their earrings and the lone woman put on a skirt before they rode the elevator to the third floor of the company's American headquarters. Brandishing their walkie-talkies, they approached a secretary and warned her that the building was being evacuated. Mistaking them for security guards, she departed. The intruders barricaded themselves inside an empty office facing the highway and called a press conference.

Their outside support team met the media politely and professionally, with full explanations about the human cost of the drug company's greed. It was a great story for quiet North Carolina: handsome young activists dying of AIDS invade local corporate headquarters.

Peter grabbed the lead-in on the nightly news. He had no impact whatsoever on the price of AZT.

Sixteen AIDS groups, including ACT UP, sat down with Burroughs Wellcome months later — at a safe distance from their headquarters. Despite threats of a boycott of BW's over-the-counter drugs, including Sudafed, the company wouldn't budge on the price.

So that September morning, they went to Wall Street, blew fog-horns to drown out the morning trading bell and chained themselves to the VIP balcony. Trading was suspended and the progress of American commerce came to a halt. "Die, faggots!" incensed traders yelled. "Mace them!" When Peter was led away by police, he smiled at the sweetness of revenge.

Four days later, Burroughs Wellcome lowered the price of AZT by 20 percent. It was not, corporate spokesmen declared emphatically, a result of ACT UP's demands.

The organizers of the Sixth International Conference on AIDS in San Francisco didn't need their computers and high-tech diagnostic equipment to know they were next. ACT UP seemed to be everywhere. The year before, at the fifth AIDS conference, in Montreal, the opening ceremonies had been delayed two hours when Peter Staley and a few dozen Canadian and American AIDS protesters seized the stage and refused to budge until they were promised entry to all sessions. Then, seated in chairs reserved for dignitaries, they'd waved signs denouncing Canadian Prime Minister Brian Mulroney for doing nothing about AIDS and hissed when Zambian President Kenneth Kuanda, who was not up to speed on PC jargon, referred to "*victims* of AIDS."

Less than two months before the San Francisco meeting, ACT UP members had stormed the National Institutes of Health demanding swifter drug testing. Peter wound up on the roof of Building 1 leading the crowd of more than one thousand demonstrators. As he was taken away by police, he passed Dr. Anthony Fauci, head of NIH's AIDS research program. "See you next week," Peter said, reminding Fauci that they had an appointment scheduled.

Despite the angry protests and the frequent public rants, Fauci had already opted for appeasement of the treatment activists. A consummate politician, he'd invited them into his office and later gone to New York to meet them on their turf. He had some difficulty cajoling his colleagues into similar cooperation, but the scientists planning the San Francisco meeting had followed his lead. They invited an ACT UP representative to speak at the opening ceremony and hired a leading San Francisco AIDS activist to work with conference organizers. They wined and dined activists at luncheons and cocktail parties. They consulted with them earnestly on scientific issues. They even prevailed upon the police to treat them with kid gloves.

The much feared ACT UP riot against researchers turned into a love-in between the AIDS establishment and leading activists. "Activists have shown us some of the old rules no longer apply and policies must change to conform to the urgency of the situation," said Dr. John Ziegler, head of the AIDS Clinical Research Center at the University of California at San Francisco. "To the scientists and clinicians I ask: Listen to our patients. They are our advocates."

Ziegler and other leading scientists and federal officials energetically, repeatedly — almost desperately — credited activists with forcing down drug prices, increasing federal spending on AIDS research, speeding the pace of drug approval and designing a new, more humane approach to drug trials. The policy of appeasement didn't prevent ACT UP from staging a mock trial of five researchers — the so-called Gang of Five — or disrupting the speech of Secretary of Health and Human Services Louis Sullivan at the closing ceremony of the conference.

Most of the scientists secretly enjoyed the pranks; many, in fact, agreed with the sentiments. Even those who did not had been lobbied by their colleagues: Don't alienate the activists, include them. They can help increase our funding. They can be our allies against Congress. They can be coopted.

In San Francisco, activists were finally offered a seat at the table. Doris Feinberg and Jon Greenberg stayed outside yelling. Peter Staley accepted the invitation.

Doris returned from San Francisco filled with ACT UP attitude. At last Body Positive was energized with a force beyond grief. Politics would be the antidote to the endless round of support groups and AIDS information meetings. Fliers and stickers and posters were printed and handed out by a small cadre who'd caught Doris's excitement — and who wanted to feel part of the scene New York had made chic.

Few of the men and women who joined with Doris knew much about AIDS; even fewer thought that made any difference. They didn't want to do research; they wanted to run through the streets yelling. They weren't interested in local problems that afflicted Miami AIDS patients daily: seventeen-hour waits at the emergency room of the only public hospital in town; AIDS physicians who dropped long-time patients if they lost their insurance; the lack of housing for people with AIDS; the total indifference of the city to AIDS education, prevention and awareness. Unraveling bureaucracies was no fun, after all.

"Let's stop talking and do something," someone shouted at the first meeting. Most people there agreed.

Finally, the head of AIDS research at the National Institutes of Health declared that the institutes should limit their spending on AIDS. The next afternoon, as the downtown Miami streets filled up at lunchtime, one hundred AIDS activists marched and chanted on the steps of the Dade County Courthouse.

Doris joined the group, dressed in black and white, as it circled the courthouse carrying placards. An ACT UP member clad as the Grim Reaper struck a bell every 8½ minutes, reminding bystanders that AIDS had taken another victim. A local judge came by and ordered the police to disband the rowdy protesters. As the crowd scuffled with the cops, waving a permit in the air, Doris had a San Francisco moment — a shot of adrenaline for the grief waiting for her back at Body Positive.

Jon Greenberg returned from San Francisco ready for some fun. He and ACT UP were about to part ways; he couldn't tolerate the backbiting and pettiness that had become part of its group culture. But he wasn't ready to give up on action. Jon found it instead with the Marys, an ACT UP affinity group.

Late on the afternoon of January 22, 1991, Jon and six other men and women sat in the lobby of Channel 13, waiting nervously for their beeper to go off. Meanwhile, two friends sat at home, glued to the television screen, ready to send the signal. When Robert MacNeil, in the New York studio, went live on the *MacNeil/Lehrer NewsHour,* they passed the word. The seven, all members of the Marys, invaded the studio flashing signs declaring, "The AIDS Crisis Is Not Over," and chained themselves to MacNeil's desk. As they alternately reassured the news staff that they weren't terrorists — a wise precaution during the Persian Gulf War — and demanded that the crisis at home receive equal attention, the director switched to Jim Lehrer in Washington. Millions of Americans watched Lehrer's puzzled expression. "Robert, Robert, can you tell us what's going on there?" he asked.

"AIDS activists have broken into the studio," MacNeil answered.

Jon, who'd been initiated into group activity in his synagogue's teen club, was in heaven. "It was the most thrillingly empowering moment of my life," he declared proudly.

His work wasn't done. The following morning the Marys reassembled and joined hundreds of other activists at the World Trade Center for a Day of Desperation march through lower Manhattan. But they quickly split off from the main group because they had business uptown. As the lunchtime crowd swarmed into the CitiCorp building, the Marys dropped bloody chicken bones down onto the atrium floor. That day, they renamed themselves the Bloody Marys.

That same afternoon they delivered a casket filled with bones to Tickets/Tickets, along with a packet of fliers reading, "The AIDS Crisis Is Not Over." Then the group raced off to the last stop of the day: Grand Central Station, where they joined a rowdy mob that blocked the entrances and wrapped the station in red ribbon, chanting, "We're dying of red tape!"

Jon was giddy with delight; he was also deadly serious. "We will do anything we can possibly do to get the response that we need to the AIDS crisis," he said. And he meant it. That summer, he and the Marys led a group of activists on a Labor Day excursion to Kennebunkport, where President George Bush was relaxing. "People with AIDS don't get a vacation from AIDS," he explained.

The following November, the Marys' rituals turned grim. On a rainy afternoon, the small band gathered to dress Mark Fisher for the last time, in his favorite old jeans splattered with paint and the T-shirt he'd designed for them: "All People with AIDS Are Innocent." They helped lay out the young architect in the slip-lid casket used by ultra-Orthodox Jews, the only kind of coffin that could be closed and reopened. Then, after a short service at Judson Memorial Church, they carried him out to the street and thirty-nine blocks up Sixth Avenue, through the heart of Manhattan to the Bush-Quayle campaign headquarters. The banner preceding the cortege read, "Mark Lowe Fisher, 1953–1992, Murdered by George Bush." Police following the procession turned off their radios and removed their hats.

"I want my own funeral to be fierce and defiant, to make the public statement that my death from AIDS is a form of political assassination," Fisher had written a few weeks earlier. His friends vowed to fulfill that last request. It was Election Day.

Mark was the first, but he wouldn't be the last, the group declared as the crowd of three hundred, soaked and weeping, melted back onto the busy streets of the city. "Our plan is to drop bodies on the

White House steps because that's where the blame must be laid," they declared.

By the time he returned from San Francisco, Peter Staley was AIDS activism's poster boy, featured on *Nightline* and in *Rolling Stone* and the *Wall Street Journal*. But when he walked into the Monday night ACT UP meeting, he was not hailed as a conquering hero. The membership was furious at a form letter Peter had just sent out asking for money to support the congressional candidacy of his friend Sean Strub. The anger was no reflection on Strub, who was one of ACT UP's most successful fundraisers. It was provoked by Peter's unilateral expropriation of the group's most valuable assets: its brand image and its mailing list. "Typical Staley arrogance," activists muttered.

The mailing wasn't Peter's only sin. While on the podium in San Francisco, he had not hesitated to offer some criticism of the group. "ACT UP has made mistakes, such as choosing an inappropriate target for a demonstration or using an offensive tactic," he conceded. "Communion wafers come to mind."

The Floor — what passes for the membership of ACT UP — was out for blood.

Peter had been referring to ACT UP's most infamous action, the group's assault on New York Archbishop John Cardinal O'Connor during a mass at St. Patrick's Cathedral in December 1989. Five thousand activists from AIDS and women's groups had targeted O'Connor for his opposition to abortion and condom distribution in the schools. Most of them had remained outside the church, chanting as O'Connor celebrated mass. Several hundred entered the sanctuary and staged a die-in. One activist stood in line to take communion and threw the wafer on the floor.

ACT UP, the darling of the liberal media, was branded as villainous.

Everyone in ACT UP knew what Peter thought about the Stop the Church action. The day after, he'd risen at a meeting to denounce the antics as counterproductive. But public criticism was something else. The word used most often was treason.

Peter might have looked boyish, but he had the full arrogance of a young man raised on the Philadelphia Main Line. "I will not be silenced by ACT UP's thought police," he declared in a letter to the membership.

In fact, trouble had been brewing for months between Peter and much of the group. A Wall Street pragmatist, he didn't have much patience with radical democracy and had been lobbying for a firmer organizational structure. He echoed Larry Kramer: Forget experiments in empowerment, this is a plague. He was sick of speeches about the evils of racism and the necessity for supporting the anti-apartheid movement in South Africa. But ACT UP wasn't looking for a corporate make-over.

Peter was not deterred. He had a new vision of AIDS activism that didn't include the endless fights with ACT UP. He was already planning to create a small, disciplined group that would act simultaneously as inside-the-system lobbyists and outside agitators. If ACT UP didn't like the idea, too bad.

He and the other members of the Treatment and Data Committee already had secure positions inside the AIDS establishment. Fauci had invited them to join the AIDS Clinical Trials Group and declared them "here to stay." They were given voting membership on the executive board and on all important committees — at a cost to the taxpayer of $250,000 by 1994. They were meeting regularly with the heads of pharmaceutical companies, members of Congress and officials of the FDA.

Some accused them of being coopted. Peter declared himself ready to kiss any ass necessary to win the war against AIDS. At the same time, he aspired to turn his group into the Greenpeace of AIDS activism, a small band that would use high technology and bold strokes rather than mass demonstrations to apply pressure when negotiations failed.

He applied this one-two punch when he targeted Astra Pharmaceutical, makers of foscavir, a drug that treated the blindness caused by AIDS-related cytomegalovirus. At $22,000 a year per patient, for life, the drug was unacceptably expensive. In the fall of 1991, Peter organized a coalition of sixteen AIDS groups that asked Astra to cap the price. Astra didn't respond. In November, representing the Treatment Action Group — his new ACT UP affinity group — Peter met with company executives. To no avail.

Two months later, the Treatment Action Guerrillas invaded Astra's Massachusetts headquarters with a crew from *60 Minutes* in tow. "Astra's Greed Robs Us Blind," read the sign they unfurled along the side of their rental trucks. Peter and a dozen others chained themselves underneath the trucks and blocked traffic trying to enter the company's grounds.

Even as they were hauled off to jail, Peter was smugly self-satisfied at what he'd pulled off with his small, invitation-only band.

But Astra did not budge on the price of foscavir.

The San Francisco conference was ACT UP's last national gasp of anger. In the ensuing years, activists continued running through the streets in noisy demonstrations, but their numbers and frequency diminished inexorably. Gradually the bold outrage dissipated.

Activists long convinced that the FDA and NIH didn't know what they were doing now sit on every imaginable scientific committee. Researchers redesign drug studies to conform to activists' demands. Drug companies consult with them about the release of new compounds. The FDA approves drugs in record time. Funding for AIDS research, education and prevention continues to climb. The Ryan White Care Act provides people with AIDS all over the country access to services that are the envy of cancer patients.

But the death toll still rises.

By 1991 ACT UP meetings in New York had begun to deteriorate into tense acrimony as the utter helplessness no one wanted to acknowledge pervaded activist ranks. Demoralization bred infighting, and members slugged it out at meetings that went on hour after hour, week after week.

There were dozens of disputes about funding and priorities and who said what to whom. The cattiness was fueled by the publication of anonymous barbs in the weekly rag *TITA* (Tell It to ACT UP), published by an activist whose major contribution to the group was to turn up the volume on personal pettiness.

Underlying the bitchiness was a substantive battle fought between the members of the Treatment and Data Committee — who believed that greasing the wheels of research and drug approval were the only issues worth discussing — and their archrival Maxine Wolfe, a New York college professor and long-time activist, who was intent on keeping social issues high on ACT UP's agenda. Wolfe had brought years of activist experience — and a dedication to careful homework — to the young group.

"What good is a cure if you can't afford it?" Maxine asked endlessly. Peter Staley's group responded, "What good is egalitarian health care if you're dead?" The Treatment and Data Committee wanted to restructure NIH and consolidate its AIDS research programs; Maxine Wolfe and her supporters wanted to restructure health care delivery.

The men wanted to negotiate with pharmaceutical companies about drug access; Maxine's group wanted to fight pharmaceutical companies about the exclusion of women from drug studies.

Every Monday night, the treatment activists took their places on the right hand side of Cooper Union's cavernous Great Hall and tried to hold their own against Wolfe and her supporters on the left. The rivalry degenerated into a quagmire of backbiting, ego-tripping and political infighting. Finally, the treatment activists accused Maxine of being blinded by her seronegativity, of writing her utopian agenda on gay men's graves; she accused them of indifference to the plight of seropositives who didn't happen to be affluent, gay, white and male.

The membership of ACT UP was divided. HIV-positive men had a deep loyalty to the treatment activists. No one could deny their achievements. They had seemingly burst open the FDA pipeline, and drugs were being approved in record time. Because of their work, the price of AZT had been slashed. Because of their knowledge and persistence, AIDS activists had been included at every level of decision-making for the AIDS Clinical Trials Group. They were a wealth of information about new drugs and new trials, and had clout to help the aspiring enroll.

Sitting down with federal officials and corporate executives, however, reeked of a sellout. You're making a pact with the devil, many insisted. Watch out for the old tactics companies used to coopt union officials, others warned. Few of the treatment activists knew what they were saying. They were young — in their twenties and thirties — and had no background in radical politics. People like Maxine Wolfe and Jim Fouratt, a founder of ACT UP with a thirty-year history in radical politics, knew from experience how seductive paneled conference rooms could be.

The Treatment and Data crowd was an impatient, often arrogant lot, not fond of listening to history lectures. They bristled at the accusation of selling out. Jim Fouratt tried to explain how subtle the process could be: you sit at the table with the other side and they become human beings. They're nice guys, really. They don't sound unreasonable, and they probably aren't. In fact, as you spend more time talking with them, your old friends start to sound like the crazies. Without meaning to — without even realizing it's happening — your frame of reference begins to shift. Suddenly you stop demanding the impossible, because you have lost your sense of the possibilities.

That's what had happened to civil rights leaders offered places at the table. To union officials and feminist leaders. If you aren't incredibly careful, that's what will happen to you, Jim told them.

Fouratt and Wolfe might have been oversensitive to the problem, but the treatment activists were dismissive of their concerns. "This isn't the Pentagon and the war in Vietnam we're talking about," they said, cutting off all further discussion. They were too caught up in the science of AIDS, too convinced that if they mastered the bureaucratic and scientific technicalities, they could stop the dying. It never seemed to occur to them that it might turn out to be more complicated.

The revolution devoured itself in a dozen disputes. The concerns of the black caucus were haughtily dismissed while treatment held center stage; its members walked out. When new queer militants trying to emulate the Black Panthers sent out a broadsheet asserting, "I Hate Straights," heterosexual members of ACT UP balked at the insult. Lesbians, who'd struggled hard to fight an epidemic that wasn't theirs, felt demeaned — with good reason. At one meeting of the Treatment and Data Committee, a prominent female researcher made a long presentation on a drug the group had already declared useless. "Can't someone shut that broad up?" one of the men yelled.

Similar struggles were fought out in ACT UP chapters all over the world. ACT UP San Francisco split into two, with the treatment activists leaving the lefties to form ACT UP Golden Gate. Chicago split as well, with the HIV-positive members organizing a group for people with AIDS or HIV only. ACT UP/Germany disappeared when all of its demands were met by the federal government there. The Washington, D.C., chapter disbanded. "Out of money, out of steam, out of community support," said one spokesman for the group. It was a familiar story in most of ACT UP's one hundred chapters.

By 1992 three-quarters of the 1990 leadership were either dead or gone. Attendance at the New York meeting had fallen from 750 to 150, and money from what had seemed like the bottomless ACT UP pot was actually becoming tight.

Everyone was tired. The roster of leaders who'd been buried was shockingly long. Ronald Reagan had been a cofounder of ACT UP; with Clinton in the White House there was no energizing target. Many wondered whether activism inside or outside the system was relevant. Sure they'd forced down the price of AZT, but now no one wanted to take it. They'd gained early access to ddI and ddC, but who cared about access to bad drugs?

The New York treatment activists tried to allay the fears of the group at large by insisting that they had become more effective by working inside the system — and that they would be ready to mobilize for radical action if they were ignored.

But their fellow activists saw a different reality during a meeting of the AIDS Clinical Trials Group in November 1991. The ACTG was mounting a massive study of a combination of three drugs (AZT, ddI and ddC) which would use up one-fifth of its budget. People were angry: make the drug companies pay, Maxine Wolfe and her cadre demanded. To drive their point home, they went to the meeting and stormed a cocktail party celebrating the achievements of the ACTG. As they ran in yelling, they saw the members of the Treatment and Data Committee sipping drinks with the very people they were targeting.

The division within ACT UP reached a breaking point when a group of women proposed a moratorium on all meetings between ACT UP representatives and government officials. The women were infuriated when they heard that on the same day Fauci had dismissed their demands for more female participants in trials of AIDS drugs, a member of the Treatment and Data Committee had had dinner with him. Enough, the women screamed, sensing a cozy bond among the men that was excluding women's interests. The women's caucus lost the moratorium vote, but the treatment activists saw the handwriting on the wall.

Four years after his first moment in the limelight in San Francisco, Peter Staley sauntered into one of those anonymous meeting rooms in hotels around the nation's capital where much of the business of government is conducted. It was July 1994. As he took his place at the conference table, Dr. Daniel Hoth, the former director of NIH's Division of AIDS, now senior vice president of a biotech company, limped in on a foot still bandaged from an accident earlier in the summer. Assistant Secretary of Health Phil Lee whispered in the corner with Dr. Harold Varmus, a Nobel Prize–winning retrovirologist who'd just been appointed to head the National Institutes of Health. Peter nodded his head to greet Flossie Wong-Staal, a leading geneticist and professor at the University of California at San Diego, and stopped to chat with Dr. Steven Carter, a vice president of Bristol-Myers Squibb.

Peter looked totally at home seated at the table with Nobel Prize winners, captains of industry and senior government officials. He was a member of the National Task Force on AIDS Drug Development, appointed by President Clinton to remove barriers to the swift development and approval of drugs to treat AIDS. He flew around the country to conferences and meetings paid for by the federal government and major pharmaceutical companies. As he sent government secretaries off to fax notes and information back to New York and asked clerks to do his copying, Peter looked exactly like the young bond trader he'd been. He yelled no slogans at the government bureaucrats whom other AIDS activists continued to harangue. He wore no buttons accusing drug companies of profiteering.

Peter was there representing the Treatment Action Group, not ACT UP. Two years earlier, he and thirteen other savvy treatment activists had spun their affinity group off into a separate entity, and TAG incorporated. Membership was by invitation only, and could be revoked by the board. Activists received salaries.

"We have abandoned the politically correct form of activism," Peter explains. "We just want to get things done." He is the group's chief operating officer, and he has repeated the fundraising miracle he pulled off in ACT UP. Money is important, of course; travel to meetings and conferences, phone calls and printing and salaries don't come cheap. But this time he didn't turn to the T-shirt business or to generous artists. At a public ceremony in the summer of 1992, TAG's coffers were filled when Peter accepted a $1 million check from executives of Burroughs Wellcome, his former corporate archenemy.

The movement reeled at the image.

No one in ACT UP denies that TAG has continued to produce results — they have too much talent not to. Peter might be the group's most public face, but the real brains of the operation is Mark Harrington, who spent the years before AIDS studying German Jewish intellectuals at Harvard and slinging espressos, first in a Cambridge coffee shop, later in New York. With no background in science, he has mastered enough of the biology of AIDS to converse comfortably on technical matters with the Nobel laureate David Baltimore, Harvard virologist Bernard Fields, and NIH director Harold Varmus.

Harrington's first efforts as a treatment activist, even before he himself tested positive, were focused on beating a cure for AIDS out of the bushes. "I thought there must be a drug out there that would be a cure," he says. "Something, somewhere, existed; we just all had to put our shoulders to the wheel and shake it loose from the federal bureaucracy." Harrington has since become more skeptical. "You can't shout a cure out of the test tube," he now says.

Working with the other members of the Treatment and Data Committee, and later with TAG, Harrington turned his remarkable talent for detail to designing faster and more humane ways to conduct trials for promising drugs and to finding potential treatments for opportunistic infections.

The system caved in — but the sick kept dying.

By 1992 he and TAG had become convinced that the real problem lay in the very structure of NIH's AIDS research program, an uncoordinated project that disburses funds across fifteen institutes, nine centers and divisions. With the help of Senator Ted Kennedy's staff, they wrote a bill to solve the problem by strengthening NIH's Office of AIDS Research. Rather than turn to activists for support in Congress, they signed up two hundred prominent medical researchers as their lobbyists.

TAG members wound up doing what the scientists and policy makers they long criticized do with their time — producing research studies, attending meetings and workshops and consulting with scientists and policy makers around the globe. Guerrilla warfare wasn't part of that agenda. "Frankly, we've got our hands full doing other work," Peter says. "We don't have time for actions, and there's no great urge. We can get a great deal done by tapping into pockets of support in the scientific or political establishment. That's much more effective."

More effective for what? is the question increasingly asked in the community. Unconcerned with tenure and promotion, TAG members voice doubts and concerns that researchers have hesitated to express. As outsiders not socialized into the culture of American science, they consistently bring a fresh perspective and a sense of urgency to discussions.

Unfortunately, NIH's AIDS research program remains a swamp of academic self-indulgence in which competition, self-interest and mutual back-scratching routinely preclude urgency. Despite years of TAG membership on its executive committee, the AIDS Clinical Trials Group remains a $110 million black hole. In expanding the number of sites it includes, the ACTG has ignored scientific expertise and bowed to political pressure, and political correctness, in pulling in new hospitals. Drug companies refuse to use the multisite network, accusing it of being slow and not "user-friendly." So in order to justify the network's existence, the ACTG spends millions of dollars defining and redefining the uses of the same few compounds — even of some questionable ones — while patients die without treatments for many diseases.

By early 1995 — eight years into the ACTG's existence — no one, including TAG, was sure precisely what the trials group should be doing, what work it should leave to pharmaceutical companies, or whether it should exist at all. "Should the ACTG focus on new agents without champions, or should they acknowledge that drug companies are more expert at early trials and let the ACTG get involved when they need to mobilize patients fast?" asks Maureen Myers, former director of the ACTG and now the director of virology at Boehringer, Ingelheim Pharmaceuticals. "No one knows what they're for, or if they're necessary. The ACTG has ended up as jack of all trades and master of none."

The speed-up in the FDA approval process was the activists' most revolutionary achievement, but that victory has produced so little information that neither physicians nor patients know whether the treatments they are offered are safe and effective, whether they are better than no drugs at all. In 1994 TAG attacked the process of accelerated approval, its own stepchild, for the quandary it created, never acknowledging that researchers had warned them of that result years earlier.

What went wrong?

Many researchers believe that TAG has moved too close to the drug companies. "I can't understand why they trust industry so much," says Dr. Charles van der Horst of the University of North Carolina at Chapel Hill. "What we've got is an unholy alliance of Republicans, libertarians, the *Wall Street Journal,* the pharmaceutical companies and activists. I don't understand. Their bottom line is that they want to make money. That's it." Many people with AIDS go even further, accusing TAG of selling out to pharmaceutical companies, which after all have been extraordinarily generous to the group.

Even some TAG members are worried. In the summer of 1994, Peter Staley seemed to cross yet another line when he openly defended industry's attempts to end NIH's requirement that companies agree to charge fair prices for drugs developed collaboratively with some federal scientists. "How can he oppose fair prices?" ACT UP members asked. "Who is he working for anyway?"

Peter is unapologetic. "If we want a cure for AIDS, we have to give pharmaceutical companies incentives," he says. "After all, they're in this for the profit." Profit, once considered a dirty word, had somehow become a sympathetic rationale.

· · ·

On October 3, 1994, David Feinberg walked into an ACT UP meeting for the last time.

One of TAG's firmest defenders, Feinberg brought none of the humor that had made him a minor celebrity among New York literati — a gay Fran Lebowitz, if you will. He was frail, with the gait and grimace of the ancient. When he entered the crowd of vital, healthy young people affirming life by acting up, it was as if the reality of AIDS had come home to the heart of AIDS activism.

"I want you to know what AIDS is," he said, reading from prepared notes. His speech faltered. At times he seemed to have difficulty focusing. "I want to remind you, with my catheters, my hanging bags of TPN and drugs, my pole, my infusion pump. I lived in an awful studio in midtown Manhattan for more than ten years. Last March I moved to Chelsea. In June the city announced the water supply was corrupted. I believe I got cryptosporidiosis and mycoavium complex from the drinking water.

"I have constant diarrhea. My gastrointestinal system resembles a worm's. I have eaten a spoonful of Cheerios and voided it in a minute. My weight dropped from 145 to 118. I weighed myself today, 105. Lose 30 percent of your body weight and you're basically dead. I am a corpse."

The room was entirely still. No one could speak. Few at the meeting had known Feinberg B.C., Before the Crisis, as he measured time. He'd started out as a classic nerd, the type of skinny little guy born to ace the SATs. In the years after MIT, Feinberg, like his literary alter ego, N. H. Rosenthal, had looked for love in all the wrong places — and as many of them as possible. "I may have forgotten to use a condom five or six thousand times back in 1982, before there were rules and regulations to follow," he had quipped more than once.

Activists knew Feinberg as a darling of liberal literary critics who polished his sharp wit on the disease that was killing his immune system, cell by cell. By then, his hours at the gym had sculpted the skinny kid into the Gay Urban Clone. He showed up at all the right demonstrations, wearing all the right clothes, shouting all the right slogans. In his off moments, he held back despair with humor.

His description of his first medication, AZT: "The pills came with a highly technical pamphlet too depressing for words, listing dosage, warnings and approximately 16,457 side effects. My favorite was 'taste perversion,' which I interpreted as a strong predilection for chintz and black velvet paintings of nude large-breasted women."

In a speech delivered at the Gay Pride Rally in New York's Union Square on June 26, 1993: "I'm halfway down that HIV Highway to Hell. You know the route: Finding out you're positive, telling your friends, your first nucleoside-analogue reverse-transcriptase inhibitor, telling the folks, your second nucleoside-analogue reverse-transcriptase inhibitor, your first bad reaction to a PCP prophylactic, your third nucleoside-analogue reverse-transcriptase inhibitor, telling your prospective tricks, your diagnosis according to the recently changed CDC definition of PWLTC — Person With Lousy T Cells — your fourth nucleoside-analogue reverse-transcriptase inhibitor, telling your current boyfriend, your first infusion, your thirty-ninth arrest with ACT UP, your ninety-third placebo-controlled protocol, your forty-eighth opportunistic infection and, eventually, hopefully after the Oscars, Gay Pride, and Part Two of *Angels in America,* you achieve the status of metabolically challenged, which is a polite way of saying dead."

The ironic, whiny angst was quintessential David. The humor was not, of course, even remotely reflective of the truth.

Feinberg wrote for the same reason that he sat through endless meetings of ACT UP every Monday night, year after year. He was furious that he was dying. He was convinced that if his anger could be amassed with enough other anger, the plague would end. That if he and his friends and their lovers were arrested enough times, the virus would cease its insidious march or drugs would come pouring out of research laboratories.

Feinberg was released from St. Vincent's Hospital on October 3. It was a Monday night. ACT UP night. The word spread that he was planning to speak. He was seated alone on a wooden box in the center of the main room at the Lesbian and Gay Community Center. He continued to read:

"I was diagnosed as HIV positive in the summer of 1987. I joined ACT UP entirely out of self-interest and self-preservation. I wanted to live.

"I've been arrested inside St. Patrick's and at the FDA. At the Holland Tunnel abortion block and the Irish Lesbian and Gay Organization's counterdemo on St. Patrick's Day. I risked arrest most recently in New Jersey, at the Hoffmann–La Roche demonstration a year ago last January. I took my first pill of AZT at an ACT UP meeting. And now I've probably taken my last.

"I personally have taken AZT, ddI, ddC, d4T and 3TC, and I have absolutely no idea whether any of them produced any sustained, positive effect . . . I'm not sure, now that we have so many drugs available that may or may not work, whether introducing still more drugs of unknown efficacy would be of any value. I may try a protease inhibitor, but at this point it is almost immaterial. My T cells are so low my doctor refuses to tell me my count.

"I am impatient when ACT UP wastes precious time bickering about how many people to send to the international AIDS conference, or indulging its obsession with the Catholic Church and Cardinal O'Connor. I am at that totally self-serving stage where I want every argument and action to help save my life. I thought people joined ACT UP because we had seen too many friends die and would do anything to prevent yet another death. Obviously, we have failed.

"I am a totally self-absorbed, narcissistic pig.

"I don't care about latex dental dams.

"I don't care about AIDS in Africa, Asia, Europe, Australia, Antarctica or South America.

"I am no longer fighting with ACT UP. The stench of self-interest and egotism is too overpowering. I am fighting for my life.

"If ACT UP continues in this fashion, it may as well be plowed over into the same mass grave that already overflows with the rotting corpses of our friends who have died of AIDS."

The room was tense as Feinberg departed. There was absolute silence. Finally, the facilitator took the microphone and spoke:

"Next item on the agenda."

By 1992, Doris Feinberg was so tense and overwhelmed that she was ready to crack. AIDS service groups throughout Miami were caught up in the same fractious fights that were tearing apart communities all over the country. The federal government was channeling hundreds of thousands of dollars into community-based organizations, and civil war broke out as they fought each other for the money.

ACT UP Miami had died in its infancy. From time to time, its few members held a kiss-in or a die-in, but nobody cared. Perhaps the tropical air had sapped the energy for radical activity. Maybe the leaders were inept. Three HIV-positive men tried to take over by demanding an HIV-positive majority on the coordinating committee. They were drowned out by rage over the implication that people with AIDS might have some special stake in AIDS activism.

When ACT UP's national network received a large donation from the sale of the *Red, Hot and Blue* album, Miami received its full share,

$25,000. Its leadership bought bank certificates of deposit to ensure the group's continuing existence.

By the end of 1994, they were down to three members.

Doris reimmersed herself in caretaking. But there was nothing left but death. No anger. No hope on the horizon. She helped bury Sonia Singleton and Shirley Wilson, two black women with AIDS who had fought to broaden the community's view of the epidemic. Bruce Moore died. Then Miguel Chinchilla. It was too much. She still hadn't cleaned out her sons' bedrooms.

She finally fled to Orlando, to start again. Death pursued her. Just as she was building a new life far from AIDS, her old friend Alberto succumbed to the disease. Then Pedro Zamora and Jim Pruitt, within one month.

There was nowhere to hide.

July 16, 1993, was such a clear, bright day in New York City that even in the late afternoon the sun actually glistened off the litter along First Avenue. The Marys had posted lookouts in a small Brazilian bar on the corner of First and Houston. The bar's owner seemed oblivious to the tension of the watchers as they used his phone to announce that the coast was clear.

It was a motley crew. Lesbian and gay activists in full clone costume mixed with yuppies arriving from Madison Avenue and the United Nations. Radical Faeries — Gay America's answer to hippies — showed up in crinolines, dreadlocks and wings, beating an eerily flat tattoo on their drums. The tone was too somber for streets where the music is sirens and screams, the cadence the monotonal mumblings of the homeless and the electronic blaring of salsa.

The casket appeared out of nowhere, a blue-gray box that somehow didn't seem out of place in the midst of the decaying East Village, that strange meeting ground of the young and hip with the old and desperate. An activist crowd famous for its noisy anger was hushed as six men and women began carrying the coffin up First Avenue preceded by a blazing purple banner: "Jon Greenberg Lived with AIDS Until He Died."

Jairo Pedrazo, a Colombian AIDS activist, handed out candles in glass holders embossed with Jon's name and fliers with his creed: "The solution to AIDS is not more but less. Aggressive acceptance. Accepting the change that is happening in my body, in my biology, embracing the other as a lover, the virus is breaking down my defenses so I can learn how to live without defenses, so I can learn how to live in many, in unity with the other."

Jon had died four days earlier in St. Vincent's Hospital after years of living with the constant diarrhea and stomach cramps of crypto-sporidium, with the disfigurement of Kaposi's sarcoma, the excruciating pain of shingles, and lungs weakened by *Pneumocystis carinii* pneumonia. He was killed, in the end, by cryptococcal meningitis.

On that summer afternoon, with drums calling out a methodical chant and the drummers intoning, "There is a wind to life, there is a wind, all that falls shall rise again," the six friends carried Jon's body into Tompkins Square Park. Hispanic families wheeling baby carriages along the paths stopped in the kind of disbelief residence in New York usually makes impossible. Rollerbladers made way for the procession. Even the junkies and punks and winos paused when the casket was gently placed between the towering oaks and opened to public view. CNN and *New York Newsday* rushed in to photograph the corpse.

The remaining members of the Marys passed out fliers printed with a photograph of the thirty-seven-year-old man lying in his sickbed and his final wishes spelled out: "I don't want an angry political funeral. I just want you to burn me in the street and eat my flesh."

Jon hadn't wanted his funeral turned into a rant against Bush or Clinton. Unlike most of the young men with whom he'd demonstrated and been arrested, Jon had never believed that raving could ward off death. It was an anomalous attitude in a community that had survived ten years of plague — of social calendars filled with memorial services, of calling old friends only to discover that they had died three weeks earlier — by clinging to anger and blame as magic shields against reality.

Jon's memorial service was a ritual of grief for young men and women who'd dedicated themselves to planning new rituals of life. Actions and demonstrations, protests and sit-ins, after all, are about the future. The power those actions create might be illusory, but it is life-affirming. Anger might be cynical, but cynicism is the last bastion of hope. On that summer afternoon there was little hope left. Jon was the last HIV-positive Mary to die. In Tompkins Square Park that day, grief overwhelmed anger.

As dozens of friends rose to remember Jon, his father, Lionel, a Minneapolis attorney, sat on the ground among the youthful crowd in a white short-sleeved shirt and gray tie. He carried a package of tissues in his belt and clutched the hand of his wife, Myra, in her sweat pants and sensible shoes. John Kelly rose to the microphone and in a voice quivering with loss sang Jon's favorite Joni Mitchell song. "We are stardust, we are golden, and we've got to get ourselves back to the garden." Jon's brother Stan told stories about his younger brother, who knew the words to every song in *Bye Bye Birdie* and *The Music Man,* who could belt out an unbeatable falsetto rendition of the aria "Habanera" from *Carmen.* Then he opened a Jewish prayer book and recited the Kaddish, the prayer said at funerals:

"Glorified and sanctified be God's great name throughout the world which he has created according to his will. May he establish his kingdom in your lifetime and during your days. And within the life of the entire house of Israel, speedily and soon, and say amen.

"Be not afraid of sudden terror, nor of the storm that strikes the wicked. Form your plot, it shall fail. Lay your plan, it shall not prevail.

"May there be abundant peace from heaven and life for us and for all Israel, and say amen."

IN MEMORIAM

Stacey Baker, 33
Enrique Bertheau, 34
John Boswell, 47
Michael Callen, 38
Charles Caulfield, 38
Bob Caviano, 42
Miguel Chinchilla, 31
Charles Elder, 27
Juan Faedo, 24
Jeffrey Feinberg, 27
Lenny Feinberg, 26
Roland Funk, 46
Dann Galen, 32
Jon Greenberg, 37
Leonard Horowitz, 43
Alberto Julbe, 46
Raul Llanos, 39
Jeffrey Lyon, 38
Fr. Antonio Mendoza, 43
Paul Monette, 49
Bruce Moore, 39
Jim Pruitt, 42
Jeffrey Schmalz, 39
Randy Shilts, 42
Sonia Singleton, 37
Titti Sotto, 48
Mario Trincheria, 44
Shirley Wilson, 39
Pedro Zamora, 22

SOURCES

NOTES

INDEX

SOURCES

This book is based on almost seven years of reporting on AIDS. During that time, I interviewed patients, physicians, activists, scientists, political leaders and policy makers. I read scientific journals, the popular press, the gay press and the plethora of specialized newsletters and computer databases that AIDS has created. Most important, the AIDS wards of hospitals became my second home as I watched friends die.

INTERVIEWS

Scientists and physicians. In New York: Dr. Joseph Sonnabend, Dr. David Ho, Dr. Harvey Bialy. In Boston: Dr. Deborah Cotton. In Florida: Dr. William Reiter, Dr. Nancy Klimas, Dr. Gwendolyn Scott, Dr. Lionel Resnick, Dr. Paul Arens, Dr. Gordon Dickinson, Dr. Sanford Kuvin, Dr. Margaret Fischl, Dr. Robert Rubin. In North Carolina: Dr. Charles van der Horst. In California: Dr. Peter Duesberg, Dr. Douglas Richman, Dr. Kary Mullis, Dr. Dan Hoth. At the National Institutes of Health: Dr. Robert Gallo, Dr. Anthony Fauci, Dr. Harold Varmus, Dr. Robert Yarchoan, Dr. Samuel Broder, Dr. Jack Killen. In Washington, D.C.: Dr. Ellen Cooper, Dr. Abdul-Alim Muhammad. In Havana: Dr. Jorge Perez.

Activists. ACT UP/New York, then and now: Robert Jones, Robin Haueter, Bob Lederer, James Baggett, Joy Episalla, George Carter, Risa Denenberg, Terry McGovern, Larry Kramer, Jim Fouratt. In New York: Bob Caviano, James Scitaro, Michael Ellner. In California: Billi Goldberg and Mike McIntee of ACT UP/San Francisco, Sean Sasser and the late Michael Callen. In Detroit: Jerome Boyce. In Seattle: Paul Feldman. In Florida: Joel Rapoport, Ivan Bernstein, Doris Feinberg, the late Miguel Chinchilla, the late Sonia Singleton, John O'Hara, the late Raleigh Funk,

Alfredo Martínez-Garcia, Mary Kaplan, Lenny Kalpan, George Bergalis, Allison Bergalis, Philip Holtsberg, Jon Cullipher and the late Jim Pruitt. In Philadelphia: Julie Davids. In Baltimore: Lynda Dee of AIDS Action/Baltimore. In Cincinnati: Lisa Hernández. In Washington, D.C.: Steve Michael, Mary Fisher, Shepherd Smith, Anita Smith, Michael Petrelis. From the Treatment Action Group: Peter Staley, Rebecca Pringle-Smith, Derek Link, Spencer Cox, Garance Franke-Ruta, Greg Gonsalves, and Mark Harrington.

Politicians, attorneys and policy makers. In Washington: Hon. Barney Frank, James Guyton of Frank's office, Steve Morin in the office of Hon. Nancy Pelosi, Helen Fox and Charles Nelson of the National Minority AIDS Council, Alexander Robinson of the National Task Force on AIDS Prevention, Jeff Levi in the office of Patsy Fleming, Jane Silver of the American Foundation for AIDS Research. In Florida: Joe Gersten, Mort Laitner, Ernie Aguila. In California: Phill Wilson, Peter Lurie. In Boston: Tim Palmer, Rich Stevens. In Arizona: Walt Senterfeit. In Milwaukee: Doug Nelson and Mike Gifford.

Journalists and writers. In New York: Joey Lovett, Celia Farber, the late Robert Massa, Gina Kolata, Chuck Ortleb. In California: Hank Plante, the late Paul Monette, the late Randy Shilts, and Michelle Cochrane. In Detroit: Frank Bruni. In Washington: Chris Bull, John Crewdson. In Florida: Kevin Krausse, Don Van Natta, Justin Gillis.

GOVERNMENT AND QUASI-GOVERNMENT DOCUMENTS

I consulted the regular publications, press releases and periodic reports from the branches of the National Institutes of Health, the Food and Drug Administration, the Health Resources Services Administration, the Centers for Disease Control, the National Research Council, the Institute of Medicine, the General Accounting Office and the congressional Office of Technology Assistance, as well as the transcripts of congressional hearings devoted to AIDS research, the Ryan White Care Act and the Food and Drug Administration.

I obtained most of the government documents used under the Freedom of Information Act, a piece of legislation that is more help in theory than in practice because of the snail's pace of FOI offices and the reluctance to give up documents that belong, in fact, to the public. The Centers for Disease Control is a notable exception, making documents available in a timely fashion on microfiche. Documents and transcripts were also obtained from the Food and Drug Administration, the Federal Trade Commission, the National Institutes of Health, the U.S. Navy, the Securities and Exchange Commission, the National Task Force of AIDS Drug Development, the Office of the Surgeon General, the U.S. Senate, Dade County and the states of Florida and New York.

NEWSPAPERS AND MAGAZINES

Much of the story of AIDS is covered exclusively by the gay press. I relied on the following periodicals: *The Advocate, QW, Out, 10 Percent,* the *New York Native, POZ* and the *Washington Blade.* In the mainstream press, the finest AIDS coverage has appeared in *New York Newsday,* thanks to the work of Laurie Garrett. The other newspapers I used regularly were the *Los Angeles Times,* the *San Francisco Chronicle,* the *San Francisco Examiner,* the *New York Times,* the *Wall Street Journal* and the *Chicago Tribune.* Also invaluable were the newsletters of a variety of organizations: Project Inform in San Francisco, the Gay Men's Health Crisis, AIDS Action Council, the Treatment Action Group, and the National Minority AIDS Council. John James's *AIDS Treatment* newsletter provides perhaps the best coverage of AIDS drug and research issues in the world.

REPORTS

Scores of private groups study AIDS from dozens of perspectives. For this book, I used the dozens produced by the following groups: Treatment Action Group, AIDS Action Council, National Minority AIDS Council, the American Foundation for AIDS Research, Center for Women Policy Studies, the Gay Men's Health Crisis, the San Francisco AIDS Foundation and the U.S. Conference of Mayors.

DATABASES

Two electronic databases gave me access to a great deal of information and community sentiment: Ben Gardiner's BBS and the AIDS Education Global Information System (AEGIS). Readers interested in an excellent Internet conference on AIDS should sign on to sci.med.aids.

VIDEOTAPES

James Wentzky of New York provides an invaluable service to the AIDS community and to history by videotaping nearly every significant AIDS activist event. His videotapes allow journalists who haven't attended events to report on them with accuracy. They are available from DIVA-TV in New York.

BOOKS

The bibliography of AIDS books is extensive. The works most often used for this book were: Peter Arno and Karyn Feiden, *Against the Odds,* 1992; Ronald Bayer, *Private Acts, Social Consequences,* 1989; Charles Caulfield, *The Anarchist AIDS Medical Formulary,* 1992; Gena Corea, *The Invisible Epidemic,* 1992; Elizabeth Fee and Daniel Fox, eds., *AIDS: The Making of a Chronic Disease,* 1992; Michael Fumento, *The Myth of Heterosexual AIDS,* 1990; Stephen Joseph, *Dragon Within the Gates,* 1992; Arthur Kahn, *AIDS: The Winter War,* 1993; Jonathon Kwitny, *Acceptable Risks,* 1992; Bruce Nussbaum, *Good Intentions,* 1990; Sandra Panem, *The AIDS Bureaucracy,* 1988; Robert Root-Bernstein, *Rethinking AIDS,* 1993; Renée Sabatier, *Blaming Others,* 1988; Randy Shilts, *And the Band Played On,* 1987.

NOTES

INTRODUCTION: MAD DOGS AND MEDICINE MEN

The author was a reporter at the *Miami Herald* from 1988 to 1992. In addition to my experiences, the section on AIDS reporting is based on interviews with the late Randy Shilts, Frank Bruni of the *Detroit Free Press,* Chris Bull of *The Advocate,* Gina Kolata of the *New York Times,* the late Robert Massa of the *Village Voice,* Hank Plante of WPIX-TV, Celia Farber of *Spin* and Joey Lovett. Stuart Byron's article appeared in *The Advocate* on July 17, 1990. Robert Massa's piece on Kolata ran in the *Village Voice* on May 8, 1990. The incident at the *Washington Blade* was covered in *OutWeek* magazine on August 22, 1990.

Information on Campbell's campaign contributions is on file in the Dade County (Florida) elections office and the zoning violations by the Club Body Center are on file in the building inspector's office there. The account of the interaction between the gay activists and Laitner is based on interviews with both parties. Laitner supplied the information on Janet Reno's request for the documents on the dispute, to be submitted as part of the record for her confirmation hearing.

The response of Martin Delaney to my piece on Fischl was contained in a letter to the publisher of the *Miami Herald,* as was the echoing of his remarks by the University of Miami.

The information questioning the accuracy of the HIV tests is from Eleni Papadopoulos-Eleopulos et al. in *Bio/Technology,* June 11, 1993, and Max Essex et al. in *Journal of Infectious Diseases,* February 1994.

1: POMP WITHOUT CIRCUMSTANCE

The events and nonevents in San Francisco were witnessed by the author. The letter from the Executive Director of San Francisco Mobilization Against AIDS, Paul Bonenerg, was written on June 20, 1990.

The material on Larry Kramer is based on my years observing his work; on my interview with him; his *Reports from the Holocaust* (1994), *The Normal Heart* (1985), *The Destiny of Me* (1993); his regular column in *The Advocate;* his speeches at the memorial services of Jeff Schmalz (December 7, 1993) and Vito Russo (January 1991); his letters, published and unpublished, to the *New York Times* and letters to Harold Ickes and Bob Hattoy; interviews with many members and former members of ACT UP New York about him; and interviews with Kramer published in *The Progressive,* June 1994, and *Playboy,* September 1993. See also Robert Wachter, *The Fragile Coalition* (1991).

The material on Dr. Gallo is for the most part based on my interview with him at his home, his *Virus Hunter* (1991) and, most important, the reporting of John Crewdson of the *Chicago Tribune.* Crewdson's definitive piece on Gallo ran on November 19, 1989. Follow-ups to that story have appeared regularly in the *Tribune* since then. For selected quotes and further information, see "Say It Ain't So, Dr. Science," *Spy,* July 1990; "By AIDS Obsessed," *GQ,* August 1991; Randy Shilts's *And the Band Played On* (1987). Much of the rest of this chapter is derived from the reports of the House Committee on Commerce and Energy and the inspector general of the Department of Health and Human Services.

2: EVIDENCE TO THE CONTRARY

Much of the material in this chapter first appeared in my "HIV. Not Guilty?" *Tropic* (the *Miami Herald*), December 23, 1990.

The opening scene was taken from transcripts and news reports from April 1984. The remark about Heckler's sore throat is from author's interview with Robert Gallo in Bethesda, September 1994. For a more complete discussion of Gallo's role in the discovery of HIV, see the chapter "Pomp Without Circumstance."

The most thorough ongoing reporting on HIV dissidents appears in the *New York Native* (Chuck Ortleb, editor). For examples of the writings of nonscientist AIDS dissidents, see Stephen Caiazza, *AIDS: One Doctor's Personal Struggle* (1990); Joan McKenna, "Unmasking AIDS: Chemical Immunosuppression and Sero-Negative Syphilis," in *Medical Hypotheses* 21, 1986; John Lauritsen, *Poison by Prescription* (1990); and *The AIDS War* (1993). There are scores of books postulating various AIDS conspiracies. See, for example, Thomas Bearden, *AIDS Biological Warfare* (1988); Paul Cameron, *Exposing the AIDS Scandal* (1988); Alan Cantwell, *AIDS and the Doctors of Death* (1988). Books, articles, tapes, videos and periodicals on alternative hypotheses are reviewed in Ian Young, *The AIDS Dissidents: An Annotated Bibliography* (1993).

The positions of the scientists who question the HIV hypothesis are covered thoroughly in two British documentaries, *The AIDS Catch,* which aired in London on June 13, 1990, and *AZT — Cause for Concern,* which aired on February 12, 1990, were produced by Meditel of London. The other most helpful source is the newsletter *Rethinking AIDS,* published by the Group for the Scientific Reappraisal of the HIV/AIDS Hypothesis.

All information on Dr. Duesberg is based on extensive interviews with him, Dr. Harvey Bialy of *Bio/Technology,* Celia Farber of *Spin,* as well as Dr. Duesberg's articles: "The Last Word: A Challenge to the AIDS Establishment," *Bio/Technology,* November 1987; "Retroviruses as Carcinogens and Pathogens," *Cancer Research,* March 1987; "Human Immunodeficiency Virus and Acquired Immunodeficiency Syndrome: Correlation but Not Causation," *Proceedings of the National Academy of Sciences,* February 1989; "HIV Is Not the Cause of AIDS," *Science,* July 29, 1988; and "Duesberg Replies," *Nature,* August 30, 1990.

The quote from Dr. Jonas is from an interview with him printed in "The Big Lie about AIDS," *Penthouse,* April 1994.

Sample references for the bulleted sections outlining dissident criticisms of the HIV hypothesis include R.J.G. Cuthbert, C. A. Ludlum, J. Tucker, et al., "Five-year prospective study of HIV infection in the Edinburgh haemophiliac cohort," *British Medical Journal* 301, 1990; for a discussion of the percentage of infected T cells, Werner Green, *Scientific American,* 1993. The research from the Tulane University team appeared in *Science,* July 1, 1994. The information on HIV infection in New York prostitutes is from J. Wallace, "Case presentation of AIDS in the United States," in *AIDS and Infections of Homosexual Men,* P. Ma and D. Armstrong, eds. (1989). The seronegativity of spouses of prominent HIV-infected individuals has been widely covered in the press. The study of New York City sperm donors was published by M. A. Chiasson, R. L. Stoneburner and S. C. Joseph, "Human immunodeficiency virus transmission through artificial insemination," *Journal of AIDS* 3, 1990. The study of mice with HIV antibodies is by T. A. Kion and G. W. Hoffmann, "An idiotypic network model of AIDS immunopathogenesis," *Proceedings of the National Academy of Sciences,* April 15, 1991. The fact that AIDS is not spreading beyond the original groups in which it first arose is clear from a careful reading of the *Morbidity and Mortality Weekly Report* of the Centers for Disease Control. Case reports on Kaposi's sarcoma and *Pneumocystis carinii* pneumonia in the absence of HIV have been reported in A. E. Friedman-Kein et al., "Kaposi's sarcoma in HIV-negative homo-sexual men," *Lancet,* 335, 1990, and J. L. Jacobs et al., "A cluster of *Pneumocystis carinii* pneumonia in adults without predisposing illnesses," *New England Journal of Medicine,* January 24, 1991. For a discussion of long-term survivors, see Lawrence Altman's overview of the topic in the *New York Times,* January 24, 1995. These and other anomalies are covered thoroughly by Robert Root-Bernstein in *Rethinking AIDS: The Tragic Cost of Premature Consensus* (1993).

The tenor of the debate has been discussed, bemoaned and created by both sides. Dr. Weiss's quote appeared in his article, written with Dr. Harold Jaffe, in *Nature,* June 21, 1990. The quote from Dr. Duesberg is printed in his book, *Why We Will Never Win the War Against AIDS.* The quotations of Dr. Charles Thomas are from his remarks delivered at the annual meeting of the Pacific division of the American Association for the Advancement of Science, San Francisco State University, June 1994, and from an interview with him by G. Null, "The Big Lie about AIDS," *Penthouse,* April 1994.

The mechanism by which HIV is believed to cause AIDS is still a matter of considerable controversy. The basis for the HIV hypothesis is contained in bits and pieces in hundreds of articles. The salient points are outlined clearly in W. Blattner, R. Gallo and H. Temin, "HIV causes AIDS," *Science* 242, 1988. See also R. A. Weiss and H. W. Jaffe's responses to Duesberg in *Nature,* June 21, August 30 and September 27, 1993. Variations on and refinements of their initial hypothesis appear on a regular basis in *Science* and *Nature.* A particularly helpful guide is *Science*'s special issue entitled "AIDS: The Unanswered Questions," May 28, 1993. For a good general discussion of the hypotheses, see *Newsday,* July 28, 1992, and June 15, 1993. These and other pieces by *Newsday* reporter Laurie Garrett are the clearest and most concise popular explanations of the continuing scientific discussion of the pathogenesis of AIDS.

For further information on Robert Koch, see T. D. Brock, *Robert Koch: A Life in Medicine and Bacteriology* (1988). For the relationship of Koch's postulates to viruses, see T. M. Rivers, "Viruses and Koch's Postulates," *Journal of Bacteriology,* 1937.

For the application of Koch's postulates to HIV, see Piatek et al., "High levels of HIV-1 in plasma during all stages of infection determined by competitive PCR," *Science,* 1993. The information on HIV-negative AIDS cases was provided by the Centers for Disease Control. The inapplicability of Koch's postulates is covered most thoroughly by R. A. Weiss and H. W. Jaffe, "HIV and AIDS," *Nature,* June 21, August 30 and September 27, 1990.

The section on Dr. Root-Bernstein is based on author's interview with him and his book, *Rethinking AIDS.*

Studies cited on the overburdened immune systems of members of the highest-risk groups for AIDS include A. J. Pinching et al., "Studies of cellular immunity in male homosexuals in London," *Lancet,* July 16, 1983; J. N. Weber et al., "Three-year prospective study of HLTV-III/LAV infection on homosexual men," *Lancet,* May 24, 1986; R. M. Donohoe and A. A. Falek, "Neuroimmunomodulation by opiates and other drugs of abuse," in Bridge et al., eds., *Aspects of AIDS* (1988); C. Bartholomew et al., "Transmission of HLTV-1 and HIV among homosexual men in Trinidad," *Journal of the American Medical Association,* May 15, 1987; M. B. Hultin et al., "Controlled prospective study of factor IX concentrate therapy and immunodeficiency," *American Journal of Hematology,* May 1989. The quote on the immune status of HIV-negative gay men in the London group is from L. A. Rogers et al., "IgD production and other lymphocyte functions in HIV infection," *Clinical Experimental Immunology,* January 1989. Dr. Aronson's quote is from R. M. Henig, "AIDS: A new disease's deadly odyssey," *New York Times Magazine,* February 6, 1983.

The section on Dr. Lo is based on the author's interviews with him. See also his "Mycoplasmal Agents," in *Policy Review* 54, 1990. The quotations from Dr. Tully and Dr. Fauci are based on the author's previously published interviews with them.

The section on Dr. Montagnier is based on author's attendance at the conference cited and his publications, especially "Inhibition de l'infectiosite de souches prototypes du Vih par ies anticorps diroges contre une sequence peptidique de mycoplasme," *Comptes Rendu Academie de Science Paris,* 311, 1990. For a review in English of Montagnier's work in this regard, see M. Balter, "Montagnier Pursues the Mycoplasma-AIDS Link," *Science,* January 18, 1991. The exchange between Montagnier and Dr. Levy was witnessed by the author. The quotation from Drotman was provided in an interview with the author for a prior publication.

The section on Dr. Sonnabend was based on the author's interviews with him. "How to Have Sex in an Epidemic" was a forty-eight-page booklet first published in May 1983, now out of print. Sonnabend's article on the causation of AIDS appeared in *AIDS Research,* vol. 1, No. 1.

Duesberg's travails are covered extensively in his book, coauthored with Bryan Ellison, *Why We Will Never Win the War on AIDS* (1994). The Maddox quote is from his article "Has Duesberg the Right of Reply?" *Nature,* May 13, 1993. The results of Duesberg's application for a grant renewal were confirmed in documents provided by Duesberg.

The attacks on Dr. Rubin were described by him in a telephone interview. Dr. Gallo's criticism of Root-Bernstein appears in his book *Virus Hunter* (1991). The information on Dr. Mullis was provided by him.

The quote from Haueter is from the author's interview with him in July 1994.

3: MAGIC BULLETS AND BOTTOM LINES

The information on the approval of AZT, ddI, ddC and d4T is based on the transcripts of the FDA's Anti-Infective Drugs Advisory Committee meetings on January 16, 1987; July 18, 1991; April 22, 1992; and May 20, 1994. The described benefits of these drugs is based on information presented by a special advisory panel to the National Institute of Allergy and Infectious Diseases during a three-day meeting, June 23–25, 1993.

The section on Dr. Fischl is based on reporting the author completed for her article "The Queen of AZT," in *Tropic,* the *Miami Herald,* September 23, 1990. The interviews with Dr. Fischl, Dr. Rubin, representatives of Burroughs Wellcome, Dr. Yarchon, Dr. Sonnabend, Dr. Fogel, Ms. Dodds and Dr. Magleby were all conducted for that article.

The best overview of the approval of AZT is available from the transcript of the FDA's Anti-Infective Drug Advisory Committee or in Bruce Nussbaum, *Good Intentions* (1990). My remarks on the early search for anti-AIDS drugs owes much to Peter Arno and Karyn Feiden, *Against the Odds* (1992), and to interviews with Drs. Broder and Yarchon.

The results of the first AZT trial were published by Fischl et al. in the *New England Journal of Medicine,* July 23, 1987. The information on the breaking of the blind in that trial is based on the FDA's Drug Advisory Committee transcript, interviews with Fischl and patients on the study as well as Nussbaum's book.

The tale of Drs. Darsee and Slutsky was reported by the *Washington Post,* April 24, 1988.

The conflict between Dr. Dickinson and Dr. Fischl was reported in the *Miami News,* October 1987.

The criticisms of the AIDS Clinical Trials Group for its overemphasis on the use of AZT was covered in the Institute of Medicine, *Report of a Workshop: The Potential Value of Research Consortia in the Development of Drugs and Vaccines Against HIV Infection and AIDS* (1989) and at the hearings of the House Subcommittee on Human Resources and Intergovernmental Relations, 100th Congress, 2nd session, April 28–29, 1988, on

"Therapeutic Drugs for AIDS." The insights of activists are from my interviews with them.

The analysis of conflict of interest in the case of Drs. Cantaken and Bluestone is culled from reports published in the *Washington Post,* June 13, 1989, and September 9, 1990. The information about the t-PA investigation was covered by the *Washington Post,* September 9, 1990. The *Post* has also published a number of excellent reports on the wider issue of conflict of interest among scientists. See particularly April 24, 1988; January 13, 1989; July 6, 1989; August 26, 1991; January 14, 1992.

The cases of Salahuddin and Sarin were widely covered in the press. Salahuddin was indicted for and pled guilty to accepting illegal gratuities. Sarin was found guilty of embezzlement and lying on an NIH disclosure form. See articles in the *Washington Post,* July 20, 1989; May 1, 1990; and January 4, 1991. The dispute over the proposed federal conflict-of-interest guidelines was thoroughly covered in those articles.

The disagreement within the AIDS Clinical Trials Group is based on interviews with Drs. Anthony Fauci, Charles van der Horst, Deborah Cotton, Harold Varmus, Dan Hoth and Margeret Fischl.

The information on studies leading to the approval of AZT for early intervention is based on reporting at the time by the *Wall Street Journal,* Nussbaum's *Good Intentions,* and Paul Volberding et al., "Zidovudine in asymptomatic human immunodeficiency virus infection," *New England Journal of Medicine,* April 5, 1990. The European skepticism was voiced in *Nature,* October 26, 1989, when the Concorde group decided to continue its AZT study. Details of the Veterans Administration study were presented on February 14, 1991, at a special meeting of the FDA's Anti-Viral Drug Advisory Committee. The discussion about the relationship between AZT and lymphoma is based on statements made at press conferences at the Sixth International Conference on AIDS, San Francisco, June 1990.

The documentation of the ACTG's emphasis on AZT is derived from their periodic reports. The budgets of various departments of the National Institutes of Health were provided by the agency's press office.

The section on FIAU is derived from interviews with Dr. Deborah Cotton and Dr. Charles van der Horst; a series of *Washington Post* articles by John Schwartz on July 8, September 7 and September 28, 1993; a *New York Times* article, November 16, 1993; transcripts of the FDA hearing on the drug, September 21, 1993; the FDA report on FIAU from November 15, 1993; and the results of animal tests published in the *Journal of Antimicrobial Agents and Chemotherapy,* March 1990.

The preliminary results of the Concorde trial were previewed in April

1993 in *Lancet*. The final results of the Concorde trial were published in *Lancet* 343, 1994. The additional American reaction was covered by the *Journal of NIH Research*, July 1993. The dispute in Berlin was witnessed by the author.

The critique of clinical trials design was covered by the *Journal of NIH Research*, July 1993; *Science*, June 10, 1994; and was widely discussed at the fifteenth annual meeting of the Society for Clinical Trials, in Houston, May 1993.

The Chow hypothesis was covered extensively in the press in February and March 1993. The scientific publication was in *Nature*, February 19, 1993. The findings were disavowed both in the popular press and in *Nature* in July 1993.

The section on Dr. Cotton is based on a lengthy interview with her and the transcripts of the approval hearings for ddI and ddC. The quotes in the section on basic research are from interviews with Greg Gonzalves and Dr. Anthony Fauci. Fields's article appeared in *Nature*, May 12, 1994. See also *Business Week*, October 24, 1994.

The Johns Hopkins study on Vitamin A and maternal transmission was presented at the meeting of the American Society for Microbiology on February 2, 1995, by Dr. Richard Semba. *AIDS Treatment News* discussed the findings in its January 6, 1995, issue.

The abrupt ending of the study of AZT in children was announced by the National Institute of Allergy and Infectious Diseases on February 13, 1995.

The new research on a viral cause of Kaposi's sarcoma was published by Yuan Chang and Patrick Moore in *Science*, December 16, 1994.

The section on Dr. Paul's new committee was covered in the *New York Times*, February 3, 1995.

The investigations of Resnick and Fischl were covered by the *Miami Herald* on February 3, 1995

4: RIDING THE AIDS GRAVY TRAIN

The bulleted advertisements appeared in *The Advocate*, October 18, 1994; *POZ*, April-May, 1994; and *POZ*, August-September, 1994.

The purported cures in the section on charlatans were reported in the *St. Petersburg Times*, May 14 and 17, 1994, and in the *Miami Herald*, April 26, 1987, October 8, 1989, and May 10, 1992; *TAGLine*, February 1995.

The consumer fraud attack on the health food industry is covered thoroughly in Stephen Barrett and William Jarvis, eds., *The Health Robbers* (1993). The action by the New York City government was covered by *Newsday,* June 25, 1993. The St. Louis study is cited in *The Health Robbers.* The International White Cross case information was culled from Federal Trade Commission documents obtained under the Freedom of Information Act. The quotation from Mr. Howard is from the *St. Petersburg Times,* May 17, 1994. The quote from Ms. Hollingsworth is from my interview with her published in the *Miami Herald,* October 8, 1989.

The information on Dr. Salk and Immune Response Corporation is based on the author's presence at his presentations and press conferences at the relevant international conferences on AIDS and on stories in *Newsday,* July 21, 1992; the *Wall Street Journal,* June 16, 1988; June 9 and September 29, 1989; June 13, June 21, August 26 and November 11, 1991; July 21 and August 11, 1992; May 26 and June 10, 1993; the *Los Angeles Times,* June 10, 1993; the *Philadelphia Inquirer,* June 10, 1993, and June 29, 1991. Redfield's report was published in the *New England Journal of Medicine,* June 13, 1991. The quote from Robert Massa was from my interview with him. Salk's vaccine trial results were published in *Science,* June 3, 1994. The quote from Brandt is from his article in the *Los Angeles Times,* July 15, 1990.

The most thorough coverage of Heimlich's involvement in AIDS was published in the *Los Angeles Times,* October 30, 1994. Further documents on his purported treatments were made available to the author by Dr. Stephen Barrett.

The section on Louise Hay is based on a series of interviews with past and current members of Healing Circles. For further information on Hay, see the *Los Angeles Times,* March 2 and December 30, 1988. See also Louise Hay, *You Can Heal Your Life* (1987) and *The AIDS Book* (1988). For information on Marianne Williamson see her *Woman's Worth* (1993) and *A Return to Love* (1992). The problems at Project Angel Food were covered in the *Los Angeles Times,* February 16, July 26 and September 27, 1992. I also interviewed a number of people with AIDS who attended Williamson's lectures.

The profitability of condoms is documented by the *Wall Street Journal,* November 4, 1985; February 23, 1987; July 6, 1988; and November 24, 1992; *Marketing News,* February 24, 1984; *Forbes,* November 4, 1985.

The information on pharmacies is culled from interviews with patients who used them. Community Prescription Service advertises regularly in *POZ.* For comparative pieces, see also the *Los Angeles Times,* November 21, 1993.

The participation of companies in AIDS fundraising is reported consistently in the gay press. The Clairol campaign was reported in *PRNewswire,* September 19, 1994. The dispute over the Bennetton ad was detailed in *NYQ,* February 16, 1992. The Nike ad began to air on television in March 1995. Ads for red ribbons regularly appear in gay periodicals.

Overpricing by home health care companies was investigated by New York City's Department of Consumer Affairs and detailed in its report "Making a Killing on AIDS," May 1991. The section on T2 Medical was derived from reports in the *Atlanta Constitution,* December 13, 1992, and August 27 and 29, 1994. See the *Chicago Tribune,* October 19, 1994, and the transcript of *Prime Time Live* for February 22, 1995, for information on Caremark and the Booth case.

The section on new companies serving people with and without AIDS is culled from the *Miami Herald,* August 16, 1991; March 15, 1992; and August 2, 1994.

Viatical companies have been the topic of considerable reporting. See the *Washington Post,* August 23, 1992, and October 9, 1994; and the *Los Angeles Times,* April 14, 1993, and May 22, 1994.

5: AIDS INC.

The conflict between the Campaign for Fairness and the Ryan White service providers from large cities was reported from interviews with Douglas Nelson and Mike Gifford, Tom Sheridan, James Guyton of Barney Frank's office, the late James Pruitt of Miami, Tim Palmer and Rich Stevens of Boston, Alexander Robinson of Washington, D.C.; Jerome Boyce of Detroit and Paul Feldman of Seattle. Nelson made available to me a packet of correspondence between his office and the other members of the Campaign for Fairness, between his office and members of the CAEAR Coalition and correspondence between the CAEAR Coalition and other groups from around the country.

The section on the origins of and lobbying for the Care Act are based on interviews with Jeff Levi and Tom Sheridan, Steve Morin of Nancy Pelosi's office, and Jane Silver of the American Foundation for AIDS Research.

The problems in Newark are based on reporting in the *Star-Ledger,* March 18, 19, 23, 25; April 9, 13, 14, 17, 19; May 2 and 7; June 8, July 28, August 12 and 15, December 24, 1993; and March 25, April 8, May 22, 1994.

For further information on the Houston problems, see the *Houston*

Post; July 22 and 24, August 5, 6 and 13, and November 18, 1992; January 1, April 16 and 17, and July 8, 1993.

The section on the conflicts in Washington, D.C., is based on reporting from the *Washington Times,* June 16 and 22, and July 10, 1993; and the *Washington Post,* July 7, 10, 16 and 29, August 25, September 2, 27 and 29, and November 29, 1993; and June 16, 23, 1994. The information was supplemented by interviews with Dr. Abdul-Alim Muhammad and Jane Silver.

Documents produced by the Health Resources and Services Administration were used extensively in the preparation of this section. However, that agency's virtual refusal to make documents available under the Freedom of Information Act precluded a more intensive investigation of the problems within the agency. More helpful were a series of reports prepared by Behavioral Science Research in Miami; "Lessons from the First Two Years," a background paper prepared for the AIDS Action Foundation by Roger Doughty in May 1993; and a series of reports on the Care Act prepared by the office of the inspector general of the Department of Health and Human Services in April 1994.

The section on San Francisco is based on that city's 1992 report, "People of Color and HIV/AIDS," and that city's evaluations of Care Act service providers. The situation was summarized in a series of articles by Lisa Krieger in the *San Francisco Examiner* beginning on November 15, 1992.

The problems in Dallas were reported in the *San Francisco Examiner* on September 15, 1993, and the difficulties in Philadelphia in the *Philadelphia Inquirer,* July 23 and December 8, 1993; and April 12, November 22 and 29, 1994, and March 22, 1995.

The problems in New York have been covered in depth in the gay press. See the *Philadelphia Gay News* and *The Advocate.*

The section on La Liga is based on interviews with Jim Pruitt and Rich Stevens. The section on the Cascade AIDS Project is culled from reports in the *Oregonian,* September 30, 1994.

The information on Rapoport and on the centralization attempts in Miami are from interviews with Rapoport, Doris Feinberg, John O'Hara, Jim Pruitt and Ernie Aguila.

The information on Sheridan's lobbying fees is from his filings with the U.S. Senate. The information on AIDSPAC is from reports filed with the Federal Election Commission. Sheridan's comment about his reason for establishing the Sheridan Group was printed in the newsletter of the Chronic Fatigue Association, for which he is also a lobbyist.

The section on Shepherd Smith is based on interviews with him and with a broad range of activists.

6: COLOR BIND

The controversy over Kemron was the subject of interviews with Dr. Jack Killen of NIAID, Lenny Kaplan of Fort Lauderdale and Dr. Abdul-Alim Muhammad. It was also reported in *Newsweek,* January 4, 1993; *Nature,* November 5, 1992; *Newsday,* August 17 and 20, 1990; December 20, 1991; April 28, 1992; June 3, 1993; the *Los Angeles Daily News,* October 4, 1992; the *Los Angeles Times,* October 28, 1990, and October 9, 1992; the *Washington Times,* November 23, 1990; July 15 and December 9, 1992; the *Boston Globe,* August 24, 1992; the *Journal of the National Medical Association,* April 1994.

The first study suggesting the benefits of Kemron was published by Dr. Koech in the *East Africa Medical Journal* and in the *Journal of Molecular Biotherapy* in 1990. Overviews of the research on the drug were printed in *Treatment Issues,* published by the Gay Men's Health Crisis, June 20, 1991, and May-June 1992. The efficacy of the drug was the topic of a study published in *Lancet,* May 2, 1992. NIAID also made available to me a variety of internal documents related to Kemron, especially the results of a study by their AIDS Research Advisory Committee, finalized in April 1992. The studies sponsored by the World Health Organization are available from their office in Geneva. Reports on Kemron were pulled also from the Inter Press Service in Africa and the *Capitol Spotlight,* September 1990.

The figures from the bulleted section are from *Newsday,* April 26 and October 4, 1987; March 24, 1989; and March 24, 1991; the *Philadelphia Daily News,* November 21, 1987; June 6, 1989; and January 25, 1991; the *Los Angeles Daily News,* September 8, 1989, and November 30, 1990; the *Bergen County Record,* October 2, 1991, and September 4, 1994.

The quotes from Joseph are from his book, *Dragon Within the Gates* (1992), or from his interview with me. The quote from Koop appeared in the *Washington Post,* April 21, 1987. The quote from Mayor Reeves appeared in the *New York Times,* February 20, 1995.

The African reaction to AIDS is surveyed in Renée Sabatier's *Blaming Others* (1988). The article in the *Ghanaian Times* appeared in October 1987. The comment from the Nigerian government was quoted in the *New York Times,* November 19, 1987. The reaction to speculation that AIDS first arose in Africa is from R. C. Chirmuuta and R. J. Chirmuuta, *AIDS, Africa and Racism* (1987).

The controversy over needle exchange was covered by Joseph in *Dragon Within the Gates*. See also the *New York Times,* November 7, 1988; the *Washington Times,* May 16, 1992; and the continuing coverage in the *Amsterdam News.*

For Dalton's analysis of the problem of AIDS in the African American community, see his "AIDS in Blackface," in Nancy McKenzie, ed., *The AIDS Reader* (1991).

The reporting on AIDS as a racist plot is taken from "The USSR's AIDS Disinformation Campaign," published by the U.S. Department of State, July 1987; *Social Change and Development* magazine, September 1986; and the *African Interpreter* (Lagos), October 1986.

The statistics on black life expectancy are from the *Bergen County Record,* March 16, 1989.

The section on the dinner held by the National Minority AIDS Council was based on author's observations.

7: VAGINAL POLITICS

A number of books have been written about women and AIDS. The most thorough is Gina Corea's *The Invisible Epidemic* (1992). Also worthwhile is *Women, AIDS and Activism* (1990), from ACT UP/New York's Women and AIDS book group. The most complete study of how women contract HIV was published in the *Journal of the American Medical Association,* August 10, 1994. Another survey of the impact of the epidemic on women appeared in *JAMA,* July 11, 1990. For the risk of infection among women with partners who inject drugs, see the *American Journal of Public Health,* August 1994. The first study documenting women's decreased survival time was published in the *Journal of Infectious Diseases,* June 19, 1992. A source of continuing information on women's issues is *Women Alive: A Quarterly Publication by and for Women Living with HIV/AIDS.* For information on female-specific AIDS-related ailments, see *Lancet,* October 1, 1994, and the *Journal of the American Academy of Dermatology,* September 1994.

Internal documents from the Women's Committee of ACT UP/NY were invaluable in the preparation of this chapter. Included in those papers were transcripts of numerous meetings those women held with senior government officials.

All statistics in this chapter are from the Centers for Disease Control.

The section on Katrina Haslip was based on interviews with McGovern and Corea, *The Invisible Epidemic.*

The section on McGovern is based on author's interviews with her and with Risa Denenberg. The controversy over the definition of AIDS is based on interviews with McGovern, as well as documents she made available to the author — most particularly a copy of her lawsuit.

The section dealing with women's access to experimental drugs is based on interviews with McGovern, transcripts of meetings of the National Task Force of AIDS Drug Development and documents made available to the author by McGovern. See particularly her citizen petition filed with the FDA on December 15, 1992.

The section on Dr. Kaplan is based on an article in *New York Newsday*, March 8, 1994. The comment from Singleton was made to the author prior to her death in 1992.

The pros and cons of contact tracing have been debated extensively by ethicists specializing in AIDS. See, in particular, the work of Dr. Ronald Bayer, especially his book *Private Acts, Social Consequences* (1991). The section on the contact-tracing controversy is based on interviews and on excellent articles on women and AIDS by Nina Bernstein in *Newsday*, February 2 and 3, 1993.

The Burling case was reported in *Newsday*, October 19, 1992. Marie Tulman was discussed in Corea, *The Invisible Epidemic*. The case of the woman who discovered her infection after her infant died was reported by Bernstein and the quote from the older Hispanic woman from the Bronx is also from *Newsday*, February 2, 1992.

For studies on the risks of woman-to-woman sexual transmission, see *Genitourinary Medicine*, June 1994, and *JAMA*, August 10, 1994. The comments of Dr. Francis are from my interview with him. The account of the meeting with Secretary Shalala is from a DIVA-TV videotape of the meeting.

8: THE IMMACULATE TRANSMISSION

The interviews conducted for this chapter were with Dr. Lionel Resnick of Miami Beach; Dr. Paul Arens, former medical director of the AIDS program of the state of Florida; George Bergalis, Allison Bergalis, Dr. William Roper, Dr. Sanford Kubin, Dr. Nancy Klimas and Shepherd Smith.

The case was thoroughly reviewed by *AIDS Alert* in its July 1991 issue, by *Lear's* in April 1994, and on *60 Minutes*, June 19, 1994. The best account of the case and the backgrounds of the infected individuals was written by Laurie Garrett for *Newsday*, August 18, 1991. An excellent profile of Barbara Webb appeared in the *Miami Herald*, January 30, 1994.

The information on the CDC investigation and the case in general came from that agency in scores of microfiches obtained under a Freedom of Information Act request. The CDC's conclusions in the case were published first on January 18, 1991, and then on May 15, 1992. Dr. Harold Jaffe of the CDC also delivered his version of those findings at the Seventh International Conference on AIDS in June 1991. The agency's investigation was reviewed by the General Accounting Office in a seven-month study the results of which were released in October 1992.

The argument over mandatory testing and the risk to patients posed by HIV-infected health care workers was well covered by David Zinman in *Newsday*, September 24, 1991. For Dr. Kuvin's position, see his piece in *Newsday*, July 19, 1991. See also *JAMA*, April 14, 1993, and the *New England Journal of Medicine*, September 19, 1991. The CDC published its own analysis of the risk in February 1991. The CDC's recommendations on HIV testing for health care workers appeared in its *Morbidity and Mortality Weekly Report* in July 1991. The suggestion that Acer infected his patients on purpose has been widely debated. For Dr. Horowitz's analysis, see *AIDS Patient Care*, August 31, 1994.

The molecular epidemiology of the case was reviewed in *Science*, May 22, 1992. That work was disputed by Dr. Ronald DeBry in *Nature*, February 1993.

The section on infant testing is based on interviews with Nettie Mayersohn and Teresa McGovern. See also *JAMA*, April 3, 1991, and *Lancet*, December 13, 1992. The columns referred to were written by Nat Hentoff in the *Washington Post* on April 9, July 5, July 30 and October 1, 1994. The other columnist who devoted considerable space to the controversy was Jim Dwyer of *Newsday*. His columns appeared on May 27, June 3, June 13, July 4 and September 21, 1994.

9: LIGHTS, CAMERA . . . DEATH

I first met Pedro Zamora in the summer of 1990 and told his story in the *Miami Herald* on November 4, 1990.

The story of his last days and his relationship with Sean Sasser is based on my observations and on interviews with Sean. Over the years I have also interviewed Pedro's father; his sister Milagros; Alex Escarano, his roommate in Miami and the individuals with whom he worked at Body Positive in Miami.

Invaluable in reconstructing Pedro's story were videotapes of his appearances on MTV's *Real World*.

The clash at his memorial service comes from interviews with Ivan Bernstein, Rose Anderson and Joel Rapoport.

10: PILL PUSHERS AND POLICY MAKERS

The account of the 1988 FDA demonstration is culled from a variety of media reports at the time. See also Douglas Crimp, *AIDS Demo Graphics* (1990).

The ganciclovir disaster is extremely well covered by Peter Arno and Karyn Feiden's *Against the Odds* (1992). See also the transcripts of the FDA Anti-Infective Drugs Advisory Committee meeting of October 26, 1987, and May 2, 1989.

The discussion of the approval of pentamadine is based on *Against the Odds* and the transcripts of the relevant FDA hearings.

The debate over the role of the FDA has been the topic of numerous research studies and analyses. Perhaps the most important are Ellen Flannery, "Should It Be Easier or Harder to Use Unapproved Drugs and Devices?," *Hastings Center Report,* February 1987; David Kessler, "The Regulation of Investigational Drugs," *New England Journal of Medicine* 320, 1989; Ruth Macklin and Gerald Friedland, "AIDS Research: The Ethics of Clinical Trials," *Law, Medicine & Healthcare* 14, 1986; transcripts of the Institute of Medicine, March 12, 1990, roundtable, "Expanding Access to Investigational Therapies"; and Milton Silverman and Philip Lee, *Pills, Profits and Politics* (1974).

The political argument over the role of the FDA has been well covered in the press. See, for example, the *Los Angeles Times,* February 16, 1992; *Forbes,* November 22 and December 20, 1993; the *Washington Post,* September 7, 1993. For Dan Quayle's position on the FDA, see his piece in the *Washington Post,* December 8, 1991.

The section on Martin Delaney owes much to Jonathon Kwitny, *Acceptable Risks* (1992). Delaney is well known for his attacks on newspaper reporters. This section is culled from interviews with Gina Kolata, Celia Farber, John Crewdson and the author's personal experience. Delaney's confrontations with other activists about drug approvals were the topic of the author's interviews with Jeff Levi, Dr. Ellen Cooper, Mark Harrington, Lynda Dee, Dr. Robert Gallo and Dr. Anthony Fauci.

The information on ddC is contained in transcripts of the April 21, 1992, hearing of the Anti-Viral Drug Advisory Committee. The information on the approval of d4T is based on transcripts of the meeting held on May 20, 1994.

The 1994 debate over accelerated approval is based on transcripts of the special meeting of the FDA Anti-Viral Drug Advisory Committee on September 12 and 13, 1994.

The section on Epitope is based on interviews with Al Ferro, president of Epitope; Shepherd Smith of Americans for a Sound AIDS Policy; FDA documents, especially the FDA advisory committee transcripts from December 1992 and June 1994. The discussions and correspondence between the FDA and activists over the approval of the saliva test kit were made available to the author by Shepherd Smith, as were the FDA's statements regarding leaks to Dan Dorfman.

The section on Johnson & Johnson's home test kit is based on interviews with Bruce Decker and Chris Bull; correspondence made available to the author by Mr. Smith; the transcript of CBS *This Morning* of June 23, 1994; the transcript of NBC's *Today* show, June 30, 1994; and transcripts of the advisory committee hearing in June 1994.

11: THE ENEMIES OF THE PEOPLE

The Henrik Ibsen play was first published in 1882.

The section on Joseph is based on my interview with him; his book, *Dragon Within the Gates* (1992); and interviews with members of ACT UP New York who organized the demonstrations against him. The quotations from prominent New York figures attacking him are from the *New York Daily News*, the *New York Post* or *Newsday*. The quotation from Dr. Francis is from the author's interview with him.

The sections on Jesse Helms are based on accounts of his career that have appeared in the *Charlotte Observer*, the *Raleigh News and Observer*, the Associated Press and the *Washington Post*.

The section on Shilts is from the author's interview with him.

Kraus was quoted by Ellen Goodman in the *Washington Post*, July 9, 1983.

The demands made of President Clinton were reported by the *New York Times* on December 10, 1992. The antics of ACT UP / Presidential Project and the speech of Aldyn McKean were witnessed by the author.

The dialogue on the computer bulletin board occurred on AEGIS in July and August 1994. The report card was reported by Reuters on August 8, 1994.

The section on the relapse from safe sex is based on a 1993 report from the San Francisco health department and L. Dean's presentation on rates of unprotected sex among young gay men in New York City is from the Ninth International Conference on AIDS.

The quote from Signorile is from his article in *Out,* October 1994.

The quotations from Kirp are drawn from his two-part article in *The Nation,* July 4 and 18, 1994.

The section on Callen is drawn from interviews with him.

The section on Silver is from Randy Shilts, *And the Band Played On.*

The discussion of the 1995 bathhouse controversy comes from an interview with Duncan Osborne, my attendance at community meetings on the topic, the Consensus Statement referred to and Amy Pagnozzi's reporting on the dispute for the *New York Daily News* in March 1995.

For information on the risk of HIV transmission through oral sex, see "The Safer Sex Knowledge Base," NIH Information BBS; *Lancet,* February 13, 1993; the account of Samuel's study in the *Village Voice,* November 6, 1990; *Positively Aware,* November 1993; and the Gay Men's Health Crisis's audiotapes of its 1994 conference on the risks of oral sex.

The quote from Steve Michael is from an author's interview with him. The Rotello article appeared in *Out.* The quotes from Barney Frank and James Guyton are from my interviews with them. The flier from the PWA Army was handed out at a meeting of the AIDS Clinical Trials Group, July 23–27, 1994, which I attended.

The story of what happened to Alan Cranston was covered by Randy Shilts in the *San Francisco Chronicle,* January 2, 1988. The information on the demonstration against Cuomo was from an interview with Michael Petrelis.

12: STRIKE A POSE

This chapter is based on seven years of the author's reporting on the epidemic, from international AIDS conferences, ACT UP meetings in seven cities, demonstrations, negotiating sessions and planning meetings. In addition, I interviewed the following activists specifically for this book: Robert Jones and Robin Haueter, former media coordinators for ACT UP/NY; Bob Lederer, James Baggett, George Carter, Risa Denenberg, Maxine Wolfe, Terry McGovern and Jim Fouratt of ACT UP/NY; Doug Nelson and Mike Gifford of the Milwaukee AIDS Project; James Scitaro of New York; Michael Ellner of HEAL; Lenny and Mary Kaplan of Fort Lauderdale; Billi Goldberg and Mike McIntee of ACT UP/San Francisco; Steve Michael of ACT UP/Washington, D.C.; Jerome Boyce of Detroit; Paul Feldman of ACT UP/Seattle; Joel Rapoport, Jon Cullipher and the late Jim Pruitt of Miami; Julie Davids of ACT UP/Philadelphia; Lynda Dee of AIDS Action, Baltimore; Peter Staley, Spencer Cox, Garance Franke-Ruta, Greg Gonsalves and Mark Harrington of the Treatment Action Group; Lisa Hernandez of Cincinnati; Jeff Levi, formerly of the AIDS Action Council; Jane Silver of the American Foundation for AIDS Research; Shepherd Smith of Americans for a Sound AIDS Policy; Larry Kramer; and John Fisher of Fort Lauderdale. Finally, I also interviewed the following scientists and policy makers about the activists: Congressman Barney Frank, Dr. Dan Hoth, Dr. Harold Varmus, Dr. Anthony Fauci, Dr. Deborah Cotton, Dr. Charles van der Horst and numerous congressional staffers.

The section on the San Francisco conference is based on the author's reporting of that meeting. Sections of this chapter appeared in the *Miami Herald* in June 1990.

All information on Doris Feinberg and her sons are based on author's interviews with Ms. Feinberg.

The section on Jon Greenberg is based on author's interviews with him, as well as with Robin Haueter, Risa Denenberg, James Baggett and Joy Episalla.

The section on Peter Staley is based on author's interviews with him and many other members of ACT UP/NY.

A comprehensive history of ACT UP has yet to be written, but the group's founding, early demonstrations and expertise in the use of graphics is well reported in Douglas Crimp, *AIDS Demo Graphics* (1990). The negotiations between scientists and activists around the San Francisco meeting have been chronicled by Robert Wachter in *The Fragile Coalition* (1991).

Staley's remarks at the meeting of the the National Task Force on AIDS Drug Development are from the transcript of that meeting.

David Feinberg's farewell remarks at the ACT UP meeting are available on videotape from DIVA-TV.

The author attended Greenberg's funeral.

INDEX

Aaron Diamond Institute, 51–52
Abundant Life Clinic, Washington, 150–51, 176–77
Acer, Dr. David, 216, 218–19, 220, 221, 222, 223, 224, 226, 227, 228, 229, 232–33, 234–35
Acquired immunodeficiency syndrome. *See* AIDS
ACTG. *See* AIDS Clinical Trial Group
ACT UP, 315–47; and ACTG, 334, 336, 338, 340–41; and Burroughs Wellcome, 328–29; and Catholic Church, 333; on Clinton, 301–2; committees of, 325–26; creation of, 37–40, 322; divisions and dissolution of chapters, 337–38; and FDA drug regulations, 263, 265–66; Frank on, 312; heterosexuals in, 337; Kramer and, 37–40, 42–43, 48, 321–22; lesbians in, 337; Los Angeles chapter, 317; Miami chapter, 4; and minorities, 325–26; New York chapter, 9, 318, 331–44; Presidential Project, 301; protests by, 323–25; San Francisco chapter, 154, 317–18, 337; and Sixth AIDS Conference, 316–18, 329–30; structure of, 325–26; style of, 315–16; Treatment Action Group (*see* Treat-

ment Action Group); Treatment and Data Committee, 325, 326, 327, 334, 335, 338, 340; women in, 203
Adams, Gregory, 188
Addicts Rehabilitation Center, Harlem, 183
adult T-cell leukemia virus (ATLV), 24
Advocate, The, 47, 284, 294, 307
Africa: AIDS in, 34, 192; Kenyan Medical Research Institute, 169; origin of AIDS in, 181–82
African Americans. *See* black community
African sleeping sickness, 258
Afrique Hope, 111
AIDS: in Africa, 34, 192; battle over congressional research funding, 298–300, 301; call to revamp research on (1994), 104; conflicts of interest in research, 89–90, 282; controversy over numbers of cases, 289–91; and culture of blame, 14–16; definition of, 71–76, 194; drug research and, 77–108 (*see also* drug research); epidemiology of, 57–59, 288–91 (*see also* epidemiology of HIV/AIDS); federal funding for, 15–16 (*see also individual programs*);

AIDS *(cont.)*
  funding for research on diseases related to, 95; gay liberation and, 14–15, 21, 294–95; as growth industry, 14, 109–40 *(see also* AIDS-related profiteering); Helms's campaign on, 293–94, 296–300, 305, 306, 307; HIV's relation to, 54–61, 55, 61–63, 63–76; in Miami, 1–5, 10–11; miracle cures, 128–32; need to shift research from drug trials to basic science, 105–6; official version of causation, 61–63; politics and, 292–314; public mood and, 303–5; quack treatments, 4, 111–15; from repeated insults to immune system, 66–67; reporting on, 4–14 *(see also* media; *specific journals and newspapers)*; service programs for patients with, 141–68 *(see also* service programs); in teenagers, 242–54; vaccine research, 115–25; without HIV infection, 59; in women *(see* women, AIDS in). *See also* human immunodeficiency virus (HIV) infection
AIDS Action Council, 143, 154, 159–60, 164, 166
AIDS and Racism conference, London (1987), 186
AIDS Arms Network of Dallas, 154–55
AIDS Clinical Trials Group (ACTG), 78, 90, 104; ACT UP and, 334, 336, 338, 340–41; under attack, 104; and AZT, 87, 90–91, 94, 95, 99, 101, 103–4, 105, 107; and combination therapy, 103; disclosure policy, 90–91; and ganciclovir, 258; and pentamidine, 104; and rush to approve drugs, 107; TAG and, 340–41
AIDS czar, 16

AIDS fundraisers, 13, 38, 134–35, 145
AIDS Inc. *See* service programs
AIDS Memorial Quilt, 255
AIDS Negative Health Care Professionals, 138
AIDS Network, 27
AIDSPAC. *See* American AIDS Political Action Committee
AIDS Project Los Angeles, 147
AIDS-related profiteering, 109–40; from AZT, 83, 92, 110; entrepreneurs, 132–40; fraud and scandals in service programs, 152–58; home health care companies, 135–38; miracle cures, 128–32; pharmacies, 134; quackery, 4, 111–15
AIDS-related virus (ARV), 31
AIDS Research Advisory Committee (NIH), 175
AIDS Resource Center of Wisconsin, 141
AIDS service organizations. *See* service programs
AIDS Task Force, Philadelphia, 155
AIDSthink, 17
AIDS Walk, Washington, 150
Akhter, Dr. Mohammed, 176–77
Alacer Corporation, 112–13
Albert Lasker Prize, 20
Allegra, Dr. Joseph, 137
alpha-interferon, 169–70, 171–78
Alternative Gallery, Kent, Conn., 135
alternative medicine: ACT UP and, 327; for AIDS, 94–95; and AIDS-related quackery, 111–15. *See also* miracles
Amarillo Cell Culture, 171, 172, 173
American AIDS Political Action Committee (AIDSPAC), 159
American Association of Physicians for Human Rights, 311
American Dental Association, 226
American Enterprise Institute, 275

American Foundation for AIDS Research, 38, 72, 134, 135, 154, 265
American Medical Association: and alternative medicine, 112; and controversy over doctor-patient HIV transmission, 220, 226
American Physicians for Human Rights, 25
American Preferred Prescription, 134
Americans for a Sound AIDS Policy, 42, 165, 167, 230, 284
Americans with Disabilities Act, 301
ampligen, 275
Amsterdam: Eighth International Conference on AIDS (1992), 119–20
Amsterdam News, 172, 183–84
anal fissures, 66
anal intercourse, 10, 15, 306
And the Band Played On (Shilts): movie adaptation, 51
Anonymous Queers, 135
Ansell Corporation, 133
antibiotic abuse, 67
antiviral research, 80–2. *See also* drug research; *specific drugs*
APP Community Pharmacy, New York, 134
Aragon, Regina, 162
arap Moi, Daniel, 170
Arieff, Dr. Allen, 98
Aronson, Dr. David, 68
Art Against AIDS Gala, 13
Ashe, Arthur, 58, 135
Ashe, Jeanne Marie, 58
Astra Pharmaceutical, 334–35
AZT, 80, 81–87, 92–95, 97, 98–100, 101, 102–3, 106, 107, 170, 257, 275, 336, 342; ACTG and, 87, 90–91, 94, 95, 99, 101, 103–4, 105, 107; anemia from, 82–83; for children, 87, 107; combination therapy, 87, 94, 103, 338; Concorde trial, 99–100, 101; early intervention with, 99; hepatotoxicity of, 98; and lymphomas, 93–94; marketing of, 92; phase II study, 82; placebo tests, 83, 84, 85, 86, 92, 93; for pregnant women, 87, 107, 202–3; profits from, 83, 92, 110, 328, 329, 337; research on, 79, 81–87, 92–95, 97, 98–100, 101, 102–3, 106, 107; and surrogate markers, 101; toxicity of, 3, 82–83, 85–86, 93–94, 95, 98, 337; VA research on, 93

bacterial infections: in AIDS, 62
bacteriology, 63
Bactrim, 73, 110, 134, 257
Baltimore, Dr. David, 22–23, 108, 339
Barnes, Mark, 226
Barr, David, 231, 271
Barrio, Dr. Sergio Pérez, 127
Barry, Marion, 150
bars: revival of sex in, 308–10
bathhouses. *See* gay bathhouses
Bauer, Gary, 38
Bayh, Birch, 50
Bayview Hunters Point Foundation/American Indian AIDS Institute, 152–53
Benetton, 135
Bergalis, Allison, 221
Bergalis, Anna, 215–16
Bergalis, George, 215–16, 231
Bergalis, Kimberly, 215–25, 227–29, 230–32, 233, 234, 235, 236–37, 241, 299
Berkowitz, Richard, 308
Berlin: Ninth International Conference on AIDS (1993), 101–2, 103, 121–22, 301
Bernstein, Ivan, 254
beta-blockers, 262
Biden, Joseph, 146
Bihari, Dr. Bernard, 172

biomedical research. *See* drug companies; drug research

biotechnology: profit-making in, 110; small companies vs. pharmaceutical giants, 276; and viral-load testing, 106

bisexuality: and AIDS, 7; and AIDS epidemiology, 290; and AIDS in women, 3, 208–10; among Hispanics, 3

black community: ACT UP and, 326; AIDS activists in, 188–90, 326; and AIDS conspiracy theories, 114, 176, 181–82, 186–87; AIDS in, 13, 169–90; breakdowns in, 188; confrontations with gay activists, 185–86, 303; decline of safe sex among young, 306; denial by leaders of, 180–81; health and lifespan in, 188; homophobia in, 13; increase of AIDS in (1987–1993), 178–80; and Kemron (alpha-interferon) therapy, 170–77; and needle exchange programs, 182–84; social conservatism of, 185; struggle for control of AIDS federal funding, 148–50, 157; suspicion of white suggestions on AIDS, 184–85, 204–5

black gays, 169, 180, 182, 188–89

Black Leadership Commission on AIDS, 180

Blacks Educating Blacks about Sexual Health Issues, Philadelphia, 174

black women, 179–80, 191, 204–5

blame, culture of: and AIDS, 14–16

blood transfusions: and immune status, 67; infections from, 67

blood transmission of HIV, 54–55, 58

Bloody Marys, 332, 345–46. *See also* Marys

Bluestone, Dr. Charles, 88–89

Body Positive, Miami, 3–4, 157, 244, 246, 249, 250, 319, 326, 330

Bolognesi, Dr. Dani, 74, 123

Booth, Michael Alan, 137–38

Boston AIDS Consortium, 163–64

Brandt, Dr. Allan, 125

breast cancer, 212

Brecher, John, 4–5

Bristol-Myers Squibb, 268

Britton, Dr. Carolyn, 241

Broadway Cares–Equity Fights AIDS, 135

Broder, Dr. Samuel, 50, 80–82, 86

Brook, Dr. Itzhak, 83, 84

Bross, Daniel T., 301

Brown, Rev. Clemson, 171

Browning, Frank, 8

Bruni, Frank, 7

Bryant, Anita, 2

Bull, Chris, 284

Burling, Catherine, 208

Burroughs Wellcome, 80, 81, 82–83, 87–88, 91–92, 94, 98, 257, 274, 328, 339; ACT UP and, 328–29; AZT profits, 83, 92, 110, 328, 329. *See also* AZT

Burton, Dan, 231

Bush, Barbara, 231

Bush, George, 15, 39, 135, 167, 231, 256, 259, 267, 307, 319, 332

butyl nitrite: and AIDS, 55, 67

Byrd, Gary, 171, 172, 173, 175

CAEAR (Cities Advocating Emergency AIDS Relief), 143, 158–60, 162–65

Caiazza, Dr. Stephen, 55

Callen, Michael, 72, 308

Cambridge University, 95

Campaign for Fairness, 144, 164

Campbell, John "Jack," 11

cancer: retroviruses and, 22–23

Cantekin, Dr. Erdem, 88, 89

Care Act, 141–43, 145–47, 155–56, 158–65, 335; passage of, 145–47;

per capita formula sought for funding, 161–64; renewal of, 142, 143, 158–65; Title I, 142–43, 155, 158–65; Title II, 142–43, 164

Caremark International, 137–38

Carson, Joanne, 126, 127

Carter, Dr. Steven, 338

Carter-Wallace Corporation, 133

Cascade AIDS Project, Portland, 155

Castro, Clemente, 140

Castro, Fidel, 246, 247

Catholic Charities: AIDS housing program (San Francisco), 153

Catholic church: response to AIDS, 13, 39, 118, 288, 333, 344

Caulfield, Charles, 152

CBS, 250–51

CDC. See Centers for Disease Control

CD4 cell counts, 105; as test for drug effectiveness, 100–101, 271, 272. See also T cells

cellular immunity: vaccines and, 120

Celluloid Closet, The (Russo), 39

Center for Living: Los Angeles, 130; New York, 131

Centers for Disease Control (CDC), 25, 26, 28, 47; and controversy over doctor-patient HIV transmission, 219–20, 221, 223, 225–30, 232–36; defining AIDS in women, 191, 192–93, 194–95, 214; funding of, 293; Helms and, 297; and HIV discovery conflict, 40–41; and HIV's relation to AIDS, 60; and mandatory testing for HIV, 239; and pentamidine, 258–59; predictions on AIDS epidemiology, 57, 65; and testing of health care workers for HIV, 225–30, 232–36

cervical cancer, 195, 197

Cheng, Yung-Chi, 97, 98

Chermann, Jean-Claude, 31

Chicago: AIDS resource funding in, 161–62

Chicago Tribune, 19, 41, 44, 46

chi chong therapy, 112

Childers, Michael, 131

children and infants: AZT for, 87, 107, 202; HIV testing of, 237–41

Chinchilla, Miguel, 345

Chirac, Jacques, 36

chlamydia: among gays, 66

Chow, Yung-Kang, 103–4

Christian, Marc, 58

Christian Right: and AIDS, 8, 292

chronic fatigue syndrome, 55

Church of Religious Science, 128–29

Ciesielski, Dr. Carol, 219

CIGNA Dental Health of Florida, 224, 228

Citizens for a Sound Economy, 275

Clairol, 134

Clark, Hilton, 288

Clerici, Dr. Mario, 120

Clinton, Bill, 15, 47, 201, 244, 300–302, 305, 312, 313, 339

Clinton, Hillary, 233

closeted gays, 25

Club Body Center, Miami, 10–11

Coffin, Dr. John, 54

Cohen, Richard, 151

Colgate-Palmolive: and HIV vaccine research, 117

combination drug therapy, 87, 94, 103, 338

commercialization of caring, 135. See also AIDS-related profiteering

Community Prescription Service, 134

Competitive Enterprise Institute, 274

Competitiveness Council, 263. See also Quayle, Dan

Compound Q, 9

Concorde trial: on AZT, 99–100, 101; on CD4 cell increases and survival, 272 condoms, 132–33, 308; black opposition to, 184; controversy over distribution of, 287, 288, 293; decline in use of, 305–6

Confide, 279–80, 284

confidentiality laws, 207–8, 209; and HIV testing of newborns, 237–38; and partner notification, 206–7, 209–10

conflicts of interest: in AIDS research, 89–90, 264, 282; federal regulation of, 90–91; kickbacks, 110, 136–38; in scientific research, 88–89, 90–92

Congress: Bergalis testimony before, 230–31; elections of 1994, 164–65, 274, 284; and FDA, 260–61; and politics of AIDS, 293–307

Conlin, Kelli, 239, 288

conservatives: and AIDS policy, 167, 205; and deregulation, 263, 274–75

conspiracy theories on AIDS, 60, 114; among blacks, 141, 176, 181–82, 186–87; among gay men, 114, 295

Consumer Health Education Council, 112

contact tracing. See partner notification

Cook, Terrence Cardinal, 27

Cooper, Dr. Ellen, 83–84, 266–67, 268, 269, 273, 274

Cooper, Dr. Lou Z., 240

Copmann, Tom, 271

Corey, Dr. Lawrence, 97

Cosmopolitan, 324

Costa Rica, 111

Cotton, Dr. Deborah, 104–7

Course in Miracles, A (Williamson), 129–30

Cox, Spencer, 272

Cranston, Alan, 314

Crew Club, Washington, D.C., 309

Crewdson, John, 41–42, 50, 51, 264

Critical Path, 174

Cuban Americans: AIDS in Miami, 1–5, 8, 10–11, 246–49. See also Hispanics

Culliton, Barbara, 50

Cuomo, Mario, 240, 314

CURAS, 152

Curran, Dr. James, 27, 72

cytomegalovirus: among gay men, 66; foscavir for, 334–35; ganciclovir for, 256–58; from transfusions, 67

Dallas: AIDS service programs in, 154–55

Dalton, Harlon, 184

Dannemeyer, William, 230, 231, 307

Darsee, Dr. John, 86

Darwin, Charles, 75

Davis, Ed, 301

ddC: approval of, 79, 270–71; combination therapy, 338; toxicity of, 95, 98, 337

ddI: approval of, 79, 106; combination therapy, 103, 338; toxicity of, 95, 98, 337; for women, 197

Dear, Noach, 288

DeBry, Dr. Ronald, 234, 235

Decker, Bruce, 281, 282, 283

Delaney, Martin, 9, 12, 42, 264–74, 276

delayed-type hypersensitivity, 120

DeLeon, Dennis, 309

dentists: controversy over transmission of HIV to patients, 215–41

Destiny of Me, The (Kramer), 47

Detroit: AIDS resource funding in, 161–62

Detroit Free Press, 7

Devine Design auction, 132

Deyton, Dr. Lawrence, 178

d4T: approval of, 79, 272; toxicity of, 95

Dickinson, Dr. Gordon, 86–87

dilevalol, 270

Diller, Barry, 130
Dingell, John, 41, 45, 46, 50
Dinkins, David, 207, 291
Direct Access Diagnostics, 280–81
di Sautel, Rhonda, 139
disease causation, Koch's postulates on, 63–64
District of Columbia. See Washington, D.C.
DNA: testing to match viruses, 220–21, 232, 234
doctors. See health care workers; physicians
Dole, Robert, 230
domestic partnership laws, 304
donations: for AIDS, 134–35; AIDSPAC, 159. See also fundraising for AIDS
Dorfman, Dan, 278
double-blind testing, 85, 86
Dragon Within the Gates (Joseph), 289
Driskill, Richard, 223, 229, 235
Drotman, Peter, 71
drug abuse: among gays, 13, 66; immune suppression and, 67
drug addicts, IV: AIDS among, 3; black, 180, 181–82, 183; HIV infection among, 54, 58; in Miami, 3; needle exchange programs, 15, 181–84, 287–88; women partners, 208, 212
drug benefits/side effects in HIV/AIDS, 79
drug companies: and accelerated approval, 269–72, 274; and alpha-interferon, 171–72; and conflicts of interest in research, 89–91, 282; and deregulation, 259, 275; and funding of research, 88, 89–90, 94, 95; gay activists and, 334–35, 336; profit motivation of, 77–108, 256, 262–63; profits from AIDS, 111;

TAG and, 341. See also specific companies
drug prices: home health care profiteering, 137–38; pharmacies and, 134
drug regulation controversy, 255–85; FDA and, 259–62 (see also Food and Drug Administration)
drug research, 77–108, 255–85; accelerated approval campaign, 261, 265, 267–74; on alpha-interferon, 171–72; AZT monopolizes at expense of other drugs, 94; conflicts of interest in, 88–89, 282; FDA and, 255–85; federal funding for, 79, 88; and funding for basic science, 105–6; gay activists and, 325; profit motive in, 77–108; rush to release drugs, 106–7; small vs. large companies, 276–84; surrogate markers, 100–101; for women with AIDS, 197–200, 202–4. See also specific drugs
drug tests: ACTG and, 87 (see also AIDS Clinical Trial Group); for AZT, 82–7 (see also AZT); costs of, 77–78; double-blind, 85, 86; gay activist demand for trials and, 9, 106; on women, 199–200, 202–4. See also drug research
drug therapy: alpha-interferon (Kemron), 170–77; AZT (see AZT); combination, 87, 94, 103, 338; ganciclovir, 256–58; pentamidine, 73, 110, 258; for women with AIDS, 197–98
Duesberg, Dr. Peter, 56–57, 59, 60, 64, 71, 72, 73–74

East African Medical Journal, 170
Eclipse Enterprises, 135
Economu, Nikki, 217, 218, 228
Eighth International Conference on AIDS (Amsterdam, 1992), 119–20

Elders, Dr. Jocelyn, 188, 189
Eli Lilly, 97, 99
ELISA, 13
Elizabeth, Mary, 301
Ellis, Dr. Alonzo, 176
E-mergen-C, 112–13
Enemy of the People, The (Ibsen), 286, 292
entrepreneurial profit-making from AIDS, 132–40
Ephron, Nora, 322
epidemiology of HIV/AIDS, 57, 289–91; among blacks, 178–80; controversy over numbers, 289–91; incubation/latency, 65–66; in women, 192, 211, 239
Epitope, 276–79, 284
Epstein-Barr virus, 67
equine encephalitis treatment, 111, 115
Escarano, Alex, 253
Essex, Dr. Max, 28, 50, 123
"Etiology of AIDS, The" (Sonnabend), 73

Fabrégas, Tómas, 154
Faggots (Kramer), 20, 21
Family AIDS Network, 282
Farrakhan, Louis, 175, 182
Fauci, Dr. Anthony, 38, 47, 52, 70, 73, 92, 105, 107, 121, 123, 126, 171, 268, 329, 334, 338
FBI, 138
FDA. *See* Food and Drug Administration
federal funding for AIDS, 15–16, 298–99, 301, 304; Care Act, 141–43, 145–47, 155–56, 158–65 (*see also* Care Act); under Clinton, 301, 302; competition among AIDS agencies for, 147–68; for drug research, 79, 88; service programs, 141–68, 300, 301 (*see also* service programs; *indi-*

vidual programs); treatment research, 94–95 (*see also* drug research). *See also individual programs*
federal government: and AIDS conspiracy theories, 114; gay activists and, 312–14 (*see also* gay activists)
Federal Trade Commission: and investigation of kickbacks, 137
Feinberg, David, 327, 342–44
Feinberg, Doris, 319, 322, 326–27, 330–31, 344–45
Feinberg, Jeffrey, 319
Feinberg, Lenny, 319
Feingold, Russ, 160, 163
feminists: and AIDS activism, 205
fialuridine (FIAU), 95–98, 107
Fields, Dr. Bernard, 104, 339
Fifth International Conference on AIDS (Montreal, 1989), 117, 288, 329
Fire Island, New York, 21–22
Fischl, Dr. Margaret, 3, 12, 79–80, 82–83, 86–88, 91–93, 99, 102–3, 108; and Burroughs Wellcome, 91–92; and combination drug therapy, 101–2; commitment to AZT therapy, 102; and conflicts of interest in research, 91; under investigation, 108; training and early career of, 79–80
Fisher, John, 316
Fisher, Mark, 332–33
Fisher, Mary, 244–45, 281, 282, 289
Fleiss, Joseph, 272
Fleming, Patsy, 253, 265
Fleming, Thomas, 102
Florence: Seventh International Conference on AIDS (1991), 12, 118
Florida: AIDS quackery in, 111–12. *See also* Miami
Focus on the Family (TV), 167
Food, Drug and Cosmetic Act, 260–61

Food and Drug Administration (FDA), 25, 255–85; and accelerated drug approval, 106–7, 265–74; and AIDS in women, 193, 199–204; and alternative medicine, 112, 115; Anti-Infective Drugs Advisory Committee, 83; Anti-Viral Drug Advisory Committee, 104, 106, 270, 273; and AZT testing, 82, 83–84, 85, 90, 91, 97, 98–99; and conflicts of interest in research, 90; conservative attack on, 274–75; creation of, 260; and drug release, 37, 59, 259–63; and drug research, 77–78, 255–85; evolution of, 260–62; gay activists and, 106, 255–56, 264–74, 322, 324, 335–36; and HIV vaccine research, 117, 121, 122; and home test kit for HIV, 279–84; Kramer's attack on, 37, 38; and saliva test for HIV, 277–79; and toxicity of AZT, 98–99

Fortensky, Larry, 130

foscavir, 334–35

Foster, Wendell, 288

Fouratt, Jim, 336–37

Fourth International Conference on AIDS (Stockholm, 1988), 116

Four Title Coalition, 143, 159–60, 162, 164, 165

Fradd, Brandon, 121, 122

Franc, Mike, 230

Francis, Dr. Don, 27, 28, 31, 40–41, 51, 212, 292

Frank, Barney, 312, 313–14

Frankel, Max, 38

fraud: entrepreneurial, 132; medical (see quackery); miracle cures (see miracle cures); and profiteering (see AIDS-related profiteering); scientific (see scientific fraud)

Free Congress Foundation, 284

Freeman, Donna, 106

Freiman, Joel, 98

French scientists: and identification of HIV, 19, 28–32, 34–36, 45, 46, 54

freon enemas, 112

Friends in Deed, 131

fundraising for AIDS, 13, 38, 134–35, 145

funeral business, 139

Funk, Roland, 10

Futurebiotics, 113

Galileo, 68, 74

Gallagher, Robert, 23

Gallo, Dr. Robert, 19, 22–24, 28–32, 34–36, 40–42, 44–47, 49–52, 53, 56, 61, 67, 71, 73, 74, 81, 89, 116, 214, 264, 307; conflict over HIV discovery, 28–32, 34–36; early career of, 20, 22–24; investigated for fraud, 40–42, 44–47; Kramer and, 42–44, 52; scandals at lab of, 89; supporters and detractors of, 49–52; *The Virus Hunter,* 44, 74

Gallo, Mary Jane, 42, 49

ganciclovir, 256–58

gay activists: ACT UP (see ACT UP); appointed to HHS positions, 302; confrontations with black community, 185–86, 303; and decline of safe sex, 306–8; diversity among groups, 318–19; and drug research, 78 (see also drug research); and FDA, 106, 255–56; Frank on, 312; GMHC (see Gay Men's Health Crisis); lesbian, 204, 210–14; and media coverage of AIDS, 6–14; and need to redirect AIDS research (1994), 104–5; opposition to partner notification, 206; and politics of AIDS, 292–314; and traditional politics, 312–14. See also *individual activists and organizations*

Gay and Lesbian Activist Alliance, Washington, 148–50
Gay and Lesbian Prevention Activists, New York, 309–10
gay bathhouses: activist defense of, 10–11, 308; Kramer's attack on, 25, 33; in Miami, 10; renewed call for closure of, 308–10; and spread of infectious disease, 66–67
gay bowel syndrome, 66
gay community: advances of, 304–5 (see also gay liberation); attacks on media coverage of AIDS, 6–14; conspiracy theories on AIDS, 114; and creation of service industry for AIDS, 145–7 (see also service programs); decline in safe sex practices, 7–8, 305–11; and denial of AIDS, 14–15, 21–22; and planning councils for AIDS federal funds, 147; and service programs for AIDS, 141–68; and struggle for control of AIDS federal funds, 147–68. See also gay activists; gays; lesbians; individual communities
gay liberation, 14–15, 294–95
Gay Men's Health Crisis (GMHC), 166, 296–97; growth of, 26, 27, 147; Kramer and, 25, 33, 36–37, 39; scandals at, 155; women and, 208
gay physicians: and AIDS, 3
gay press: gay activists and, 6–10. See also specific journals
Gay Pride Day, New York (1983), 27
gay pride rallies: AIDS and, 212
gay reporters: pressures on, 6–8
gays: black, 169, 180, 182, 188–89; discrimination against, 304–5; Helms's campaign against, 293–94, 296–300, 305, 306, 307; in the military, 300; numbers of, 290; resurgence of unsafe sex among, 7–8, 305–11; STDs among, 66–67; violent crimes against, 305. See also gay activists; gay community
gay teens: AIDS in, 242–54
Geffen, David, 129, 130
Gendin, Stephen, 134
germ causation of disease, 63–64
Getty, Estelle, 127
Ghanian Times, 182
Ghia, Alex, 139
Gifford, Mike, 144, 158, 160, 161, 165
Gingrich, Newt, 167, 185, 274
Glavin, James, 119
Glick, Marion, 177
Global Black Experience, The, 171
GMHC. See Gay Men's Health Crisis
gonorrhea: and AIDS, 56, 66; among gays, 66
Gonsalves, Greg, 104–5
Gore, Al, 301
Gould, Steven, 256
Graham, Reverend Billy, 298
Grand Fury, 324
Gray, Bob, 42
Gray, C. Boyden, 266–67
Greenberg, Jon, 319–20, 322–23, 327, 330, 331–32, 345–47
Greentree, Dr. Leonard, 126
Griffith-Sandiford, Jean, 174
Group for the Scientific Reappraisal of the HIV/AIDS Hypothesis, 60
Gunderson, Steve, 19
Guyton, James, 313

Hadley, Dr. Suzanne, 45
Haiti: AIDS quackery in, 111
Haitian Americans: AIDS among, 2, 3, 28
Halberstam, Jean, 131
Hanks, Tom, 304
hantavirus, 60
Hardie, Dr. John, 233

Haring, Keith, 315, 325
Harrington, Mark, 17, 269, 270, 274, 339–40
Harris, Rod, 138
Harvey, Jim, 148, 177
Haseltine, Dr. William, 12
Haslip, Katrina, 191, 195, 196
Hassett, Dr. Joseph, 173
Hatch, Orrin, 146, 159
Hatunen, Dave, 310
Haueter, Robin, 76
Hay, Louise, 128–29
Hayashibara Biochemical Laboratories, 172
Hay House, 129
Hayrides, 128–29
Health and Human Services, Department of: Clinton appoints gays to positions at, 302; and definition of AIDS in women, 196
health care workers: controversy over transmission of HIV to patients, 215–41, 299–300; HIV-infected, 226, 300; HIV testing of, 138, 225–32. See also physicians
Health Crisis Network, Miami, 157
health food stores, 112–13
health insurance industry, 25; and billing for drugs, 134
Health Policy and Research Foundation, 281
Health Resources and Services Administration: and Care Act funds, 147–48, 152
Healy, Dr. Bernardine, 45
Heal Your Body (Hay), 129
Heckler, Margaret, 46, 50, 53, 57, 73; and discovery of HIV, 53–54
Heimlich, Dr. Henry, 125–27
Helms, Jesse, 6, 11, 15, 164, 230, 292, 293–94, 296–300, 305, 306, 307
hemophiliacs: AIDS among, 7, 54;

HIV-negative after exposure, 58; immune suppression among, 67–68
Henle, Friedrich Gustav Jacob, 63
hepatitis, 56, 65, 224; and AIDS, 66; FIAU for, 95–98; among gays, 66; testing for, 287; from transfusions, 67
Heritage Foundation, 167, 168
herpes virus: and AIDS, 55, 56, 66
Herzog, Doug, 250
heterosexuals: in ACT UP, 337; AIDS among, 4, 7, 208–9, 289; indifference to AIDS epidemic, 15. See also women
High Five Club, 138
High-Risk Pregnancy Clinic, 239
Hilts, Phil, 43
Hirsch, Dr. Charles, 207
Hirsch, Dr. Martin, 89–90, 103–4
Hispanics: and ACT UP, 326; and AIDS in Miami, 1–5, 8, 10–11, 246–49; bisexuality among, 3; CURAS (San Francisco), 152
HIV. See Human immunodeficiency virus
HL-23 virus, 23–24
Ho, Dr. David, 13, 51
Hockney, David, 130, 325
Hodel, Derek, 172
Hoffmann–La Roche, 197–99, 271
Hogan, Carleton, 272
Hollingsworth, Dotty, 115
Hollingsworth, Michael, 115
home health care industry, 110, 135–38
homeless: AIDS among, 3; in Miami, 3
home test kit for HIV, 279–84
homophobia: in black community, 13, 181, 182; and media coverage of AIDS, 5; of Nation of Islam, 150
homosexuality. See gays; lesbians
Hoofnagle, Dr. Jay, 95–96

Hopland Band of Pomo Indians, 113–14
Horowitz, Dr. Jerome, 81
Horowitz, Dr. Leonard, 233
Hoth, Dr. Daniel, 120, 338
housing programs for AIDS patients: ACT UP and, 325; Shanti Project, 153
Houston, 147
Howard, Tom, 115
"How to Have Sex in an Epidemic" (Sonnabend), 72
Hudson, Rock, 4, 58, 135
human immunodeficiency virus (HIV), 16–17; in Africa, 181–82; antibodies to, 68–70, 71; conspiracy theories on spread of, 141, 176, 181–82, 186–87; controversies over role in AIDS, 54–76; DNA testing to match, 220–21, 232, 234; false positives, 13; funding for research on, 95; Gallo investigated about his research on, 40–42, 44–47; home testing kit, 110; identification of, 19, 28–32, 34–36, 45, 46, 53–54; incidence of doctor-patient transmission, 227; incubation time, 65–66; infection with (see human immunodeficiency virus [HIV] infection); Koch's postulates and, 64; mandatory testing controversy, 223, 224, 225–32; need to redirect research on, 104–5; positive conversion to negative, 58; relation to AIDS, 54–61, 63–76, 104; relative virulence of, 59; royalties on test patent, 45; skeptics of relation to AIDS, 55–61, 63–76; supporters of relation to AIDS, 61–63, 71–72; tests for, 13–14, 166, 276–84 (see also testing for HIV); transmission of, 12, 54–55; vaccine research, 41, 53–54, 115–25; viral-load testing, 105–6

human immunodeficiency virus (HIV) infection: AIDS vs. (defining conditions), 194; controversies over, 57–59; controversy over numbers, 289–91; defining conditions in women, 191–205 (see also women, AIDS in); epidemiology of, 57 (see also epidemiology of HIV/AIDS); funding for research on diseases related to, 95; in health care workers, 226; latency, 65–66; in lesbians, 211; lifespan with, 57; New York registry plan, 288–89; official version of, 61–63; oral sex and, 311–12; partner notification (see partner notification); responsibility of infected vs. uninfected, 307–8; "right to know" controversy, 236–41; U.S. ban on foreigners with, 302. See also AIDS
human leukemia virus, 19, 23
Human Rights Campaign Fund, 38
human T-cell leukemia virus (HTLV), 24, 28–32, 34–36; HTLV-3, 28–32, 34–36, 41, 44, 47
Hunter, Nan, 302
hyperbaric therapy, 112

Ibsen, Henrik, 286, 292
ICN, 275, 284
Illinois mandatory testing program for marriage applicants, 239
immigrants: AIDS among, 4, 166, 302
Immune+ PLUS, 113
Immune Response Corporation, 116, 117–18, 119, 121–22, 124; stock value, 119, 121–22, 124. See also Salk, Dr. Jonas
immune system: AIDS from repeated insults to, 66–67, 73; fraudulent therapy offers, 112–13; HIV attack on, 61–63; of HIV negatives and positives, 67

Immunetech Pharmaceuticals, 118
Immunex, 174, 176–77
Immunizer Pak Program, 113
immunology: funding for research in, 94–95
ImmunoViron, 177
incubation period of HIV, 65–66
infusion therapy, 136–37
Innovative Therapeutics Ltd., 172
Inside Edition, 112
Institute for Justice, 285
Institute of Medicine: and ACTG, 87
interferon, 169–70, 171–78
International AIDS Society, 87
International Conference on AIDS: Fourth (Stockholm, 1988), 116; Fifth (Montreal, 1989), 117, 288, 329; Sixth (San Francisco, 1990), 8, 12, 19, 39, 54, 70–71, 80, 316–19, 329–30, 335; Seventh (Florence, 1991), 12, 118; Eighth (Amsterdam, 1992), 119–20; Ninth (Berlin, 1993), 101–2, 103, 121–22, 301; Tenth (Tokyo, 1994), 104, 301–2
International White Cross, 113, 114
IntraCare, 137
Irene (AIDS patient), 196–97
Irving, Amy, 127
Iskowitz, Michael, 159

Jackson, Jean, 317
Jackson, Jesse, 182
Jaffe, Dr. Harold, 59, 233–34
Japanese scientists: and retrovirology, 24, 28
Jauregg, Julian Wagner von, 126
Johnson, Earleatha, 58
Johnson, Earvin "Magic," 58, 62, 119, 133, 135
Johnson, Sherry, 235
Jonas, Dr. Steven, 57
Jones, Grace, 325
Jordan, Dr. Wilbert, 173, 176

Joseph, Dr. Stephen, 180, 183–84, 286–92
Journal of Tropical Medicine, 69
Justice, Dr. Barbara, 171, 173, 175–76

Kaplan, Dr. Gilla, 204
Kaposi's sarcoma, 195, 219; fraudulent cure promises, 111, 170; in HIV negative people, 59, 68; viral source of, 55, 107–8
Karpas, Dr. Alexander, 40
Kassebaum, Nancy, 165, 188
Katabira, E. T., 178
Katz, Melinda, 238
Kaul, Dr. Aditya, 239–40
Kawata, Paul, 188
Kefauver, Estes, 261
Kelly, John, 347
Kelly, Sharon Pratt, 150, 151
Kemri News, 171
Kemron, 170–77
Kennedy, John F., 303
Kennedy, Ted, 144, 146, 159, 160, 165, 188, 230, 340
Kenya: AIDS treatment research in, 169–70
Kenyan Medical Research Institute, 169
Kessler, Dr. David, 98–99, 200, 201, 203, 214, 269, 270, 274, 283
kickbacks: in AIDS-related practice, 110, 136–38. *See also* conflicts of interest
Kimberly Bergalis Patient and Health Providers' Protection Act, 230
Kinsey report, 290
Kirp, David, 307
kissing: and HIV transmission, 12
Koch, Ed, 25, 26, 27, 33, 34, 39, 183–84, 289
Koch, Robert, 63–64, 69
Koech, Dr. Davey, 169–70, 171–72, 173, 176

Kohl, Herb, 160
Kolata, Gina, 8–10, 12
Koop, Dr. C. Everett, 133, 180–81, 240, 281–82, 284
Kramer, Larry, 19–22, 24–28, 32–34, 36–40, 42–44, 47–49, 52, 114, 316, 326–27, 334; and ACT UP, 37–40, 42–43, 48, 321–22; *The Destiny of Me,* 47; early activism of, 25–26; early career of, 20, 21–22; finds a lover, 49; and Gallo, 42–44, 52; and GMHC, 25, 33, 36–37; *The Normal Heart,* 33–34, 36, 48; notoriety and access to media, 38–39, 47–49; *Reports from the Holocaust,* 326
Kraus, Bill, 295
Krim, Dr. Mathilde, 38, 72
Kuanda, Kenneth, 329
Kuromuya, Kiyoshi, 174
Kuvin, Dr. Sanford, 224, 227, 230

La Liga Contra SIDA, Dade County, 155
Lancet, The, 100, 311
LaRouche, Lyndon, 55
Latino Commission on AIDS, 309
Lauritsen, John, 55
Lee, Dr. Phil, 201, 338
Lehrer, Jim, 331
Leibovitz, Annie, 243, 325
Lemon, Dr. Stanley, 84
Leonard, Karen, 139
lesbians: in ACT UP, 337; AIDS activists, 204, 210–14; AIDS in, 211; in government, 304; physicians, 3, 210
Levi, Jeff, 265, 267
Levine, Dr. Alexandra, 122–23
Levy, Dr. Jay, 31, 71
Lewis, Sinclair, 260
life insurance: viaticals, 139–40
LifeStyle Urns, 139
Link, Derek, 272

Living Benefits, 139–40
Lo, Dr. Shyh-Ching, 68–70, 71, 72
London: AIDS and Racism conference (1987), 186
Loren, Sophia, 4
Los Angeles: AIDS Project, 147; AIDS service funding in, 163; gay bathhouses in, 309
Los Angeles Times: coverage of AIDS, 5, 294
Lucey, Mary, 213–14
Ludington, Pierre, 153–54
Lyme disease, 127
lymphadenopathy-associated virus (LAV), 29–32, 34, 41, 47
lymph nodes, 61–62
lymphoma: AZT therapy and, 93–94
Lymphomed, 258, 259
Lynch, Catherine, 208

MacNeil, Robert, 331
MacNeil/Lehrer NewsHour, 331
Maddox, John, 73
Mahoney, Roger Cardinal, 118
malaria-induction therapy: for AIDS, 125–27
mandatory testing for HIV, 166; for health care workers, 223, 224, 226–32; for marriage, 239; of newborns, 237–41
Mankiewicz, Frank, 50
Many Feathers, R. Morgan, 131
March of Dimes, 303–4
March on Washington for Lesbian and Gay Rights (1987), 323
Marys, 331–32, 345–46
Massa, Robert, 9, 124
Massachusetts General Hospital, Boston, 103
Maximum Immune Support, 113
Mayersohn, Nettie, 237–41
McGovern, Terry, 192–93, 194, 195–205, 210, 213

McGuire, Jean, 143, 158
McKean, Aldyn, 301
McKenna, Joan, 55
McQueen, Steve, 111, 128
media: and AIDS in black community, 186; gay images in, 304; reporting on AIDS, 4–14, 25. *See also individual newspapers*
Medicare: and home health care industry, 137
medications. *See* drug research
Medley, Raan, 326
Medoff, Dr. Gerald, 175
Meier, Dr. Paul, 271
Mellor, William, III, 285
Memorial Sloan-Kettering Hospital, New York, 324
Merck, 275
Mercy Hospital, Miami, 244
Merkatz, Ruth, 201
Mexican clinics, 111
Miami: ACT UP in, 4, 344–45; AIDS in, 1–5, 8, 10–11, 242–50, 330–31, 344–45; AIDS service program scandals in, 155, 156; antidiscrimination laws in, 2; Body Positive in, 3–4, 157, 244, 249, 250, 319, 326, 330; Club Body Center, 10–11; gay bathhouses and clubs in, 10–11, 309; Little Haiti, 2–3; local news coverage of AIDS, 4–5, 7, 8; Pedro Zamora's celebrity, 242–54; People with AIDS Coalition, 4, 10; revival of South Beach, 1–2; service programs for AIDS in, 142; sex clubs in, 3–4, 157, 244, 246, 249, 250, 309
Miami, University of, 11
Miami Herald: reporting on AIDS, 4–5, 7–8, 10, 11–12, 108, 249
Michael, Steve, 312
Michaelides, Dr. K. Mike, 137
microsporidiosis, 95

Midler, Bette, 130
Milk, Harvey, 294
Millenson, Elliot, 279–80, 284
Miller Brewing Company, 6
Milloy, Courtland, 151
Milwaukee: AIDS resources in, 141–44, 161, 163
Minnesota AIDS Project, 161
minority groups: ACT UP and, 325–26; conflicts with gays in Washington, 150–51; and federal funding for AIDS, 151; services in San Francisco, 152–53. *See also* blacks; Hispanics
Minsky, Leonard, 89
Minuto, Maurice, 111
miracles: and AIDS, 128–32
Mobilization Against AIDS, 154
Molecular Pharmacology, 97
Montagnier, Dr. Luc: and discovery of HIV, 28–32, 34–35, 36, 47; and HIV relation to AIDS, 57, 70–71, 75
Montgomery, Robert, 221–22, 224–25, 227, 228, 229, 230, 236–37
Montreal: Fifth International Conference on AIDS (1989), 117, 288, 329
Moore, Bruce, 345
Moses, Hamilton, III, 225
movies: gay images in, 304
Moynihan, Daniel Patrick, 25
MTV, 244, 245, 250–54
Muhammed, Dr. Abdul-Alim, 150, 175
Mullis, Dr. Kary, 56, 75
Murray, Laura, 241
mycoplasma: and HIV/AIDS, 69–71
Myers, Dr. Maureen, 341

National Abortion Rights Action League (NARAL), 239, 240
National Academy of Sciences: and investigation of Gallo, 41

National AIDS Awareness Catalog, 135

National AIDS Clearinghouse, 145

National AIDS Information Center, 110

National Alliance of Gay and Lesbian Health Clinics, 283, 284

National Association of People with AIDS, 167–68, 284

National Cancer Institute, 19, 22, 25, 53; AIDS task force, 29–32, 80–82

National Empowerment Television, 284

National Foundation on Infectious Diseases, 227

National Institute of Allergy and Infectious Diseases (NIAID), 69, 177, 178, 272; Community Program for Clinical Research on AIDS, 178. *See also* AIDS Clinical Trials Group; Fauci, Dr. Anthony

National Institutes of Health (NIH): ACT UP and, 329; AIDS symposium (1984), 34–35; and demands of gay activists, 9, 38, 264; and drug testing in women, 202; and funding for research, 88–89, 94–95; funding of, 293; and HIV relation to AIDS, 60; and investigation of Gallo, 41, 44–47; and Kemron, 175; Office of AIDS Research (*see* Office of AIDS Research); Office of Research Integrity, 41, 46; and racist charges, 175–76; regulating conflicts of interest in research, 88–89. *See also* AIDS Research Advisory Committee

National Insurance Marketing, 140

National Lesbian and Gay Task Force, 265

National Medical Association, 177

National Minority AIDS Council: "Our Place at the Table," 188–89

National Organization for Women (NOW), 240

National Public Radio: coverage of AIDS, 8, 73

National Task Force on AIDS Drug Development, 104, 338–39

National Task Force on AIDS Prevention, 151

Nation of Islam, 185; and Abundant Life Clinic, Washington, 150–51; and Kemron, 174, 175, 176

Native Americans: and AIDS-related quackery, 113–14; Bayview Hunters Point Foundation/American Indian AIDS Institute, 152–53

Native Americans AIDS conference, Tulsa (1990), 114

Natural Organics, 113

Nature, 34, 45, 73

needle exchange programs, 15, 287–88, 289, 293, 325; black community's response to, 182–84; in New York City, 182–83, 287–88, 289

Nelson, Doug, 141–44, 158–65

Nevirapine, 103

Newark: HIV Health Services Planning Council, 147; incidence of AIDS in, 148; struggle for control of AIDS federal funds in, 147–48

newborns: AZT for, 202; HIV testing of, 237–41

New England Journal of Medicine, 25, 30, 82, 85, 118

New Orleans, 147

Newsweek, 41

New York: Empire State Pride Committee, 314

New York City: ACT UP in, 9, 318, 324, 327–28, 341–44; AIDS in, 286–91, 341–44, 345–47; controversy over distribution of condoms, 287, 288; Department of Consumer Affairs, 137; gay bathhouses in, 10, 309; Kramer's advocacy in, 25–27; laws on deceptive advertising, 113; needle exchange program, 182–83, 287–88, 289; numbers of gay men in, 290–91; service programs for AIDS in, 141, 142, 161, 163

New York Daily News, 287–88

New York Native, 21, 26, 35–36, 55, 171

New York Newsday: coverage of AIDS, 5, 38, 180

New York State AIDS conference (1993), 48

New York Times: coverage of AIDS/HIV, 5, 8–10, 25, 36, 38, 42, 43, 103, 169, 235, 294, 321, 324

Ng'weno, Hilary, 169

NIAID. *See* National Institute of Allergy and Infectious Diseases

Nichols, Mike, 131

NIH. *See* National Institutes of Health

Nike, 135

Ninth International Conference on AIDS (Berlin, 1993), 101–2, 103, 121–22, 301

Nixon, Richard, 22

Nobel Prize, 20, 23, 36, 42, 55–56, 63, 75, 95

Noble, Gary, 284

Normal Heart, The (Kramer), 33–34, 36, 48

nucleoside analogues: toxicity of, 95–99

nutritional supplements, 112

Obel, A. O., 170

O'Connor, Joseph Cardinal, 39, 118, 288, 333, 344

Office of AIDS Research, NIH, 15–16, 105, 108, 272, 331, 338–42; TAG and, 339–41

Office of Alternative Medicine (NIH), 94

O'Neal, Cynthia, 130–31

oral sex: in bathhouses, 10; controversy over safety of, 10–11, 311–12

OraSure, 110, 275, 276–79, 283, 284

Ortleb, Chuck, 55

Osborne, Duncan, 310

Oscar Wilde Bookstore, New York, 21

Ostreicher, Dr. Paul, 198

Out, 307

OutWeek, 40

Owens, Reverend D. Lee, 184

oxygen therapy, 112

Palmer, Tim, 151, 163–64

Panetta, Leon, 283

papilloma virus, 66

Paras, Melinda, 153

Parsons, Edward, 233

partner notification, 166, 205–10, 287, 288–89, 292; opposition to, 206

Pasteur, Louis, 115

Pasteur Institute, Paris, 28–32, 35, 46–47, 54

Pataki, George, 237, 240, 314

Paul, Dr. William, 105, 108

Pedrazo, Jairo, 345–46

pelvic inflammatory disease, 194, 195, 196

pentamidine, 73, 110, 258; profits from, 110

People with AIDS Coalition, 4, 10, 135, 157, 265

People with AIDS Health Group, 172

Perkins, Anthony, 129, 130

Perkins, Berry, 130

Peter Claver Community, 153

Petrelis, Michael, 314, 316

pharmaceutical companies. *See* drug companies

Pharmaceutical Manufacturers Association, 271

pharmacies: and profits from AIDS, 134

Phelps, Reverend Fred, 245, 253

Philadelphia: AIDS service programs in, 155; Blacks Educating Blacks about Sexual Health Issues, 174

Philadelphia (film), 48, 304

physicians: AIDS practice, 110; black, 174; controversy over HIV transmission to patients, 215–41, 299–300; and home health care industry, 136–38; referrals for AIDS patients, 110

Pittsburgh Children's Hospital, 88–89

placebo tests: and AZT, 83, 84, 85, 86, 92, 93; and HIV vaccine, 120–21

planning councils: and Care Act funds, 147–48

Pneumocystis carinii pneumonia, 195, 216, 219; in HIV negative people, 59, 68; prophylaxis and treatment, 110, 134, 258

polio: public response to, 303–4; vaccines, 116–17, 118–19, 124–25

political action committees: AIDSPAC, 159

politics: and AIDS, 292–314; gays in, 304–5, 312, 313–14

poppers: and AIDS, 55, 67

Portland: Cascade AIDS Project, 155

POZ, 110, 139, 244, 281, 283, 308

pregnant women: AZT for, 87, 107, 202–3, 240; HIV negative offspring of, 202–3; HIV screening for, 167, 237–41

Presidential AIDS Commission, 38

President's Task Force on Regulatory Relief, 259

priests: gay, 13

Prim, Dr. Beny, 180

Pringle-Smith, Rebecca, 274

Priority Pharmacy, San Diego, 134

profiteering. *See* AIDS-related profiteering

Progress and Freedom Foundation, 274

progressive multifocal leukoencephalopathy (PML), 251; funding for research on, 95

Project Angel Food, 130

Project Inform, San Francisco, 173–74, 175, 263, 264. *See also* Delaney, Martin

prostitutes, 58; HIV infection among, 58

Pruitt, Jim, 345

public mood: and response to AIDS, 303–5

quackery: and AIDS treatment, 4, 111–15; miracle cures, 128–32

Quayle, Dan, 256, 263, 269, 332

racism: and AIDS among Haitian Americans, 3; and AIDS conspiracy theories, 114, 176; and approaches to AIDS, 174–75. *See also* black community

Radical Faeries, 345–46

Rainbow Curriculum, 291

Ramseier, Gordon, 118

Rapoport, Joel, 156–57, 245–46

Rauschenberg, Robert, 13, 325

Ray, Donald, 114

Reagan, Nancy, 297

Reagan, Ronald, 11, 14, 15, 25, 27, 36, 38, 39, 135, 240, 255, 297, 303, 307, 323, 337

Real World (MTV), 244, 245, 250–54

Redfield, Dr. Robert, 42, 118, 230; and vaccine research, 118

Red Ribbon Foundation, 135

Reeves, Kenneth, 181

Reno, Janet, 11, 233

Reports from the Holocaust (Kramer), 326

Republican party: and AIDS policy, 167–68; blacks and, 185; and deregulation, 256, 263, 269, 274–75, 276; gays in, 316. *See also* Bush, George; conservatives; Helms; Reagan, Ronald

Resnick, Dr. Lionel, 108, 234, 235

Rethinking AIDS: The Tragic Cost of Premature Consensus (Root-Bernstein), 66

reticulose, 111

retrovirology, 20, 22–24, 28–32, 74; and identification of HIV, 28–32, 34–36; retroviruses in humans, 56

Return to Love, A (Williamson), 130

reverse transcriptase, 23, 24

ribavirin, 275

Richards, Dr. Alan, 171

Richman, Dr. Douglas, 9, 82, 97

Rickman, Herb, 26

Risk (bar), Miami, 309

Robinson, Alexander, 151

Rodriguez, Freddie, 309

Root-Bernstein, Dr. Robert, 65–66, 68, 74–75

Rosenman, Howard, 131

Ros-Lehtinen, Ileana, 245

Rotello, Gabriel, 312

Rous, Francis Peyton, 22

Rubenstein, Hal, 249

Rubin, Dr. Harry, 75

Rubin, Dr. Robert, 80, 102, 103

Russo, Vito, 39, 255

Ryan, Caitlin, 150, 151

Ryan White Comprehensive AIDS Resources Emergency Act. *See* Care Act

Sabin, Dr. Albert, 118–19, 124–25

Sackett, Dr. David, 102

Safer Sex Comix, 296–97

safe sex: controversy over, 305–12; decline in, 7–8, 13, 305–11; Helms and, 296–97; Kramer's campaign for, 25; Sonnabend on, 72–73; surgeon general's campaign for, 133; teaching, 15. *See also* unsafe sex

St. Louis: AIDS resource funding in, 162

St. Louis encephalitis, 223

St. Mary's Hospital, London, 67

Salahuddin, Firoza, 89

Salahuddin, Syed Zaki, 89

saliva: and HIV transmission, 12

saliva test for HIV, 276–84

Salk, Dr. Jonas, 36; and HIV vaccine research, 115–25

salt water infusions, 112, 115

Samuel, Michael, 311

San Diego: Priority Pharmacy, 134

Sandiford, Cedric, 171, 172–73, 174

San Francisco: gay bathhouses in, 10; gay liberation in, 294–95, 304; gay population in, 290; HIV blood samples from 1970s, 65–66; misuse of AIDS federal funds in, 152–54; Mobilization Against AIDS, 20; Project Inform, 173–74, 175; service programs for AIDS in, 141, 142, 151, 152–54, 161, 163; Sixth International Conference on AIDS (1990), 8, 12, 19, 39, 54, 70–71, 80, 316–19, 329–30, 335

San Francisco AIDS Foundation, 154, 160–61

San Francisco Chronicle, 5

Sarandon, Susan, 325

Sarin, Prem, 89

Sasser, Sean, 242–43, 250–52, 253

Saturday Evening Post, 38

Sawyer, Eric, 325

Schmid Laboratories, 133

Schram, Dr. Neil, 271

Schulte, Steve, 131–32

Schwartz, Maxime, 46

Schwarz, Dr. M. Roy, 220
Science, 29, 35, 93
scientific fraud: fabrication of data, 86; Gallo investigated for, 40–42, 44–47
scientific research: conflicts of interest in, 88–89
Search Alliance, 173
Seligman, Dr. Maxime, 100
semen transmission of HIV, 55, 58; in oral sex, 311
Senate: and AIDS, 297–98. *See also* Congress; Helms, Jesse
Septra, 257
service programs, 141–68; competition for federal funds, 148–58; fragmentation and duplication in, 156–58; funding under Care Act, 141–43, 145–47, 155, 158–65 (*see also* Care Act); infighting among, 3–4; number of (1992), 145; resistance to centralization of, 157; salaries of directors, 154. *See also individual programs*
Seventh International Conference on AIDS (Florence, 1991), 12, 118
sex clubs: revival of, 308–10
sexual abstinence: among blacks, 185; for teens, 300
sexually transmitted diseases (STDs): among gays, 66–67
sexual promiscuity: and contact tracing, 206–7; and spread of infectious disease, 66–67. *See also* gay bathhouses
Shalala, Donna, 8, 48, 213–14
Shanti Project, San Francisco, 153
Shearer, Dr. Gene, 120
Sheridan, Tom, 159–63, 164, 168
Sheridan Group, 159
Shilts, Randy, 40, 51, 253; attacks on, 6, 295
Shoemaker, Lisa, 229, 235

Shriver, Mike, 154
Signorile, Michelangelo, 305–6, 310
Silver, Carol Ruth, 308
Silver, Sheldon, 241
Simon, Mark J., 119, 122
Simpson, Carole, 189
Singleton, Sonia, 3, 204–5, 345
Sissifag, Luke, 313
Sisters of Perpetual Indulgence, 318
Sixth International Conference on AIDS (San Francisco, 1990), 8, 12, 19, 39, 54, 70–71, 80, 316–19, 335; ACT UP and, 39–40, 316–17, 329–30
Slutsky, Dr. Robert, 86
Smart, Theo, 312
Smith, Anita, 165–66, 167
Smith, Shepherd, 42, 165–68, 230
Snow, Daniel, 256
Social Security Administration: and AIDS in women, 192, 193, 196
Sondheim, Stephen, 131
Sonnabend, Dr. Joseph, 30, 56, 66, 72–73, 75, 92; and AZT research, 84–85, 86
Sowell, Joe, 140
Spiegel, Dr. Robert, 171
spousal notification. *See* partner notification
Stadtlanders, 134
Stahl, Lesley, 296
Staley, Peter, 320–21, 323, 327–29, 330, 333–35, 338–39, 340, 341
Steinhart, Dr. Corklin, 245
steroid abuse, 67
Stockholm: Fourth International Conference on AIDS (1988), 116
stock market: ACT UP demonstrations at, 324, 327–28; and AIDS-related investments, 110, 119, 121, 122
Stoddard, Tom, 209–10

Stop AIDS Now or Else, 154
Straus, Dr. Stephen, 257
Streep, Meryl, 130
Streisand, Barbra, 48–49
Strub, Sean, 110, 139, 281, 282, 283, 284, 285, 333
sulfonamide, 260
Sullivan, Louis, 90, 92, 175, 192, 196, 330
support groups, 128–32. *See also specific agencies*
suramin, 265
surrogate markers: for drug effectiveness, 100–101, 267–68, 271; and HIV vaccine, 121; viral-load testing, 105–6
swine flu, 60
Syntex Corporation, 256–58
syphilis: and AIDS, 55, 56, 66; among gays, 66; testing for, 287; Tuskegee experiment, 175

TAG. *See* Treatment Action Group
Tate, Larry, 174, 175
tat inhibitors, 197
Taylor, Elizabeth, 13, 135, 154
T cells: of hemophiliacs, 67–68; HIV infection of, 58. *See also* CD4 cell count
television: gay images in, 304. *See also* MTV
Temin, Dr. Howard, 22–23
Tenth International Conference on AIDS (Tokyo, 1994), 104, 301–2
testing for HIV, 13–14, 166; home test kit, 279–84; requiring (*see* mandatory testing for HIV); saliva, 276–84
thalidomide, 198, 204, 261, 262
Thomas, Dr. Charles, 60
Tiffany's, 135
Tijuana clinics, 111
Timpone, Sallie, 127

tissue plasminogen activator (t-PA), 89
TITA, 335
Tokyo: Tenth International Conference on AIDS (1994), 104, 301–2
Tolver, Keith, 150
Tony Brown's Journal (TV), 180
Toomey, Dr. Kathleen, 209, 210
Toon, Dr. Phyllis, 236
Treatment Action Group (TAG), 48, 105, 272–74, 334, 339–42
T2 Medical, Atlanta, 136–37
tuberculosis: testing for, 287
Tully, Dr. Joseph, 70
Tulman, Marie, 208
Tuskegee experiment, 175, 186

Uganda: Kemron testing in, 177–78
Umoja Sasa Products, 133
uña de gato therapy, 112
University Hospital Laboratories Corporation, Bethesda, 279–80
unsafe sex: in bathhouses, 10–11, 308–10; response to, in Miami, 10–11; resurgence of, 7–8, 13, 305–11
Urban Inc., 150
urns, 139

vaccines: HIV research, 41, 53–54, 115–25; polio, 116–17, 118–19, 124–25; principle of, 68; therapeutic, 116
vaginitis, recurrent, 191, 195, 196
van der Horst, Dr. Charles, 91, 341
Varmus, Dr. Harold, 46, 201, 338, 339
Veterans Administration: AIDS research team, 93; and AZT research, 93
viaticals, 139–40
Village Voice: AIDS Forum, 38; coverage of AIDS, 9, 36, 124

violence against gays, 305
viral-load testing, 105–6
Vironc, 108
viruses, 16–17
Virus Hunter, The (Gallo), 44, 74
vitamin A therapy, 107; for pregnant women, 240
vitamin therapies, 112, 113
Volberding, Dr. Paul, 93, 99, 100

Wadlington, Curtis, 174
Wain-Hobson, Dr. Simon, 34–35
Wainwright, Basil, 111
Wall Street: ACT UP demonstrations on, 324, 327–28
Wall Street Journal, 5, 92, 110, 117, 118, 259, 333
Ward, Ben, 183
Washington, D.C.: Abundant Life Clinic, 150–51, 174, 176; Agency of HIV/AIDS, 150; and insurance for HIV positive people, 293; Office on AIDS Activities, 151; struggle for control of AIDS federal funding in, 147, 148–51
Washington Blade, 6
Washington Legal Foundation, 274
Washington Post: coverage of AIDS/HIV, 38, 42, 151, 294
Waxman, Henry, 165
Webb, Barbara, 223–24, 229, 235
Webster, David, 49
Weekly Review (Kenya), 169
Weiss, Dr. Robin, 59, 123
Weiss, Dr. Stanley, 236
Weiss, Ted, 27, 89, 91, 265
Welsing, Dr. Frances, 186–87
Western Blot, 13, 278
Westheimer, Dr. Ruth, 133
Westmoreland, Tim, 301
Weyrich, Paul, 284
White, Jeanne, 158
White, Ryan, 146, 160

Whitman-Walker Clinic, Washington, 147, 148–50
Williams, Esther, 128
Williams, Reverend Reginald, 183
Williamson, Marianne, 129–32
Willowbrook School, New York, 204
Wilson, Shirley, 345
Wilson, Reverend Willie, 184
Winchell, Paul, 127
Wineck, Judd, 252
Winfrey, Oprah, 130
Wisconsin: AIDS resources in, 141–44
Wisconsin Hospital Rate Control Program, 142
Witte, Dr. John, 221
Wolfe, Maxine, 335–36, 337, 338
women, AIDS in, 191–214; AZT for pregnant, 87, 107; black, 179–80, 191, 204–5; CDC and, 191, 192–93, 194–95; Cuban, in Miami, 2–3; defining conditions, 191–205; epidemiology, 192, 211, 239; FDA and, 193, 199–204; Kimberly Bergalis case, 215–41; lack of HIV infection among spouses, 58; lesbians (*see* lesbians); partner notification, 166, 205–10; prostitutes, 58; Terry McGovern and, 192–93, 194, 195–205, 210, 213; transmission, 211
Wong-Staal, Dr. Flossie, 50, 74, 338
Woodcock, Janet, 203
World Health Organization: and alpha-interferon treatment, 172, 173, 177

Yarchoan, Dr. Robert, 82–83
Yecs, John, 229, 235
You Can Heal Your Life (Hay), 129
Young, Dr. Frank, 258, 259, 264–65, 266, 269

young people: resurgence of HIV infection in, 305–6

Zagury, Daniel, 44, 116, 119
Zamora, Pedro, 242–54, 345
Zamora family, 246–47, 248

Zeiger, Dr. David C., 134
Ziegler, Dr. John, 330
Zonana, Victor, 8, 48, 302
Zone DK, New York, 310
Zuckerman, Diana, 91
Zwilling, Joseph, 288